Key Clinical To

Critical Care

Key Clinical Topics in

Critical Care

Sara-Catrin Cook MB BCh FRCA EDIC DICM
Consultant in Intensive Care and Anaesthesia, Royal Gwent Hospital
Newport, UK

Matt Thomas MB ChB MRCP FRCA
Consultant in Intensive Care, Bristol Royal Infirmary
Bristol, UK

Jerry Nolan FRCA FCEM FRCP FFICM
Consultant in Anaesthesia and Intensive Care Medicine, Royal United Hospital
Bath, UK

Michael Parr FRCP FRCA FANZCA FCICM
Director of Intensive Care, Liverpool Hospital and Macquarie University Hospital
University of New South Wales and Macquarie University
Sydney, Australia

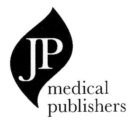

JP
medical
publishers

London • Philadelphia • Panama City • New Delhi

ISBN: 978-1-907816-67-3

British Library Cataloguing in Publication Data
A catalogue record for this book is available from the British Library

Library of Congress Cataloging in Publication Data
A catalog record for this book is available from the Library of Congress

JP Medical Ltd is a subsidiary of Jaypee Brothers Medical Publishers (P) Ltd, New Delhi, India

Commissioning Editor: Steffan Clements
Editorial Assistant: Sophie Woolven
Design: Designers Collective Ltd

Indexed, typeset, printed and bound in India.

Preface

There have been significant developments within the world of critical care over the last few years. Evidence generated from high-quality research has underpinned major changes in clinical practice and has created a need for up-to-date textbooks in critical care. In the United Kingdom, the creation of new intensive care exams is also driving the need for succinct and current information for clinicians training in this field.

Key Clinical Topics in Critical Care has been written to ensure full coverage of the specialty of intensive care medicine. Topics are presented alphabetically, with cross references to other related topics to allow easy navigation. Each topic provides a succinct overview of its subject, with reference to current key papers and guidelines in the field and including a further reading section at the end of the topic.

The topics have been written by well-established and new authors from across the globe. They have created an invaluable reference for trainees working in critical care units, enabling them to obtain a full range of key information from a single text. The book also provides a valuable revision resource for readers who are studying for exams in intensive care medicine or for the critical care elements of surgical, medical, emergency medicine and pre-hospital care exams. It will also be of interest to critical care nurses who want to expand their understanding of their field.

We hope that you will find *Key Clinical Topics in Critical Care* effective as a reference source in day-to-day practice, as well as during study and revision.

Sara-Catrin Cook,
Matt Thomas
Jerry Nolan
Michael Parr
February 2014

Acknowledgements

We thank all the authors for their very hard work. We thank our families, friends and colleagues for their invaluable support during the writing of this book. Thank you to Dr Timothy Hooper and Dr Christine Weaver for their advice.

Thank you to the authors of the forerunner to this book, *Key Topics in Critical Care,* last published in 2004, whose chapters have been revised for this book: Tim Cook, Jonathan Hadfield, Jeff Handel, Stephen Laver, Caleb McKinstry, Cathal Nolan, Andrew Padkin, Minh Tran, Jenny Tuckey, Nicky Weale.

We dedicate this book to the memory of our friend and colleague Guy Jordan (1972–2013).

SCC
MJCT
JPN
MJAP

Publisher Acknowledgements

The publishers wish to thank Series Advisors Dr Tim M. Craft and Dr Paul M. Upton for their assistance during the planning of the *Key Clinical Topics series.*

Contents

Contributors

Isabel Baker FRCPath
Topic 56
Specialist Registrar, Southmead Hospital,
Bristol, UK

Michelle Barnard BMBS BMedSci FRCA EDIC
FFICM
Topic 77, 92, 106
Consultant in Anaesthesia and Intensive Care
Medicine, Derriford Hospital, Plymouth, UK

Justine Barnett MB ChB FRCA
Topic 81
Specialty Registrar in Anaesthesia and Intensive
Care Medicine, Royal United Hospital, Bath, UK

Chris Bourdeaux MA MBBChir FRCA DICM EDIC
Topic 30
Consultant in Intensive Care Medicine, University
Hospitals Bristol NHS Foundation Trust, Bristol,
UK

Lorna Burrows MBBS BSc MRCP FRCA
Topics 35, 41, 114
Specialty Registrar in Anaesthesia and
Intensive Care, University Hospitals Bristol NHS
Foundation Trust, Bristol, UK

Adrian Clarke BM BSc MRCP FRCA DICM FFICM
Topics 11, 47, 65
Consultant in Anaesthesia and Intensive Care
Royal Gwent Hospital, Newport, UK

Emma Clow MBChB FRCA
Topics 66, 67
Specialty Registrar in Anaesthetics and Pain
Medicine, University Hospitals Bristol NHS
Foundation Trust, Bristol, UK

Alex Cochrane PhD MRCP FRCPath
Topic 55
Clinical Lecturer in Infection and Specialist
Registrar in Infectious Diseases and
Microbiology, University of Bristol, Bristol, UK

Sara-Catrin Cook MBBCh FRCA EDIC DICM
FFICM
Topic 38
Consultant in Intensive Care and Anaesthesia
Royal Gwent Hospital, Newport, UK

Matt Dallison MBBCh FRCA FFICM EDIC
Topics 51, 64, 101
Consultant in Intensive Care Medicine and
Anaesthesia, Abertawe Bro Morgannwg
University Health Board, Swansea, UK

Alia Darweish MBChB MSc MRCS (Eng) FRCA
FFPMRCA
Topics 66, 67
Clinical Research Fellow, North Bristol NHS
Trust, Bristol, UK

Keith Davies BA (Cantab) MA MBBS FRCA
Topics 19, 49, 113
Specialty Registrar in Anaesthesia and Intensive
Care Medicine, University Hospitals Bristol NHS
Foundation Trust, Bristol, UK

Richard Eve MBChB FFICM FRCA EDIC
Topics 79, 80, 82
Consultant in Intensive Care Medicine and
Anaesthesia, University Hospitals Bristol NHS
Foundation Trust, Bristol, UK

Giorgia Ferro MD MDM
Topic 57
Consultant in Anaesthesia and Intensive Care
Medicine, San Camillo Forlanini Hospital, Rome,
Italy

Stephen Fletcher FRCA MRCP(UK) FFICM FCICM
Topic 87
Director of Critical Care, Bradford Teaching Hospitals, Bradford, UK

Abby Ford BSc MBChB MRCP FRCA
Topics 1, 96, 112
Specialty Registrar in Anaesthesia and Intensive Care Medicine, Severn Deanery, Bristol, UK

Claire Fouque MBBS DCH FRCA FFICM
Topic 99
Consultant in Anaesthesia and Intensive Care Medicine, Southmead Hospital, Bristol, UK

Dan Freshwater-Turner MA MBBChir MRCP FRCA DICM FFICM
Topics 5, 9, 42, 71
Consultant in Anaesthesia and Intensive Care Medicine, University Hospitals Bristol NHS Foundation Trust, Bristol, UK

Ben Gibbison MBBS BSc FRCA
Topics 10, 27, 72
Research Fellow in Cardiac Anaesthesia and Intensive Care, Bristol Heart Institute, Bristol, UK

Alex Goodwin MBBS FRCA FFICM
Topics 12, 13
Consultant in Anaesthesia and Intensive Care Medicine, Royal United Hospital, Bath, UK

Tim Gould MBChB(Bristol) MRCP FRCA
Topic 115
Consultant Anaesthesia and Intensive Care Medicine, University Hospitals Bristol NHS Foundation Trust, Bristol, UK

Kim Gupta MBChB FRCA FFICM
Topics 58, 69, 60
Consultant in Anaesthesia and Critical Care Medicine, Royal United Hospital, Bath, UK

Pablo Hasbun MD
Topics 24, 107
Senior Registrar, Liverpool Hospital, Sydney, Australia

Mark Haslam BMBS BMedSci(Hons) MRCP FRCA DICM EDIC FFICM
Topics 6, 63, 97
Consultant in Anaesthesia and Intensive Care Medicine, Cheltenham General Hospital, Cheltenham, UK

Csilla Hasovits BSc(Med) MBBS (Hons 1) FRACP
Topic 22
Medical Oncologist Kolling Institute of Medical Research, New South Wales, Australia

Clare Hommers BM BS MRCP DTM&H FRCA EDIC DICM
Topic 50
Consultant in Anaesthesia and Intensive Care Medicine, Royal United Hospital, Bath, UK

S. Kim Jacobson MB ChB MSc MRCP MRCPath
Topic 56
Consultant Medical Microbiologist, Southmead Hospital, Bristol, UK

Dominic Janssen BA BSc(Med) MBBS FRCA DICM *Topic 62*
Consultant in Anaesthesia and Intensive Care Medicine, Frenchay Hospital, Bristol, UK

Myrene Kilminster MBBS FANZCA FFICANZCA
Topics 16, 18
Intensive Care Specialist, Lismore Hospital, New South Wales, Australia

James Low MBBCh DCH FRCA DICM FFICM
Topics 59, 60
Associate Clinical Director, Royal Derby Hospital, Derby, UK

Rachel Markham MBChB FRCA FFICM *Topic 36*
Consultant in Anaesthesia and Intensive Care
Medicine, Royal Lancaster Infirmary, Lancaster,
UK

Matthew Martin MB ChB BSc(Hons) MRCP
FRCA
Topic 20
Specialty Registrar in Anaesthesia, Southmead
Hospital, Bristol, UK

Paddy Morgan MBChB FRCA Dip IMC (RCSEd)
Topics 7, 8, 31
Advanced Trainee, Intensive Care Medicine
Royal United Hospital Bath NHS Trust, Bath, UK

Sian Alys Moxham BA(Oxon) MBBS FRCA
Topic 104
Specialty Registrar in Anaesthesia & Intensive
Care Medicine, Great Western Hospital,
Swindon, UK

Tim Murphy MA (Oxon) MBBS FRCA
Topic 53
Consultant Congenital and Paediatric
Cardiothoracic Anaesthetist, Freeman Hospital,
Newcastle, UK

Susan Murray PhD FRCPath
Topic 55
Clinical Microbiologist, Southmead Hospital,
Bristol UK

Jerry Nolan FRCA FCEM FRCP FFICM
*Topics 14, 29, 74, 75, 76, 85, 86, 90, 105, 108, 109,
110*
Consultant in Anaesthesia and Intensive Care
Medicine, Royal United Hospital, Bath, UK

Matt Oram MBBCh FRCA DICM (UK) FFICM
Topics 93, 94, 95
Consultant in Critical Care and Anaesthesia
Cheltenham General Hospital, Cheltenham, UK

Cynthia Parr MBBS FAChPM
Topic 44
Consultant in Palliative Medicine, Royal North
Shore Hospital, Sydney, Australia

Michael Parr MBBS FRCP FRCA FANZCA FCICM
Topics 17, 21, 28, 32, 34, 38, 40, 83, 91, 98, 111
Director of Intensive Care, Liverpool Hospital
and Macquarie University Hospital, Sydney,
Australia

Richard Protheroe MBBS MRCP FRCA FRCP
FFICM
Topic 52
Consultant in Critical Care Medicine and
Anaesthesia, Salford Royal NHS Foundation
Trust, Salford, UK

Kieron Rooney BSc MBBS MRCP FRCA FFICM
DICM EDIC PGCMEd
Topics 37, 78
Consultant in Anaesthesia and Intensive Care
Medicine, University Hospitals Bristol NHS
Foundation Trust, Bristol, UK

Edward Scarth BMedSci BMBS MRCP(UK) FRCA
EDIC
Topics 48, 60, 103
Specialty Registrar in Anaesthesia and Intensive
Care Medicine, University Hospitals Bristol NHS
Foundation Trust, Bristol, UK

Martin Schuster-Bruce MRCP FRCA DICM FICM
Topics 25, 46
Consultant in Critical Care, Royal Bournemouth
NHS Foundation Trust, Bournemouth, UK

Sanjoy Shah MD (Ind) MRCP EDIC MD FFICM
Topics 15, 68, 70, 84
Consultant in Intensive Care Medicine
University Hospitals Bristol NHS Foundation
Trust, Bristol, UK

Mike Slattery MB BCh
Topic 61
Specialty Registrar in Intensive Care Medicine
and Anaesthesia, Royal Gwent Hospital,
Newport, UK

Jas Soar BA MBBCh MA FRCA FFICM
Topics 23, 26, 88
Consultant in Anaesthesia and Intensive Care
Medicine, Southmead Hospital, Bristol, UK

Wade Stedman BSc (Hons) MBBS FCICM
PGDipEcho
Topics 2, 102
Senior Registrar in Intensive Care Medicine
Liverpool Hospital, Sydney, Australia

Anthony Stewart MBBS FANZCA FCICM
Topic 43
Senior Intensivist, Liverpool Hospital, Sydney,
Australia

Victor Tam MBBS FRACP FCICM
Topic 33
Senior Intensivist, Liverpool Hospital, Sydney,
Australia

Matt Thomas MBChB MRCP FRCA DICM EDIC
DIMC FFICM
Topics 39, 89, 100
Consultant in Intensive Care and Anaesthesia
University Hospitals Bristol NHS Foundation
Trust, Bristol, UK

James Walters MBBS MRCP DICM
Topics 3, 4, 73
Consultant in Acute and Respiratory Medicine
Royal United Hospital, Bath, UK

James Williams MBBCh FRCA FFICM
Topic 45
Specialist Registrar in Anaesthesia and
Intensive Care Medicine, Royal Gwent Hospital,
Newport, UK

Jonathan Whelan BM BSc(Hons) LLM FRCA
FFICM FIMC.RCS(Ed)
Topic 35, 45
Consultant in Anaesthesia and Intensive Care
Aneurin Bevan University Health Board, UK;
Medical Director, Welsh Ambulance Services
NHS Trust

Abdominal compartment syndrome

Key points

- Intra-abdominal hypertension and abdominal compartment syndrome are under-recognised conditions associated with a high mortality
- Intra-abdominal pressure measurements are key to diagnosing abdominal compartment syndrome as clinical examination has a low sensitivity
- Medical management is aimed at improving abdominal perfusion pressure, when unsuccessful surgical decompressive laparotomy may be necessary

Epidemiology

Intra-abdominal hypertension (IAH) and abdominal compartment syndrome (ACS) are common but under-recognised conditions seen in critically ill patients. Mortality approaches 100% with untreated ACS. The incidence is variable depending on the underlying cause but can be very high.

Pathophysiology

The abdomen can be considered as a closed box with rigid (costal arch, spine and pelvis) and flexible walls (abdominal wall and diaphragm). Intra-abdominal pressure (IAP) is determined by the compliance of the flexible walls and the volume of the intra-abdominal contents. IAP has a direct impact on both venous drainage and arterial blood supply to abdominal organs. Abdominal perfusion pressure (APP) can be calculated as APP = MAP - IAP (where MAP = mean arterial pressure).

Normal IAP is 5–7 mmHg. Intra-abdominal hypertension is defined as sustained or repeated pathological elevations in IAP > 12 mmHg. ACS is a sustained IAP >20 mmHg (with or without APP <60 mmHg) that is associated with new organ dysfunction or failure.

ACS is classified according to whether the causative process is caused by injury or disease within the abdomino-pelvic region (primary ACS, e.g. pancreatitis) or not (secondary ACS, e.g. severe burns).

There are several risk factors associated with the development of abdominal hypertension and ACS:

1. **Diminished abdominal wall compliance:** respiratory failure and positive pressure ventilation; abdominal surgery/trauma/burns; obesity; patient position especially prone
2. **Increased abdominal contents:** intraluminal: ileus and pseudo-obstruction; extraluminal: ascites, blood and pneumoperitoneum
3. **Capillary leak:** severe sepsis; trauma or pancreatitis exacerbated by hypotension; hypothermia and/or acidosis; massive transfusion; fluid resuscitation

Clinical features

Physical examination has a low sensitivity for the diagnosis of ACS. Maintain a high index of suspicion in patients at risk, with prompt serial measurement of intra-abdominal pressure.

Intra-abdominal hypertension or ACS leads to multiorgan dysfunction via several different mechanisms:

Respiratory: Diaphragmatic splinting leads to difficulties with spontaneous breathing and mechanical ventilation, basal atelectasis, hypoxia, increasing oxygen requirements and hypercarbia. Higher ventilator pressures used to overcome this may predispose to barotrauma and ventilator associated lung injury.

Cardiovascular: A reduction in venous return decreases cardiac output, further compromising blood supply to vital abdominal organs.

Renal: The raised IAP may directly reduce both the blood supply to the kidneys and the filtration gradient, compromising renal function. This is compounded by a reduction in cardiac output further reducing renal blood flow. Oliguria is a common feature of ACS.

Gastrointestinal system: Hepatic and splanchnic blood flow is reduced by direct pressure and reduction in cardiac output. This results in liver dysfunction, acidosis, ileus and loss of gut integrity with translocation of bacteria.

Central nervous system: Intra-abdominal hypertension increases intracranial pressure through decreasing venous return, which may be of relevance in patients with co-existing brain injury.

Investigations

IAP may be measured directly or indirectly. Direct measurement with a catheter and transducer may cause iatrogenic injury to intra-abdominal structures. Indirect measurements correlate well to direct measurements and are therefore preferred. The most common indirect measurement is intra-vesical, although intra-gastric, intra-uterine and rectal measurements have also been described. IAP measurement should be at end-expiration with the patient in the supine position with absent abdominal contractions. Saline 25 mL is instilled into the bladder and a pressure transducer attached to the catheter. Take the reading after 30–60 s to eliminate detrusor contraction, with the zero point for calibration taken at the pubic symphysis or the iliac crest at the midaxillary line. This is reproducible and reliable in the majority of patients. This enables only intermittent measurement as the catheter must be clamped at the time, therefore measurements are made 4–6 hourly depending on the patient's condition.

Diagnosis

The diagnosis is confirmed by IAP measurement. Further imaging/ investigations may elucidate the underlying pathology. Surgery may be both diagnostic and therapeutic.

Treatment

The management principles of intra-abdominal hypertension and ACS treatment include serial monitoring of IAP in patients at risk; medical treatments to reduce IAP and optimise perfusion pressure and organ function; and surgical decompression for refractory ACS.

Medical treatments are aimed at increasing APP (APP = MAP-IAP; target APP 50–60 mmHg) with fluids, vasopressors and inotropes.

IAP may be reduced by managing pain, agitation and ventilatory dyssynchrony with sedation and analgesia, and by optimal positioning. The best position for patients with IAH/ACS is unknown, however, any head of the bed elevation will increase IAP, especially when > 20° elevation. Prone positioning is also associated with high IAP. Neuromuscular paralysis may be required to aid ventilation and reduce intrinsic abdominal muscle tone. Evacuation of intraluminal contents with NG aspiration, prokinetics and laxatives may help as well as evacuation of extraluminal contents, such as ascites and blood. Correction of an excessively positive fluid balance may be achieved with diuretics, haemofiltration or dialysis.

Surgical decompression remains the definitive treatment for refractory ACS, however, concerns about long term morbidity from the procedure often delay implementation, particularly in secondary ACS. Primary ACS is more commonly treated with an 'open-abdomen' approach from initial surgery if raised IAP post-operatively is anticipated. No prospective trials have shown the best method and/or time for abdominal closure once ACS has resolved, and there is a significant morbidity and mortality associated with an open abdomen including fluid management, infection, bowel perforation and enterocutaneous fistula formation. The National Institute for Health and Care Excellence recommendations support the use of negative pressure wound therapy to manage open abdominal wounds (laparostomy).

Complications

Untreated ACS is associated with a mortality approaching 100%. Complications are multisystem and are dependent on the severity and duration of the intra-abdominal hypertension.

Further reading

Berry N, Fletcher S. Abdominal Compartment Syndrome. Contin Educ Anaesth Crit Care Pain 2012; 12:110–117.

Cheatham ML, Malbrain ML, Kirkpatrick A, et al. Results from the International Conference of Experts on Intra-Abdominal Hypertension and Abdominal Compartment Syndrome II. Recommendations. Intens Care Med 2007; 33:951–962.

Kirkpatrick AW, Roberts DJ, De Waele J, et al. Intra-abdominal hypertension and the abdominal compartment syndrome: updated consensus definitions and clinical practice guidelines from the World Society of the Abdominal Compartment Syndrome. Intens Care Med 2013; 39:1190–1206.

Malbrain MLNG, Cheatham ML, Kirkpatrick A et al. Results from the International Conference of Experts on Intra-abdominal Hypertension and Abdominal Compartment Syndrome I. Definitions. Intens Care Med 2006; 32:1722–1732.

National Institute for Health and Care Excellence (NICE). Negative pressure wound therapy for the open abdomen. NICE interventional procedure guidance 467. London; NICE, 2013. http://www. nice.org.uk/IPG467

Related topics of interest

Acute coronary syndrome

Key points

- High-sensitivity troponin assay has a negative predictive value approaching 100% when repeated at 3 h
- All patients with acute coronary syndrome should receive aspirin, with intermediate and high risk patients also benefiting from the addition of an ADP-receptor blocker
- Percutaneous coronary intervention is preferred over fibrinolysis if performed within 120 min

Epidemiology

Cardiac chest pain is one of the most common reasons for emergency admission to hospital. The term acute coronary syndrome (ACS) encompasses a range of acute myocardial ischaemic states. ACS is divided into non-ST-elevation ACS (NSTE-ACS) which includes non-ST segment elevation myocardial infarction (NSTEMI) and unstable angina (UA) and ST segment elevation MI (STEMI). The mortality of acute myocardial infarction (MI) has been markedly reduced with early diagnosis and treatment.

Pathophysiology

ACS share common pathophysiology. Most commonly atherosclerotic plaque rupture exposes a highly thrombogenic core. This is followed by thrombus formation or distal embolization, which decreases myocardial blood flow. Less commonly, non-atherosclerotic processes such as dissection, spasm including from cocaine abuse, arteritis or trauma can cause ACS.

When ischaemia is severe enough to cause myocardial necrosis, detectable quantities of biomarkers (e.g. troponin) can be found in blood. Myocardial necrosis in the presence of ischaemia is myocardial infarction.

Clinical features

The typical presentation is with heavy chest pain radiating to the neck, left arm or jaw. This is often associated with nausea, diaphoresis and dyspnoea. Atypical presentations are more common in women, chronic renal failure, diabetics and the elderly.

Investigations

If ACS is suspected an urgent 12-lead-ECG is recorded and followed by serial records.

Elevated cardiac troponins reflect myocardial injury and are more sensitive and specific than creatinine kinase and its isoenzymes.

Important differential diagnoses (e.g. aortic dissection or pneumonia) can be detected or excluded with clinical examination, chest X-ray and echocardiography. Echocardiography should ideally be performed in all patients with MI but should not delay urgent management.

Prior to discharge, testing for residual ischaemia is recommended in stable patients whose condition was treated conservatively. This can be done by stress imaging or more commonly exercise stress testing.

Diagnosis

Diagnosis of ACS is based on history, physical examination, 12-lead-ECG, biomarkers and imaging. 12-lead ECG should be performed within 10 minutes of medical contact and separates patients into NSTE-ACS and STEMI.

Symptoms suggestive of ACS and ST elevation > 0.2 mV in two adjacent chest leads or > 0.1 mV in two or more adjacent limb leads, or new left bundle branch block is diagnostic of STEMI. Confirmatory laboratory results should not be waited for to diagnose STEMI.

A rise in troponin with ischaemic chest pain, ECG changes or a new wall motion abnormality diagnoses myocardial infarction. ST-segment depression, T wave inversion and/or transient ST-elevation can be seen in NSTE-ACS. Elevated biomarkers distinguish NSTEMI from unstable angina (UA). A fall in troponin may also indicate earlier ischaemia in people with no or non-specific symptoms presenting with a raised troponin level that subsequently decreases to their baseline level.

Treatment

STEMI requires urgent revascularisation.
Treatment of NSTE-ACS is guided by quantifying risk of short-term adverse cardiovascular events. Most centres have ACS pathways which include early risk stratification. Accepted scoring systems include the Global Registry of Acute Cardiac Events or Thrombolysis in Myocardial Infarction.

Immediate management

- Assess and stabilise airway, breathing and circulation
- Supplemental oxygen if SaO_2 <95%, dyspnoea or heart failure; attach continuous cardiac and SaO_2 monitoring
- 12-lead ECG: Repeat ECG if recurrent or ongoing pain (CXR later)
- Focused clinical exam
- Aspirin: 300 mg chewed then swallowed. Use clopidogrel if allergic to aspirin
- Blood tests: FBC, urea, Creatinine and electrolytes, glucose and troponin (high-sensitivity assay if available)
- Nitrates: Sublingual glyceryl trinitrate (GTN) 0.3–0.4 mg every 5 min up to three times can reduce ischaemic pain. Intravenous should be considered if ongoing pain
- Pain control: Morphine i.v. titrated to effect with an antiemetic
- Beta-blockade: Start orally within 24 h unless contraindicated (e.g. asthma, heart failure, bradycardia, first-degree or left bundle branch block). Use intravenous only in severe hypertension and tachycardia
- Disposition: Cardiac high dependency care area for bed rest, monitoring and ongoing management

Revascularisation

Early reperfusion strategies reduce myocardial damage and decrease mortality.

STEMI

Reperfusion improves outcomes when performed within 12 h of symptom onset. Timely primary percutaneous coronary intervention (PCI) can save up to 20 more lives per 1000 patients compared with thrombolysis. In general, give thrombolytics if PCI cannot be performed within 120 min of presentation.

Thrombolytic therapy

Thrombolytic drugs given early can save up to 30 lives per 1000 STEMIs. Benefit is greatest if given within 3 h of the symptom onset, and can be given pre-hospital if delays to hospitalisation. Transfer all patients post thrombolysis to a PCI-capable centre.

- *Absolute contraindications.* Active haemorrhage. Recent major trauma/surgery/head injury. Any CNS haemorrhage/vascular lesion/malignancy. Aortic dissection. Recent CNS infarction or gastrointestinal haemorrhage. Non-compressible punctures within 24 h
- *Relative contraindications.* Coagulopathy. Pregnancy or <7 days post partum. Prolonged or traumatic resuscitation. Severe uncontrolled hypertension (systolic >180 mmHg or diastolic >130 mmHg)

Choice of thrombolytics

Fibrin-specific (alteplase, reteplase and tenecteplase) and non-fibrin specific drugs (streptokinase) improve outcomes in STEMI. Both classes increase conversion of plasminogen to plasmin, which promotes clot lysis. Streptokinase can cause systemic fibrinolysis and is antigenic. Fibrin-specific agents compared to streptokinase save an additional 10 lives per 1000 treated.

NSTE-ACS

Thrombolysis is not beneficial in NSTE-ACS. PCI evaluation followed by revascularisation improves outcome in the high risk patient.
Patients with refractory angina, arrhythmias, heart failure, new or worsening

mitral regurgitation or haemodynamic instability should have urgent PCI. If troponin positive without any of the above features, angiography and/or revascularisation, in UK NICE guidelines, are recommended within 96 h, while other international guidelines recommend within 72 h.

Antiplatelet therapy

Thromboxane A_2 promotes the aggregation of platelets. Aspirin inhibits its synthesis, reduces the incidence of MI and improves the survival of patients with ACS. Given early enough, aspirin will save 20–30 lives per 1000 infarcts. Aspirin is continued indefinitely at 75 mg daily.

Glycoprotein IIb/IIIa receptor inhibitors (tirofiban and abciximab) and ADP-receptor blockers (e.g. clopidogrel, ticagrelor or prasugrel) inhibit platelet aggregation.

Ticagrelor (loading dose 180 mg) or prasugrel (loading dose 60 mg) over clopidogrel (loading dose 300—600 mg) are recommended in most patients with ACS. Clopidogrel remains the drug of choice post fibrinolysis.

Anticoagulants

Anticoagulants are used to decrease thrombin generation. All patients with ACS should receive anticoagulant therapy early after diagnosis. Choice is dependent on treatment strategy.

Low molecular weight heparin (LMWH) reduces mortality and MI events compared to unfractionated heparin (UFH) in STEMI. UFH is preferred when using fibrinolysis.

In NSTE-ACS receiving PCI, UFH, LMWH or bivalirudin are options. In no PCI, fondaparinux is preferred over LMWH over UFH. Once started, changing anticoagulant may increase bleeding risk.

Beta-blockade

Treatment can help relieve symptoms and decreases morbidity and mortality in all patients with ACS. Beta-blockers decrease the odds of death by 23% over 2 years in patients with MI.

ACE inhibitor/ARB

An angiotensin converting enzyme inhibitor (ACE-I) or receptor blocker (ARB) improve mortality in ACS. Start within 24 h of presentation. Patients with heart failure, LVEF <40%, diabetes or anterior infarction have most benefit.

Spironolactone

Spironolactone should be commenced prior to discharge in addition to ACE inhibitors for those patients with LVEF <40% (≤35% in NSTE-ACS), New York Heart Association (NYHA) grade 3 or 4 heart failure or diabetes.

Statins

Statin therapy should be commenced as soon as possible in patients with ACS. In the CARE trial pravastatin 40 mg showed an absolute risk reduction of 3% in coronary deaths and nonfatal MI over 5 years. Discontinuing a regular statin can worsen outcome.

Glycaemic control

Acute management should be insulin based and aim for a blood glucose level of less than 10 mmol/L. This includes patients with and without a previous diagnosis of diabetes. Following hospital discharge anti-hyperglycaemic therapy should aim for a haemoglobin A1C of less than 7%. Hypoglycaemia has been associated with poor outcomes and should be avoided.

Rehabilitation

Survivors should complete a cardiac rehabilitation programme and be given advice about their modifiable risk factors (family history, smoking, hyperlipidaemias, hypertension and diabetes mellitus).

Complications

Complications of myocardial infarction depend on the size and location of the infarct. They include arrhythmias, cardiac failure, mitral regurgitation, cardiac rupture and systemic emboli.

Further reading

Libby P. Mechanisms of acute coronary syndromes and their implications for therapy. N Engl J Med 2013; 368:2004–2013.

National Institute for Health and Clinical Excellence (NICE). Unstable angina and NSTEMI, quick reference guide. London; NICE, 2010.

Hamm CW, Bassand J, Agewall S, et al. ESC Guidelines for the management of acute coronary syndromes in patients presenting without persistent ST-segment elevation. Eur Heart J 2011; 32:2999–3054.

Steg PG, James SK, Atar D, et al. ESC Guidelines for the management of acute myocardial infarction in patients presenting with ST-segment elevation. Eur Heart J 2012; 33:2569–2619.

Thygesan K, Alpert JS, Jaffe AL, et al. Third universal definition of myocardial infarction. Circulation 2012; 126:2020–2035.

Trost JC, Lange RA. Treatment of acute coronary syndrome: Part 1: Non-ST-segment acute coronary syndrome. Crit Care Med 2011; 39:2346–2353.

Trost JC, Lange RA. Treatment of acute coronary syndrome: Part 2: ST-segment elevation myocardial infarction. Crit Care Med 2012; 40:1939–1945.

Related topics of interest

- Cardiac pacing (p 88)
- Cardiopulmonary resuscitation (p 100)
- Post-resuscitation care (p 269)

Acute respiratory distress syndrome (ARDS) – diagnosis

Key points

- ARDS is under-diagnosed and a low clinical index of suspicion is required
- The categories of the Berlin definition correlate with mortality and length of ventilation
- Evaluation of cardiac function is only required if no known risk factor for ARDS is apparent

Diagnosis

The initial definition for ARDS was published in 1967 by Ashbaugh and colleagues and was based on a case series of 12 patients. There were several modifications made to this diagnosis, until an agreed definition was published by the American-European Consensus Conference (AECC) in 1994.

The AECC definition described four key aspects to ARDS; acute onset, hypoxaemia (as defined by a ratio of partial pressure of oxygen to fraction of inspired oxygen (Pao_2/Fio_2) ≤200 mmHg), bilateral infiltrates on chest radiograph and no clinical or measurable [Pulmonary Artery Wedge Pressure (PAWP) ≤ 18 mmHg] evidence of left atrial hypertension. Acute lung injury (ALI) was defined to include patients with a less severe degree of hypoxaemia (Pao_2/Fio_2 ≤ 300 mmHg). There are a number of limitations to this definition: poor inter-observer reliability in diagnosing the chest radiograph criteria, lack of consideration for the level of PEEP and other ventilator settings, the need to measure PAWP when this is now measured with increasing rarity, inability to factor for fluid resuscitation and other reasons for increased PAWP.

A Task Force was recently formed to modify the AECC definition and to develop a more reliable, valid and feasible syndrome definition. The Berlin Definition was published in 2012 and is described in **Table 1**. ALI no longer exists. ARDS is divided into mild, moderate and severe, with the definition for each group showing an improved correlation with mortality.

Epidemiology

The incidence of ARDS quoted varies and is dependant on the definition used. It is widely accepted that clinicians underestimate the true incidence of ARDS. Recent studies have

	Table 1 The Berlin definition of ARDS with associated mortality and mean ventilator duration		
	ARDS		
	Mild	Moderate	Severe
Timing	Within 1 week of known clinical insult or new/worsening respiratory symptoms		
Chest imaging	Bilateral opacities – not fully explained by effusion, lobar/lung collapse or nodules		
Origin	Respiratory failure not fully explained by cardiac failure or fluid overload; need objective assessment (e.g. echocardiography) to exclude hydrostatic oedema if no risk factor present		
Oxygenation	$200 < Pao_2/Fio_2 ≤ 300$ with PEEP or CPAP ≥ 5 cmH$_2$O	$100 < Pao_2/Fio_2 ≤ 200$ with PEEP ≥ 5 cmH$_2$O	$Pao_2/Fio_2 ≤ 100$ with PEEP ≥ 5 cmH$_2$O
Mortality (%)	27	32	45
Mean duration of ventilation	5	7	9

suggested that the incidence could be as high as 75 cases per 100,000 people per year. Further studies are now needed with the new definition being applied.

The causes of ARDS are traditionally divided into direct and indirect causes, reflecting the fact that ARDS can occur as a result of diseases of the lung such as pneumonia or by a systemic inflammatory response to a disease outside the lung such as pancreatitis. However, as there is significant overlap in the presentation and treatment of these two groups the new consensus group does not divide the causes. Risk factors that can lead to the development of ARDS are:

- Pneumonia
- Non-pulmonary sepsis
- Aspiration of gastric contents
- Major trauma
- Pulmonary contusion
- Pancreatitis
- Inhalational Injury
- Severe burns
- Non-cardiogenic shock
- Drug overdose
- Multiple transfusions or transfusion-associated acute lung injury (TRALI)
- Pulmonary vasculitis
- Drowning

Pathophysiology

Diffuse alveolar damage results from inflammatory cytokines or exogenous agents, leading to increased pulmonary capillary permeability and leak of protein rich fluid into the alveoli and interstitium. Endothelial injury may also result in the destruction of the pulmonary microvascular bed. As well as endothelial damage, the inflammatory process also affects the epithelium, further exacerbating the formation of pulmonary oedema and disrupting the production and function of surfactant. Dysregualtion of the coagulation and fibrinolytic cascades leading to the formation of microthrombi and alveolar fibrin deposition also occurs.

These changes lead to reduced compliance, increased dead space and severe hypoxaemia. Whilst in some patients these changes resolve with treatment, in others they progress to a fibrotic stage, possibly due to dysfunctional fibroproliferative repair.

The damage does not occur in a uniform manner throughout the lung, but in a patchy distribution that occurs predominantly in the dependant areas.

Clinical features

The clinical features of patients with ARDS are variable and depend on the underlying risk factors that have led to its development.

Although significant hypoxaemia is a key feature of ARDS, patients do not usually die from this. The majority die from multi-organ failure and therefore care should be taken to look for complications of ARDS and any underlying conditions that can be treated.

Investigations

Whilst it is important to perform investigations to identify and classify the ARDS, the majority of investigations performed are aimed at diagnosing and assessing the underlying condition which has led to the development of ARDS while also identifying associated complications.

There is considerable variability between clinicians in the interpretation of chest radiographs and therefore a supplement was added to the Berlin definition that contains a set of chest radiographs illustrating the spectrum of changes that are consistent, equivocal and inconsistent with the definition of ARDS. The addition of other chest radiograph criteria, such as the number of quadrants affected, does not improve the predictive validity for mortality. The Berlin definition recognises that radiological changes of the chest can be identified by X-ray or computed tomography (CT).

Although the need to exclude left atrial hypertension as a cause of the observed radiologiacal changes has been removed from the new definition, an echocardiogram is still required if there is no known risk factor present that would lead to the development of ARDS.

Further reading

Ranieri VM, Rubenfeld GD, Thompson BT, et al. Acute respiratory distress Syndrome. the Berlin Definition. JAMA 2012; 307:2526–2533.

Ferguson ND, Fan E, Camporota L, et al. The Berlin definition of ARDS: an expanded rationale, justification, and supplementary material. Intens Care Med 2012; 38:1573–1582.

Ware LB. Pathophysiology of acute lung injury and the acute respiratory distress syndrome. Semin Respir Crit Care Med 2006; 27:337–349.

Related topics of interest

- Sepsis – pathophysiology (p 333)
- Pneumonia – community acquired (p 263)
- Pancreatitis – acute severe (p 243)

Acute respiratory distress syndrome (ARDS) – treatment

Key points

- Recognise and treat promptly the underlying condition
- Prevent complications but treat rapidly if they occur
- Adhere to lung protective strategies

Treatment

There is no specific treatment for acute respiratory distress syndrome (ARDS). Treatment strategies are therefore aimed at the underlying condition, providing the best environment to allow recovery and preventing and treating complications.

Prevention of complications

Apply the strategies used to prevent complications in all critical care patients. These include stress ulcer prophylaxis, venous thromboembolism prophylaxis, management of pressure areas, catheter related blood stream infection prevention and adequate nutrition.

The recognition and prompt treatment of infection, especially ventilator-associated pneumonia (VAP), are particularly important. Consider using VAP bundles and other novel therapies such as subglottic secretion drainage and silver-coated endotracheal tubes. A low index of suspicion is required for diagnosing VAP several of the markers commonly used, such as chest radiograph changes and raised inflammatory markers will often already be present.

Ventilation and lung protective strategies

While mechanical ventilation is usually required in the presence of significant hypoxia associated with ARDS, it can also exacerbate lung injury by a combination of volutrauma (overdistension of alveoli), barotrauma (increased pressure), atelectrauma (repeated opening and closing of alveoli) and biotrauma (release of cytokines associated with high-volume ventilation). ARDS management aims to obtain adequate oxygen delivery and carbon dioxide removal while minimising further lung damage. The landmark clinical trial by the ARDS Network, demonstrated a significant mortality reduction by using lower tidal volumes (6 mL kg^{-1} versus 12 mL kg^{-1} of predicted body weight) and limiting plateau pressure to ≤ 30 cmH$_2$O. The ideal tidal volume is unknown and undoubtedly varies between patients. Low tidal volumes inevitably lead to hypercapnia and a respiratory acidosis. Unless there is a concurrent traumatic brain injury, this is less harmful than increasing tidal volume and plateau pressure, leading to the term permissive hypercapnia. A pH > 7.2 is acceptable, though many patients tolerate lower levels while others show cardiac compromise at higher values.

The ARDSnet trial also highlighted the importance of higher levels of PEEP with higher oxygen requirements. Higher PEEP leads to increased lung recruitment, improving oxygenation and preventing atelectrauma. However, it can also lead to overdistension of healthy lung, potentially worsening lung injury and cause haemodynamic compromise by reducing venous return, particularly as patients are often hypovolaemic, either secondary to the initial insult or fluid manipulation. A meta-analysis of various trials has identified a mortality benefit to a high PEEP strategy in severe ARDS.

Paralysis

Neuromuscular blocking drugs have generally been used only sparingly because they have been associated with critical care neuromyopathies, a major cause of morbidity in ARDS survivors; however, this view has been challenged recently. A trial using cisatracurium infusion for 48 h in early, severe ARDS conferred a survival benefit and reduced the duration of ventilation. This may have been due to a reduction in ventilator-associated lung injury and it is unclear if all neuromuscular blocking drugs have the same effect.

Fluid management

The ARDS definition task force recognises that while by definition, pulmonary oedema in ARDS must have a cause that is not hydrostatic, the cause for increased lung water is often multifactorial. ARDS patients often have multiple co-morbidities, including ischaemic heart disease, and they have frequently had significant fluid as part of their initial resuscitation. A conservative fluid management strategy reduces the length of ventilation and ICU days but not mortality. However, the timing of when to switch from fluid resuscitation to a conservative approach is often difficult.

Steroids

As ARDS is an inflammatory condition, it has been postulated that corticosteroids may be beneficial. However, they also have the potential to increase complications such as infection and critical care neuromyopathy.

High-dose steroids for a short period of time, as used in earlier trials, increase risk without conveying a benefit. However, there is conflicting evidence about the use of low-dose steroids (<1 mg kg^{-1} day^{-1} methylprednisolone) for prolonged (2–4 weeks) periods with two systematic reviews presenting conflicting conclusions. Low-dose steroids, instigated after the onset of ARDS but before 14 days, may improve mortality and reduce ventilator free days.

Alternative ventilatory strategies

Prone ventilation improves ventilation to the dorsal parts of the lungs and reduces ventilation-perfusion mismatching. This mechanism combined with several others enables prone ventilation to improve oxygenation in ARDS. Complications of prone ventilation include accidental line removal, facial oedema and pressure sores. A 2013 French randomised controlled trial showed improved survival for patients with severe ARDS treated with prone ventilation (for periods of at least 16 h a day) versus those ventilated supine.

High-frequency oscillatory ventilation improves oxygenation and lung recruitment by maintaining a higher mean airway pressure than is used in conventional ventilation while oscillating around this high pressure; effectively using very small tidal volumes thereby reducing volutrauma and atelectrauma. It also separates oxygenation from ventilation.

Alternative strategies for refractive hypoxia

Inhaled nitric oxide improves oxygenation by causing vasodilatation in vessels adjacent to ventilated lung units thereby reducing ventilation-perfusion mismatch. Whilst trials show a transient improvement in oxygenation, no long-term mortality benefit has been shown and it is therefore normally reserved as a bridging strategy for more definitive treatment.

Further reading

Ventilation with lower tidal volumes as compared with traditional tidal volumes for acute lung injury and the acute respiratory distress syndrome. The Acute Respiratory Distress Network. N Engl J Med 2000; 342:1301–1308.

Pipeling MR, Fan E. Therapies for refractory hypoxemia in acute respiratory distress syndrome. JAMA 2010; 304:2521–2527.

Peek GJ, Mugford M, Tiruvoipatti R, et al. CESAR trial collaboration. Efficacy and economic assessment of conventional ventilatory support versus extracorporeal membrane oxygenation for severe adult respiratory failure (CESAR): a multicentre randomised controlled trial. Lancet 2009; 374:1351–1363.

Guérin C, Reignier J, Richard JC, et al. Prone positioning in severe acute respiratory distress syndrome. N Engl J Med 2013; 368:2159–2168.

Related topics of interest

Adrenal disease

Key points

- The hypothalamic-pituitary-adrenal axis is central to the physiological stress response
- Adrenal crisis is a medical emergency and can present insidiously
- The measurement of adrenal function in critical illness is extremely difficult and does not impact on outcomes

Adrenal gland function

The adrenal glands consist of two distinct parts – the medulla, which secretes catecholamines, and the cortex, which secretes steroid hormones: glucocorticoid (cortisol), mineralocorticoid (aldosterone), and sex hormones (mainly testosterone).

Control of medullary catecholamine release

The adrenal medulla acts as a modified ganglion of the sympathetic nervous system. It receives pre-synaptic inputs from the sympathetic chain and, in response, secretes adrenaline and smaller amounts of noradrenaline and dopamine into the bloodstream. This neuronal control enables a very rapid response to sympathetic stimulation.

Control of mineralocorticoid release

This is mediated via the renin-angiotensin-aldosterone system. Low blood pressure or decreased circulating volume decreases blood flow to the juxtaglomerular apparatus in the macula densa of the kidney, stimulating renin secretion. This enzyme cleaves angiotensinogen (produced in the liver) to angiotensin I, which is subsequently converted to angiotensin II by angiotensin converting enzyme in the lungs. Angiotensin II is a potent vasoconstrictor and causes aldosterone release. Aldosterone acts in the distal convoluted tubule to cause retention of sodium and water, expanding the plasma volume.

Control of glucocorticoid activity – the hypothalamic-pituitary-adrenal axis

The hypothalamic-pituitary-adrenal axis (HPA axis) is central to the body's response to stress. Stressors act on the hypothalamus to release corticotrophin-releasing hormone (CRH), causing adrenal corticotrophin hormone (ACTH) release from the anterior pituitary. ACTH makes the adrenal cortex release cortisol, and in its absence cortisol is almost completely inhibited. Cortisol has a negative feedback effect on the HPA axis, and low circulating concentrations seen in adrenal disease lead to high concentrations of CRH and ACTH. Complex interactions exist between the HPA axis and the sympathoadrenal system. Inflammatory cytokines also play an important role in regulating the HPA axis in severe illness, with both positive and negative feedback effects seen at every level (**Figure 1**).

Cortisol is essential in the maintenance of normal vascular tone and increases the expression of adrenoceptors in vascular endothelium. Its effects on the immune system are generally anti-inflammatory and immunosuppressive. It is normally secreted in pulses showing diurnal variation with peak values seen around 08.00 h. It is highly protein-bound, mainly to cortisol-binding globulin (CBG) and albumin, with 5% existing as free cortisol in the plasma. Only free cortisol has biological activity. CBG is cleaved by elastase, which is released in inflammation, increasing local free cortisol concentrations. Free cortisol is highly lipid soluble and rapidly crosses the cell membrane to bind cytosolic glucocorticoid receptors, subsequently entering the nucleus and altering gene expression.

In certain tissues, expression of the enzyme 11-β hydroxysteroid dehydrogenase (11β-HSD) converts cortisol to its inactive metabolite, cortisone. This is important primarily in tissues with mineralocorticoid receptors, to prevent cortisol acting on them, but also plays a role in tissue resistance

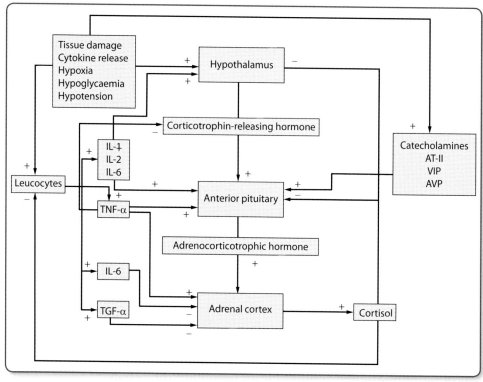

Figure 1 The interactions between the HPA axis, the sympathoadrenal system and the inflammatory response in severe illness. IL-1 = interleukin-1; IL-2 = interleukin-2; IL-6 = interleukin-6; TNF-α = tumour necrosis factor alpha; TGF-α = transforming growth factor alpha; AT-II = angiotensin II; VIP = vasoactive intestinal peptide; AVP = arginine vasopressin

to cortisol during severe illness. A silent version of the glucocorticoid receptor, that binds cortisol but is inactive, has also been described. Expression of this receptor may also be important in cortisol resistance.

Adrenocortical excess

Cushing's syndrome

Exogenous steroids used to treat other medical conditions are the most common cause of glucocorticoid excess (iatrogenic Cushing's syndrome). Endogenous glucocorticoid excess is caused by an ACTH-secreting pituitary adenoma in 70% of cases (Cushing's disease) but adrenal gland disease including tumours and hyperplasia is also important (adrenal Cushing's syndrome).

Rarely, tumours secrete ACTH-like substances (ectopic Cushing's disease).

Features of Cushing's syndrome

These include moon face, thin skin, easy bruising, hypertension (60%), hirsutism, obesity with a centripetal distribution, buffalo hump, muscle weakness, diabetes (10%), osteoporosis (50%), aseptic necrosis of the hip and pancreatitis (especially with iatrogenic Cushing's syndrome). Immune function and wound healing are impaired and the patient may exhibit resistant hypokalemia.

Conn's syndrome

Conn's syndrome (primary hyperaldosteronism) can be caused by adrenal hyperplasia or an aldosterone-secreting adenoma. Symptoms and signs include hypokalemia, hypernatraemia, muscle weakness and hypertension.

Adrenal insufficiency

Adrenal insufficiency is when inadequate amounts of cortisol are produced. Aldosterone production may also be impaired but is of secondary importance. It can be primary (disease of the adrenal glands themselves), secondary (decreased ACTH secretion) or tertiary (decreased CRH production).

Primary adrenal insufficiency is caused most commonly by Addison's disease (autoimmune adrenalitis) but other causes include surgical adrenalectomy, congenital adrenal hyperplasia, adrenal gland tumours (primary or metastatic), adrenal gland infections (including tuberculosis and fungi) and adrenal gland haemorrhage (e.g. Waterhouse-Friderichsen syndrome following meningococcal septicaemia).

Secondary adrenal insufficiency is most commonly due to HPA axis suppression from exogenous steroids. Patients on doses of >5 mg prednisolone per day may need replacement steroid treatment during surgery. Pituitary tumours or pituitary damage secondary to craniopharyngioma are rare causes, as is postpartum pituitary infarction (Sheehan's syndrome).

Diagnosis of adrenal insufficiency

The standard test of adrenal function is the Synacthen test, where cortisol concentrations are measured before and after injection of synthetic ACTH. Failure of cortisol to increase beyond a threshold value at 30 min indicates adrenal insufficiency. Further tests (e.g. ACTH concentrations, CRH concentrations, circulating renin concentrations, etc.) can be used to identify the likely cause. Variation in free cortisol fraction, increased tissue cortisol resistance and loss of the natural diurnal rhythm make the estimation of adrenal function very complex in critical illness.

Effects of glucocorticoid deficiency

Chronic adrenal insufficiency causes weakness, tiredness, orthostatic hypotension and characteristic biochemical abnormalities including low sodium, high potassium and a metabolic acidosis. Increased skin pigmentation may occur with high circulating ACTH values. Adrenal insufficiency may develop insidiously and be diagnosed only during an adrenal crisis, triggered by an intercurrent illness or trauma. In this situation, urgent intravenous fluid resuscitation and hydrocortisone replacement is required to prevent coma or death.

Critical illness-related corticosteroid insufficiency

Cortisol measurements in individuals with septic shock cover a wide range of values, from very low concentrations consistent with absolute adrenal failure to extremely high values. Some display concentrations considered normal in health that may be low in the context of severe illness. It has been proposed that both absolute and relative adrenal failure in sepsis be replaced by the term critical illness-related corticosteroid insufficiency. However the measurement of adrenal function in sepsis is problematic and there is no evidence that treating patients based on measurements of adrenal function improves outcome.

Steroids in sepsis

The use of steroids to treat severe sepsis and septic shock remains controversial. While high-dose steroids increase mortality, lower doses (200–300 mg hydrocortisone per day) may have some benefits. Large trials and meta-analyses have failed to show improved mortality but suggest that steroids increase the number of patients with refractory shock exhibiting shock reversal. The 2012 Surviving Sepsis guidelines suggest using steroids in patients who remain hypotensive on increasing doses of vasopressor, but do not recommend basing the decision on measurements of adrenal function.

Catecholamine excess – phaeochromocytoma

Rare tumours of the chromaffin cells of the adrenal medulla (10% bilateral and 10% malignant) secrete catecholamines (usually noradrenaline, but also adrenaline or dopamine) leading to intermittent symptoms of anxiety, sympathetic signs and hypertension. Prior to surgical excision, tight blood pressure control is required with alpha- and later beta-blockade. The patients are dehydrated because of chronic vasoconstriction and benefit from critical care admission post-operatively to ensure optimal management of their fluid balance and blood pressure.

Further reading

Bersten A, Soni N (Eds.) Oh's Intensive Care Manual, 6th edn. Philadelphia: Butterworth Heinemann, 2009: 647–652.

Marik PE, Pastores SM, Annane D, et al. Recommendations for the diagnosis and management of corticosteroid insufficiency in critically ill adult patients: consensus statements from an international task force by the American College of Critical Care Medicine. Crit Care Med 2008; 36:1937–1949.

Wallace I, Cunningham S, Lindsay J. The diagnosis and investigation of adrenal insufficiency in adults. Ann Clin Biochem 2009; 46:351–367.

Gibbison B, Angelini GD, Lightman SL. Dynamic output and control of the hypothalamic pituitary-adrenal axis in critical illness and major surgery. Br J Anaesth 2013; 111:347–360.

Related topics of interest

- Pituitary disease (p 255)
- Sepsis – management (p 329)
- Hypertension (p 179)

Airway complications on the intensive care unit

Key points

- Airway complications are more frequent on the intensive care unit than in the operating room and more likely to cause permanent harm or death
- Use capnography routinely
- Tracheal stenosis is a complication of prolonged tracheal intubation and percutaneous tracheostomy

Epidemiology

Tracheal intubation is more difficult on the intensive care unit (ICU): success at the first attempt is between 63% and 91%. Unplanned or accidental extubation occurs in 3–16% of ventilated patients. Failed extubation (need for reintubation within 72 h of extubation) occurs in 10–15% of ICU patients. Significant laryngeal oedema occurs in 3–30% of ventilated adults in ICU.

Long-term airway complications include tracheal stenosis which occurs in 12% of patients who are intubated for more than 11 days; after percutaneous dilatational tracheostomy, tracheal stenosis of ≥ 10% occurs in 40% of patients – symptomatic stenosis occurs in 6%.

Pathophysiology

Tracheal intubation and airway management on the ICU has a higher complication rate than during elective anaesthesia. Airway management is undertaken more frequently out-of-hours with less experienced staff available, the patients are more likely to be unstable with a reduced time from onset of apnoea to development of hypoxaemia, cardiovascular instability is common before and after induction, and availability and familiarity with advanced airway equipment may not match that of the operating room environment. Severe hypoxaemia and hypotension occurs in 20% of patients undergoing tracheal intubation in the ICU. A third of intubations are required because of problems with an existing airway, a failed trial of extubation or following accidental extubation.

Airway dislodgment is disproportionately frequent in obese patients and is also associated with patient movement and rolling. Delirium increases the risk of self-extubation or dislodgement of an airway; the frequency is higher in medical and lightly sedated patients.

Reasons for failed extubation include: the patient may not be ready to be weaned completely from mechanical ventilation, unresolved or pathology progression, inadequate muscle strength and weak cough leading to secretion retention and laryngeal and upper airway oedema causing airway obstruction. Failed extubation increases morbidity, mortality, costs and length of ICU and hospital stay.

Long-term complications of artificial airways may result from events at the time of placement, from prolonged resistance in the airway or because of abnormal healing of the injured airway mucosa. Mucosal ischaemia is central to the development of long-term complications. Use of large-volume low-pressure cuffs reduces the incidence of tracheal stenosis. Laryngeal ulceration and damage increases with duration of intubation, though tracheal tube size, shape, movement and local infection are also important factors. The damaged mucosa and underlying tracheal chondritis causes granuloma formation and fibrosis resulting in stenosis. The site of stenosis can be supraglottic, glottic or subglottic alone or in combination.

Clinical features

Failed intubation should be recognised immediately and appropriate airway management algorithms followed. Capnography must be used when attempting tracheal intubation – it helps to confirm successful tracheal tube placement.

Incomplete airway dislodgment can be more difficult to diagnose and a high index of suspicion is needed. Real-time waveform capnography provides vital information about the patency and position of a tracheal tube or tracheostomy tube before life threatening hypoxaemia develops. Warnings that an airway is becoming dislodged include the development of a cuff leak, return of the patient's voice, difficulty passing suction catheters, deterioration in gas exchange, alteration in airway pressures, abnormal chest movement or capnography waveform, or surgical emphysema developing due to tracheostomy dislodgement.

Laryngeal oedema can present as a spectrum from complete airway obstruction post-extubation or stridulous respiratory compromise to less obvious respiratory impairment.

Tracheal stenosis can present late with limited respiratory reserve, chronic cough or symptoms precipitated by subsequent respiratory tract infections. Presentation is dependent on the site and rate of progression of the stenosis. Patients are typically asymptomatic until the lumen is narrowed by 50–75% or the diameter less than 5 mm. Severe stenosis can generate inspiratory stridor or a monophasic expiratory wheeze.

Investigations

Routine use of capnography for airway management and monitoring of ventilated patients is recommended.

If dislodgement of the tracheal tube is suspected, perform a laryngoscopy to confirm its position. Fibreoptic bronchoscope examination of a tracheal tube or tracheostomy tube enables definitive confirmation of tube placement.

If stridor occurs after extubation, fibreoptic nasendoscopy will enable laryngeal oedema to be diagnosed. Tracheal stenosis can usually be investigated as an outpatient involving upper airway examination and imaging, e.g. computed tomography, which has a sensitivity of 93% and specificity of 94%. Flow-volume loops may demonstrate fixed airway obstruction but sensitivity is low.

Treatment

Ensure difficult airway algorithms are displayed in the ICU and difficult airway equipment is immediately available to deal with failed intubations and displaced tracheal tubes or tracheostomies. These algorithms should be regularly rehearsed and all staff familiar with the difficult airway kit available.

Patients at risk of requiring intubation should have risk factors for difficulty identified in advance and appropriate plans made. Patients can deteriorate very rapidly – maintain oxygenation and call for senior help early. Intubation bundles or emergency intubation checklists reduce the morbidity associated with intubation attempts on the ICU.

Intravenous steroids given before extubation decrease the incidence of laryngeal oedema and reintubation rate although they are not given routinely.

Patients identified with suspected tracheal stenosis following intensive care treatment require ENT assessment. Most patients with tracheal stenosis remain asymptomatic and never require treatment. Surgical options depend on the site and degree of stenosis and symptoms experienced.

Complications

Airway complications in the ICU are associated with significant morbidity and mortality. The 4th UK National Audit Project (NAP4) documented 14 cases of accidental dislodgement of a tracheostomy in the ICU, with seven patient deaths and four patients left with hypoxic brain injury.

Further reading

Cook TM, Woodall N, Harper J, et al. Major complications of airway management in the UK: results of the Fourth National Audit Project of the Royal College of Anaesthetists and the Difficult Airway Society. Part 2: intensive care and emergency departments. Br J Anaesth 2011; 106:632–642.

Jaber S, Jung B, Corne P, et al. An intervention to decrease complications related to endotracheal intubation in the intensive care unit: a prospective, multi-center study. Intensive Care Med 2010; 36:248–255.

Sue RD, Susanto I. Long-term complications of artificial airways. Clin Chest Med 2003; 24:457–471.

Nolan JP, Kelly FE. Airway challenges in critical care. Anaesthesia 2011; 66:81–92.

Related topics of interest

Airway management in an emergency

Key points

- Emergency airway procedures performed outside the operating theatre are associated with more complications
- Airway assessment and calling for help early in predicted difficult situations can reduce the possibility of complications
- Briefing the team and use of checklists reduces system errors and complications

Basic airway management

Initial management aims to establish and maintain a patent airway enabling oxygenation and ventilation to occur passively or with assisted ventilations. Simple manoeuvres include:

- Suctioning of foreign materials from within the oropharynx and/or nasopharynx
- Patient positioning, i.e. pillows, ramping and recovery position. The latter allows natural drainage of fluids
- Head tilt, chin lift, jaw thrust or a combination of all three. This can be a one or two-person task; occasionally, for example, if the patient is very obese, three people are required
- Insertion of nasopharyngeal and/or oropharyngeal airways
- Pharmacological: for example nebulised adrenaline in upper airway inflammation

If the above manoeuvres are insufficient and the patient is obtunded, consider insertion of a supraglottic airway device. This may enable oxygenation while preparation is made to establish a definitive airway using drug-assisted intubation.

Indications for definitive airway

Intubation of critically ill patients often has to be achieved urgently; these patients often have little or no physiological reserve and are frequently hypoxaemic.

Indications include:

Airway: Actual or impending airway compromise (not relieved with simple measures). For example, facial trauma, anaphylaxis, inhalational injury and laryngeal injury.

Breathing: Actual or impending respiratory failure or inability to oxygenate. For example, pneumonia with increased work of breathing and fatigue signified by rising $Pa\text{CO}_2$, or flail chest with hypoxaemia despite supplemental oxygen.

Circulation: Cardiac arrest, predicted deterioration due to continued haemorrhage – anaesthesia will reduce myocardial demand via reduction in sympathetic tone.

Disability: Altered conscious level. For example, agitated head injury requiring radiological investigation. A common reason seen in critical care is the septic patient with significant acidosis whose conscious level is falling.

Other indications: Some patients will benefit from intubation and anaesthesia due to their predicted clinical course or for humane reasons, e.g. multiple open limb fractures requiring manipulation and surgery in the near future.

Adverse outcomes in emergency airway management

The 4th National Audit Project (NAP4) of the Royal College of Anaesthetists, studied all serious airway complications that occurred in the intensive care unit (ICU), theatres and emergency departments over a given period of time. Less than 20% of all airway complications occurred on the ICU, but they were more likely to lead to death or persistent neurological injury compared with complications occurring in the operating room or emergency department.

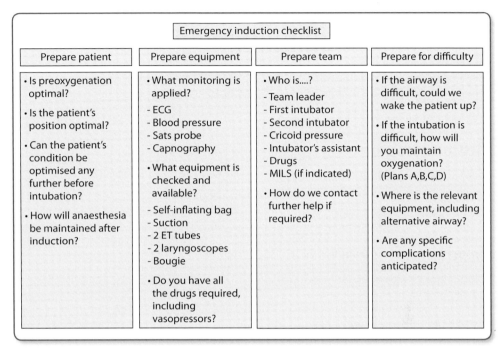

Figure 2 Emergency induction checklist. Reproduced with the permission of RTIC Severn.

Factors relating to adverse outcomes included:

- Pulmonary aspiration: In an emergency there is high risk of aspiration of blood or gastric contents and rapid sequence induction of anaesthesia is usually required. Cricoid pressure may reduce the risk of aspiration but it can distort the airway resulting in difficulty with oxygenation and laryngoscopy. The risk of aspiration should be assessed and acted upon before induction. Ensure that suction is available and switched on; consider use of a head-up position, and pharmacological interventions such as sodium citrate and metoclopramide
- Inability to establish/maintain the airway: Several cases reported to NAP4 were associated with predictably difficult airways that were not recognised as potentially difficult prior to induction; in many cases, there was no plan B when the initial attempt failed, and some were performed out of hours by junior staff with no immediate support available from seniors and other specialities (e.g. ENT). Cases included unrecognised displacement of a tracheal tube or tracheotomy during transfer and sedation holds

- Difficult, failed or unrecognised oesophageal intubation
- Iatrogenic airway trauma

The following interventions would have prevented some of these adverse outcomes:

Waveform capnography: Identifies oesophageal intubation and will also rapidly indicate displacement of a tracheostomy or tracheal tube. Practitioners should be aware of the different waveforms. Use continuous capnography in all ventilated critical care patients.

Airway equipment: Ensure that difficult airway trolleys are available in all areas where induction of anaesthesia occurs. The contents must be consistent in all areas and familiar to staff.

Intubation checklist (Figure 2)

Back-up planning: Ensure that every airway intervention has a plan B and plan C. Display and follow algorithms that include indications for calling senior or more experienced help. The presence of a second intubator decreases the incidence of complications.

Cricothyroidotomy: The most successful method of gaining front of neck access is emergency surgical tracheostomy rather than needle cricothyroidotomy.

Identification of at risk patients and at risk events: Those with potentially difficult airways, obese patients, transfers and rolling.

Further reading

Benger J, Nolan J, Clancy M. Emergency airway management. New York: Cambridge University Press, 2008.

Cook TM, Woodall N, Harper J, Benger J. Major complications of airway management in the UK: results of the Fourth National Audit Project of the Royal College of Anaesthetists and the Difficult Airway Society. Part 2: intensive care and emergency departments. Br J Anaesth 2011; 106:632–642.

Intensive Care Society. Standards for Capnography in Critical Care. London: Intensive Care Society, 2009.

Henderson JJ, Popat MT, Latto IP, Pearce AC. Difficult Airway Society guidelines for management of the unanticipated difficult intubation. Anaesthesia 2004; 59:675–694.

Related topics of interest

Airway obstruction – upper and lower

Key points

- Airway obstruction can occur anywhere from the mouth to the large bronchi
- Management is determined by site of the lesion and urgency of the case
- Complex airway obstructions require multidisciplinary approaches

Epidemiology

The true incidence of all upper and lower airway obstructions is unknown. There is a spectrum of severities, e.g. only 5% of laryngeal tumours will present with dyspnoea and stridor.

Pathophysiology

The airway can be obstructed from within the lumen or from external compression (**Table 2**). Objects within the lumen include inhaled foreign bodies and iatrogenic causes such as an obstructed tracheal tube. The airway anatomy can be affected by lesions within the tissues, e.g. abscess, angioedema or trauma from airway instrumentation. External lesions will cause compression because of their physical bulk, e.g. malignancies, thyroid cysts or haematomas.

The site of obstruction can be divided into upper and lower airway, defined by being above or below the thoracic inlet. The upper airway can be further subdivided into whether it is supraglottic, laryngeal or subglottic. This is an important distinction as it influences management if anaesthesia is required. The obstruction can be partial or full.

Clinical features

Increased work of breathing: this is evident when there is tachypnoea, tachycardia, hypoxaemia and/or hypercapnia, use of accessory muscles, see-saw breathing and inability to complete sentences. Pulmonary oedema from excessive negative intrathoracic pressures may occur.

Inspiratory to expiratory ratio: a prolonged expiratory phase indicates a lower airway obstruction; a prolonged inspiratory phase indicates an upper airway obstruction that is dynamic, e.g. a soft tissue lesion that is sucked into the lumen during inspiration and is pushed away during exhalation.

Stridor: this is a high-pitched noise created when the diameter of the airway has been reduced by at least 50%. As the resistance to flow increases so does the velocity of the gas, which becomes turbulent producing noise and increased work of breathing.

Laryngospasm: this may occur on extubation, emergence or in an inadequately anaesthetised patient.

Increased ventilatory pressures: occur during positive pressure ventilation, which reduces gas flow.

Hypoxaemia: presents as agitation/panic, reduced consciousness, cyanosis or respiratory arrest.

Other clinical features of airway obstruction include noisy respiration (gurgling and snoring), wheeze, decreased air entry on auscultation, chocking, drooling of saliva and dysphagia.

Serial observations will indicate whether there is a need to expedite management. Signs and symptoms associated with the underlying pathology may also be present in addition to the obstructive symptoms, e.g. cachexia with malignancies.

Investigations

The appropriate investigations are determined according to findings on examination, the degree of obstruction, the urgency of the situation, and whether a tissue diagnosis (preferably under local anaesthesia) is needed.

Chest radiography (posterior-anterior, lateral and/or thoracic inlet views) may

Table 2 Causes of upper and lower airway obstruction		
Upper – *Stridor usually inspiratory, or biphasic*		
Within lumen	Iatrogenic	Blocked/kinked endotracheal tube or supraglottic airway Displaced tracheal stent Foreign body, e.g. peanuts, fish bones and teeth
	Soft tissue	Pedunculated lesions, e.g. tonsils 'ball valve effect' Tongue falling back
	Fluid	Blood, gastric contents, excess secretions
In the construct	Laryngospasm	Cord dysfunction Anaesthesia associated
	Infective	Laryngotracheobronchitis Epiglottitis Croup Tonsillitis+/– abscess
	Inflammatory	Anaphylaxis Smoke inhalation, chemical burns
	Tracheomalacia/ strictures	Iatrogenic Genetic
External to airway	Haematoma	Secondary to trauma of vasculature/erosion by malignancy Within glands, e.g. Thyroid
	Infective	Retropharyngeal abscess
	Malignant	Amyloidosis Tumours of the tongue/oropharynx Thyroid lesions Perilaryngeal tumours
Lower – *expiratory stridor/wheeze*		
Within lumen	As per upper airway plus	Mucus plugging/blood clots
In the wall	Inflammatory	Brochospasm – asthma/irritant gases
	Tracheomalacia	Iatrogenic Malignancy
External to airway	Masses	Retrosternal goitre Lymphoma Other malignancies
	Vascular	Arterial aneurysms

demonstrate significant lesions such as enlarged thyroids, foreign bodies (if radio-lucent) or a pneumothorax.

Computed (axial) tomography (CT) can determine the level and extent of an obstruction (including measurement of airway patency) but the patient must be able to lie flat. CT is less useful for supraglottic lesions.

Magnetic resonance imaging is useful for soft tissue.

Pulmonary flow-volume loops (maximal inspiratory/expiratory flow-volume curves)

assist in quantifying impairment and site of obstruction: extrathoracic or intrathoracic.

Awake flexible nasendoscopy, facilitated by lidocaine and a vasoconstrictor such as epinephrine, is used to visualise the larynx from above. Supplemental oxygen enables most patients to tolerate the procedure unless full airway obstruction is imminent.

Bronchoscopy and laryngoscopy are useful diagnostic techniques, but require sedation or anaesthesia with the associated potential complications.

Full blood count, C-reactive protein and blood cultures are indicated if there is concern about an infective cause such as croup, tonsillitis, retropharyngeal abscess or epiglottis (only when the patient and airway is stable).

Capnography will assist with diagnosing an obstructed, displaced or removed endotracheal tube or tracheostomy.

Diagnosis

Diagnosis is made from the history, examination, investigations and tissue diagnosis (if applicable).

Treatment

Specific treatment depends upon the cause of obstruction. Involve other specialities such as ENT, cardiothoracic surgery and radiology at an early stage.

Simple measures such as head tilt, chin lift, jaw thrust and suctioning may help with causes such as an obstructing tongue, blood in the oropharynx or a mucus plug.

In foreign body airway obstruction, encouragement of coughing and abdominal thrusts dislodges the object in many cases. Laryngoscopy or bronchoscopy may be required.

Antibiotics, IV steroids, nebulised adrenaline and nebulised steroids may be effective for upper airway oedema, epiglottitis and croup. Give nebulised bronchodilators for lower airway bronchospasm and adrenaline (IV or IM) for suspected anaphylaxis.

Fluid-filled lesions may be drained radiologically or surgically. Obstructing masses such as a goitre or aneurysm will need surgical removal and malignant lesions chemo or radiotherapy if not amenable to surgery.

In the anaesthetised and positive pressure ventilated patient, identify and treat causes of increased airway pressure such as pneumothorax, inadequate muscle relaxant, coughing or endobronchial intubation.

Where the airway obstruction may get worse, e.g. airway trauma or smoke inhalation, or the patient is in extremis, a definitive airway, in the form of a tracheal tube or surgical airway, is required. A robust airway management plan with back-up strategies is required (see **Table 3**).

Table 3 Points to consider when constructing an airway management strategy for a patient with an obstructing airway lesion
• Where is the lesion? Does it require a front of neck procedure as 'plan A' or is it a valid option as a 'plan B'?
• Consider awake nasal flexible nasendoscopy to reassess prior to committing to anaesthesia.
• How urgent/compromised is the situation/patient?
• What are the equipment/ resources and technical capability of personnel?
• Can spontaneous ventilation or a local anaesthetic procedure be tolerated? General anaesthesia with or without muscle relaxants is associated with various problems and controversy exists as to 'best practice'.
• If general anaesthesia is required, consideration must be given to how induction of anaesthesia will be performed. The optimal technique is controversial: gas induction versus IV induction with/without muscle relaxant.
• Is cardiopulmonary bypass available or should the patient be transferred to a centre with this?
• First attempt at intubation should be the best: multiple attempts at direct laryngoscope should be avoided due to high risk of complete obstruction.
• Is an awake fibreoptic intubation possible and appropriate?
• How will anaesthesia be maintained – is helium/oxygen low density gas ventilation available?
• ENT surgical presence – rigid bronchoscopy/ emergency front of neck procedure? Investigations jointly reviewed by surgeon and critical care team?
• What is the plan 'B', 'C' etc in the case of failure?

Complications

The complications of airway obstruction progress in the following sequence:

Reduced airway patency leads to reduced airflow with increased work of breathing, fatigue, hypercapnia and hypoxia, eventually leading to cardiovascular collapse and respiratory/cardiac arrest. Depending upon the stage at which the obstruction is resolved sufficiently to enable adequate oxygenation and ventilation, the patient may sustain brain injury or other ischaemic consequences of hypoxia.

Other complications will be specific to the cause:
- Significant or complete obstruction (e.g. laryngospasm, foreign body and malignant tumour) can cause pulmonary oedema from the negative pressure generated within the lung during attempts to breath when the airway is obstructed
- Mediastinal masses may compress not just the airway, but also the great vessels, e.g. vena cava or aorta, or the heart causing cardiovascular compromise, or surrounding nerves, e.g. recurrent laryngeal nerve (causing vocal cord dysfunction)

Further reading

Cook TM, Woodall N, Frerk C. Topic 18; Head and Neck Pathology in 4th National Project of the Royal College of Anaesthetists and Difficult Airway Society. Major complications of airway management in the United Kingdom Report and Findings. London: Royal College of Anaesthetists, 2011.

Nethercott D, Strang T, Krysiak P. Airway stents: anaesthetic implications. Contin Educ Anaesth Crit Care 2010; 10:53–58.

Cook TM, Morgan PJ, Hersch PE. Equal and opposite expert opinion. Airway obstruction caused by a retrosternal thyroid mass: management and prospective international expert opinion. Anaesthesia 2011; 66:828–836.

English J, Norris A, Bedforth N. Anaesthesia for airway surgery. Cont Educ Anaesth Crit Care 2006; 6:28–31.

Related topics of interest

- Airway complications on the intensive care unit (p 18)
- Airway management in an emergency (p 21)
- Tracheostomy (p 368)

Analgesia in critical care – advanced

Key points

- Unrecognised pain is an important cause of delirium in ICU
- Epidurals can provide excellent analgesia but require careful monitoring and access to vasopressor support
- Adequate analgesia to enables mobilisation and optimises respiratory function in post-operative patients

Pain scoring and assessment

Sedated or unconscious patients may respond to pain with autonomic disturbance (tachycardia, hypertension and sweating). Untreated pain can produce agitation and delirium. Assess awake patients regularly using pain scores to enable analgesia to be titrated. Ensure adequate analgesia so that the patient can mobilise, breathe deeply and cough effectively.

Simple analgesia

Give paracetamol regularly unless contraindicated. Non-steroidal anti-inflammatory drugs can be very effective, but their side effects of coagulopathy, renal dysfunction and gastro-intestinal bleeding make them suitable only in low-risk patients and only for a short course (perhaps less than 3 days).

Opioid drugs

Opioids have powerful anti-sympathetic effects, reducing tachycardia, hypertension and anxiety, but cause anticholinergic side effects such as constipation, dry mouth, sedation and nausea as well as profound respiratory depression. They are given orally or parenterally, either as infusions or as patient-controlled infusions with a patient-delivered bolus and 5-min lockout period [patient-controlled analgesia (PCA)]. These are safer than continuous infusions because

they reduce the risk of drug accumulation and respiratory depression. Patients need to be sufficiently alert to use a PCA and are advised to anticipate painful stimuli (e.g. physiotherapy) rather than waiting for pain to become intense.

Specific opioids

Morphine has good oral bioavailability and can be given in long-acting preparations. Its metabolites accumulate in renal impairment, causing respiratory depression and seizures.

Fentanyl is fast-acting and often added to epidurals. It accumulates if given over a prolonged period, but is safer in renal impairment than morphine. Alfentanil is similar to fentanyl but with less accumulation when infused.

Remifentanil is ultra-short acting and metabolised by non-specific blood esterases. Its half-life is around 5 min even after prolonged infusion. It is ideally suited to sedation and procedural analgesia when rapid wake-up is required. It may cause wind-up of pain pathways causing increased pain after discontinuation.

Epidural analgesia

Mode of action

Epidural analgesia is used following major abdominal, thoracic or lower limb surgery. A catheter is inserted under sterile conditions into the epidural space at an appropriate spinal level, and local anaesthetic and/or other drugs are infused. Small, non-myelinated pain fibres are blocked preferentially to motor fibres at the level of insertion and 4–5 spinal levels above and below. A well-positioned epidural provides excellent analgesia while allowing full motor function and avoiding the systemic effects of opioid drugs.

Local anaesthetic drugs are infused (e.g. bupivacaine 0.1% at 12–20 mL/h for a mid-thoracic epidural) with opioids added to increase block density and allow lower local anaesthetic concentrations to be used (e.g. fentanyl 2 mcg/mL). Other drugs such as clonidine and ketamine can also be added. Patient-controlled epidural infusions enable the patient to deliver a bolus as required with a longer (approximately 20 min) lock-out period, with or without a background infusion rate.

Sympathetic blockade leads to peripheral vasodilatation and hypotension. There is also loss of splanchnic vasoconstriction, and blockade of the cardiac accelerator fibres if the block is high enough (T1–T4 level). This can be opposed by giving intravenous fluid but a vasopressor infusion may be required.

Benefits and complications

These are summarised in **Table 4**. There is consensus that epidurals provide superior quality analgesia and reduce serious respiratory complications, but the other benefits listed are more controversial. The report of the Royal College of Anaesthetists 3rd national audit project into the complications of central neuraxial blockade estimated the risk of permanent injury as the result of epidural use to be between 8.2 and 17.4 cases per 100,000 epidurals sited.

The report made several recommendations to improve epidural safety: that robust mechanisms be put in place to reduce the risk of wrong-route administration of local anaesthetic infusions; that epidurals be offered only where there is the facility to provide vasopressor therapy for hypotension; and that referral systems must ensure that cases of vertebral canal haematoma are operated on within 12 h of diagnosis. It also noted that leg weakness was an early sign of severe neurological injury, but was often mistaken for the effect of the epidural itself; staff caring for patients with epidural infusions should be appropriately trained in the signs and symptoms of vertebral canal haematoma and protocols should be used to guide the management of epidural infusions.

Monitoring an epidural block

Since pain and cold are transmitted through the same fibres, loss of cold sensation is used to map affected dermatomes. If the block is inadequate a bolus can be given; if one side is blocked, preferentially positioning the unblocked side dependent helps spread to the missed areas. Sitting a patient up promotes caudal spread. Concentrated bupivacaine solutions (0.25% and 0.5%) can

Table 4 Benefits and complications of epidural anaesthesia		
Potential benefits	**Minor/moderate complications**	**Major complications (potential for permanent harm)**
Excellent analgesia	Urinary retention	Catheter migration into subarachnoid space
Decreased respiratory complications	Pruritis	Local anaesthetic toxicity/wrong route administration
Possible decreased mortality	Nausea and vomiting	Wrong site injection
Decreased perioperative complications, blood loss, DVT and arrhythmias	Inadequate/unilateral/patchy block	Cardiovascular collapse
Faster return of GI function	Dural puncture headache	Nerve injury
Shorter duration of hospital stay when used as part of the Enhanced Recovery Protocol	Superficial infection	Epidural abscess
	Hypotension	Vertebral canal haematoma
	Motor block	Spinal cord infarction
	Sedation	
	Respiratory depression	

be used if the block cannot be established with a low concentration infusion.

Epidural removal

Epidurals are usually removed after 72 h, and by day 5 the risk of infection increases significantly. Remove the catheter at least 10 h after low molecular weight heparin administration (6 h after unfractionated heparin) and at least 2 h before the next dose. Other anticoagulants including clopidogrel contraindicate epidural use.

Nerve blocks and infusions

Local anaesthetic infusions can be used as nerve blocks, for instance paravertebral infusions following thoracic surgery or rectus sheath catheters following laparotomy. The analgesic effects of an epidural can be obtained without the haemodynamic side effects. However, the use of such techniques is not widespread and care must be taken not to confuse nerve block infusions with epidurals.

Procedural analgesia on the ICU

As well as the opioid drugs already mentioned, ketamine has a role in sedoanalgesia for painful procedures on ICU. Other sedative agents such as clonidine and dexmedetomidine may also be useful as may the use of Entonox in selected patients.

The difficult pain patient on the ICU

Drug abusers may be habituated to the effect of opioid drugs and may require very high doses to achieve adequate analgesia. Alternative drugs such as ketamine and clonidine can be very effective in addition to modified PCA regimes with higher bolus doses of opioid.

Chronic pain patients may be established on high doses of opioids and other adjunctive analgesia such as gabapentin or amitriptyline. It is usual practice to continue their usual drugs including their long-acting opioids and to administer extra opioid analgesia sufficient for pain control.

Further reading

Cook TM, Counsell D, Wildsmith JA. Major complications of central neuraxial block: report on the Third National Audit Project of the Royal College of Anaesthetists. Br J Anaesth 2009;102:179–190.

Werawatganon T, Charuluxanun S. Patient controlled intravenous opioid analgesia versus continuous epidural analgesia for pain after intra-abdominal surgery. Cochrane Database Syst Rev 2005: CD004088.

Peck T, Hill S. Pharmacology for Anaesthesia and Intensive Care, 3rd Edn. Cambridge University Press, 2008.

Related topics of interest

Anaphylaxis

Key points

- Anaphylaxis is a serious allergic reaction that is rapid in onset and may cause death
- Foods are the most common trigger in children. Medications are the most common trigger in adults
- Immediate management follows the ABCDE approach

Anaphylaxis is defined as a serious allergic reaction that is rapid in onset and may cause death. It is characterised by life-threatening airway and/or breathing and/or circulatory symptoms and signs usually associated with skin and/or mucosal changes that develop rapidly. In the initial stages of an anaphylactic reaction, the mechanism and cause of the reaction are not as important as correct recognition and treatment.

Epidemiology

The epidemiology of anaphylaxis has been difficult to quantify, but the incidence is thought to be increasing.

Key figures

- Incidence: 10–20 per 100, 000 population
- About 25% of these require admission to hospital
- Around 300 cases per year are admitted to UK critical care units
- Anaphylaxis accounts for at least 20 deaths per year in the UK (an underestimate)
- In adults, there is a female preponderance
- In children, the male: female ratio is much more evenly balanced (possibly males predominate)

Pathophysiology

The final end pathway of anaphylaxis, which is common to all mechanisms, is mast cell degranulation.

Classical pathway

Previous exposure to an allergen causes the production of allergen specific IgE.

Subsequent exposure to the same allergen causes cross-linking of the IgE and activates high-affinity IgE receptors on mast cells (and to a lesser extent basophils). IgE production also upregulates expression of these high-affinity IgE receptors, which enhances and amplifies the anaphylaxis response.

Other immunological mechanisms

Immune aggregates, T-cells, IgG, IgM, platelets and leukotrienes can all cause mast cell degranulation.

Other non-immunological mechanisms

Exercise, cold, alcohol, insect venom, radio-contrast media and vancomycin all cause mast cell degranulation via non-immunological mechanisms.

Common end pathway

This is an amplification system involving activation of several inflammatory pathways. Activation of mast cells triggers the release of histamine, proteases (mainly tryptase), leukotrienes, prostaglandins, cytokines and chemokines from vesicles within the cells.

Histamine causes Ca^{2+}-mediated production of nitric oxide via the constitutively produced endogenous nitric oxide synthase (eNOS) (rather than the inducible iNOS-mediated pathway of sepsis), which causes detrimental vasodilatation.

Fluid shifts can be massive, with up to 35% of the intravascular volume leaking into the interstitium within 10 minutes of the reaction.

Anaphylactic reactions may resolve spontaneously in minutes to hours if there is sufficient production of compensatory mediators such as adrenaline, angiotensin II and endothelin. They may also progress rapidly to cardiorespiratory arrest if unchecked and untreated.

Up to 20% of reactions are biphasic, i.e. a secondary reaction occurs. This will usually occur within 8 h of the initial reaction, but can occur up to 72 h later. The mechanism behind this is unclear but may include inadequate treatment, repeated IgE stimulation of mast cells, secondary mediators or prolonged antigen absorption.

Triggers

- Food (particularly peanuts) is the most common trigger in children
- Medications are the most common triggers in adults
  - Non-steroidal anti-inflammatory drugs (NSAIDS) and antibiotics are the most common out of hospital
  - Antibiotics, muscle relaxant and other anaesthetic drugs are the most common in hospital
- Insect bites are also a common cause
- Those with atopy and asthma may be at increased risk of anaphylaxis

Clinical features

Anaphylaxis affects the following organ systems:

- Respiratory (70% of cases)
  - Bronchospasm, stridor and airway obstruction, wheeze
- Cardiovascular (45% of cases)
  - Haemodynamic disturbance is *not* required for the diagnosis of anaphylaxis
  - Hypotension, tachycardia, coronary artery spasm, oedema and direct myocardial depression
- Central nervous system (15% of cases)
  - Confusion and loss of consciousness (caused by hypoxaemia and poor cardiac output)
- Skin (90% of cases)
  - Urticaria, angio-oedema, conjunctivitis and rhinitis
- Gastro-intestinal (45% of cases)
  - Nausea, vomiting, abdominal pain and diarrhoea

The smooth muscle effects of mast cell degranulation can cause uterine contraction and may mimic labour, or lead to premature delivery in pregnant patients.

Diagnosis

In an emergency, diagnosis is based on the clinical history, symptoms and probability. The mechanism and triggering factor can be elucidated when the patient is stable. However, anaphylaxis is likely when ALL three of the following criteria are met:

- Sudden onset and rapid progression of symptoms
- Life-threatening airway and/or breathing and/or circulation problems
- Skin and/or mucosal changes

Treatment

Immediate management

Treatment of the acute situation follows the ABCDE approach. The basic principles of management are the same regardless of age group.

- Remove the trigger if possible
- Immediate treatment follows the Resuscitation Council (UK) algorithm:
  - Adrenaline is the first line treatment and has direct effects to prevent mast cell degranulation
  - Anti-histamines and hydrocortisone are second line
- Start CPR immediately if required, following current guidelines
- Consider early intubation – there is a risk of upper airway obstruction and bronchospasm may make it difficult to ventilate the lungs
- Use the doses of adrenaline recommended in the guideline
- Give salbutamol nebulisers and/or infusion for persistent bronchospasm.

Subsequent management

- Continue vasoactive medications as needed, usually an adrenaline infusion but noradrenaline and vasopressin can be considered if hypotension is unresponsive to adrenaline. Cardiovascular instability may persist for several hours
- Continue regular antihistamines
- Continue regular hydrocortisone

- Check for the presence of a leak around the tracheal tube cuff prior to extubation

Investigations

Take a blood sample for mast cell tryptase:
- As soon as possible after emergency treatment has been started
- 1–2 h after the onset of symptoms

Refer the patient to a specialist allergy or immunology centre for further investigations. Do not discharge home without advice about further episodes of anaphylaxis and where appropriate, an adrenaline injector is provided.

Further reading

Soar J, Pumphrey R, Cant A, et al. Emergency treatment of anaphylactic reactions – guidelines for healthcare providers. Resuscitation 2008; 77:157–169.

National Institute for Health and Care Excellence (NICE). Initial assessment and referral following emergency treatment for an anaphylactic episode, Clinical Guidance CG134. London: NICE, 2011.

Association of Anaesthetists of Great Britain and Ireland. AAGBI Safety Guideline: Suspected Anaphylactic Reactions associated with Anaesthesia. London: AAGBI, 2009.

Resuscitation Council (UK). Anaphylaxis Algorithm. Resuscitation Council; London, 2008.

Related topics of interest

Antibiotics, antivirals and antifungals

Key points

- Antibiotics are a key part of the management of sepsis, although they must be used appropriately to avoid increasing resistance rates
- Reducing time to administration of antibiotics reduces mortality from severe sepsis
- Antifungal and antiviral drugs are becoming more important in treatment of critically ill patients

Appropriate antibiotics are essential in the management of sepsis; however, resistance is increasing and there are few new drugs with new mechanisms of action in development. Optimisation of the therapeutic concentration and duration of treatment will help to maintain the effectiveness of current drugs. Classes of antibiotic drugs are listed in **Table 5**.

General principles of antibiotic usage

1. Where possible, obtain all appropriate microbiological specimens before starting therapy. In some cases, antibiotics must be given immediately, regardless of whether specimens have been obtained, e.g. severe sepsis from any site, meningitis or necrotising fasciitis.
2. Give antibiotics without delay once appropriate specimens have been obtained.
3. Choice of empiric therapy is guided by the site of the suspected infection, community versus hospital acquired infection, recent previous antibiotic usage and knowledge of local common organisms. Immediate Gram staining will guide empiric therapy and should be done where possible. Surveillance is important in determining commonly encountered bacteria or resistance patterns in local ICU or ward environments.
4. Initiate empiric therapy with broad-spectrum antibiotics, but rationalise when culture results are available. Use narrow spectrum antibiotics as often as possible.
5. Antibiotic stewardship is selecting the correct drug, optimising dose and duration, minimising toxicity and conditions for selection of resistant bacteria. Monitor serum values of potentially toxic antibiotics.

Antibiotic resistance

Antibiotic resistance is of major concern, with emergence of extended-spectrum β-lactamase positive Gram-negative bacteria (e.g. *Klebsiella* and *Citrobacter*), MRSA or vancomycin-resistant enterococci (VRE). Antimicrobial stewardship and rigorous infection control are the mainstays of prevention of development and spread of resistance. ICUs are common sites of antibiotic resistance for several reasons. These include:

- Use of broad-spectrum antibiotics for empiric therapy, leading to selection pressure
- Numerous invasive devices
- Immunocompromised patients
- High intensity care for each patient, allowing cross-contamination between patients or of the environment by lapses in infection control precautions

Mechanisms of antibiotic resistance are detailed in **Table 6**.

Pharmacokinetics and pharmacodynamics of antibiotics in critically ill patients

The minimal concentration at which an antibiotic prevents replication is the minimal inhibitory concentration (MIC). Critically ill patients have altered volume of distribution (due to ascites or oedema) and clearance, which will affect the peak concentration of drug available. Antibiotics can be broadly split into two groups depending on

Table 5 Classes of antibiotics		
Class and example	**Mechanism**	**Activity/resistance notes**
β-lactams (e.g. penicillins and cephalosporins)	Inhibit cell wall synthesis by inhibiting cross-linking of polymer peptidoglycans	Three potential mechanisms of resistance; (1) alteration in target site, e.g. MRSA produces different polymer peptidoglycans with low affinity for β-lactams, and are therefore less effective; (2) production of β-lactamase enzymes which hydrolyse the antibiotic before being effective and (3) Gram-negative bacteria alter the cell membrane structure, which reduces uptake of the β-lactamase antibiotic.
Carbapenems (e.g. meropenem and imipenem)	Another β-lactam antibiotic, although resistant to the hydrolase enzyme and therefore useful in resistant infections	Bacteria producing the New-Delhi Metallo-β-lactamase (NDM-1) enzyme, which provides resistance to carbapenems have been isolated. There has been a rapid continental and global spread of resistant bacteria carrying the gene encoding this enzyme, within both hospital and community environments. Given the last-resort nature of carbapenem antibiotics this has raised significant cause for concern.
Glycopeptides (e.g. vancomycin and teicoplanin)	Interfere with peptidoglycan assembly, but at a different site than β-lactams.	Effective only against Gram-positive bacteria, including MRSA, although there are strains of vancomycin-resistant *Staphylococcus aureus*. Vancomycin has renal and ototoxicity, requiring monitoring of serum levels.
Aminoglycosides (e.g. gentamicin and tobramycin)	These drugs block protein synthesis by interfering with the translational process, leading to errors in gene transcription.	Active against some Gram-positive and many Gram-negative organisms. They are bactericidal, and have synergy with β-lactams.
Macrolides (e.g. clarithromycin and erythromycin)	These drugs bind to the 50S subunit of ribosomal RNA and prevent protein synthesis.	Active against most Gram-positive organisms, but many coliforms are resistant.
Fluoroquinolones (e.g. ciprofloxacin and levofloxacin)	These drugs inhibit bacterial DNA gyrases, which are responsible for supercoiling (folding and unfolding) of DNA during synthesis. Therefore, DNA cannot be replicated, preventing multiplication.	More sensitive against Gram-negative than Gram-positive bacteria, no effect on anaerobes.
Oxazolidinone (linezolid)	Binds to bacterial ribosome and prevents protein synthesis	Active against MSSA, MRSA and VRE. Bacteriostatic. Good penetration into the lung field so may become more useful in MRSA pneumonia.
Glycycline derivative (tigecycline)	Binds to 30S unit of ribosome to inhibit protein synthesis	Broad spectrum of action against Gram-positive organisms and many Gram-negative organisms, except *Pseudomonas aeruginosa* and *Proteus miribilis*.
Lipopeptides (daptomycin)	Binds to the bacterial cell membrane in a calcium-dependent process. Multiple molecules coalesce (oligomerise) on the membrane to form an ion pore, causing depolarisation and rapid cell death.	Active against majority of Gram-positive bacteria. Appears to be well tolerated at higher dosages, which may be needed to treat some organisms. Ineffective in lung tissue as inactivated by surfactant.

Table 6 Mechanisms of antibacterial resistance	
Natural resistance	Bacteria lack transport mechanism necessary for antibiotic to enter cell; or Bacteria lack the target of the antibiotic; or Gram-negative bacteria have a thick cell wall which is impermeable to the antibiotic
Vertical gene transfer	Sporadic mutations every $1 \times 10^{8-9}$ replications, which encode new resistant genes are then transferred to progeny during further replication
Horizontal gene transfer • Conjugation • Transformation • Transduction	Transfer of plasmids through direct cell-cell contact One bacteria takes up DNA from external environment from other bacteria that have died Bacteriophage (viruses specific for bacteria) transfer DNA directly

pharmacokinetic characteristics – either concentration-dependent or time-dependent action. Concentration-dependent agents (e.g. aminoglycosides and quinolones) require high target concentrations (8–10 times greater than MIC) to be maximally effective. Effectiveness may require using significantly higher dosages and shorter duration than in current practice. For time-dependent drugs (e.g. β-lactams, carbapenems and vancomycin), it is the time that drug concentration is above MIC that is important for maximal effectiveness. Consequently, current interest is focusing on continuous infusions of these drugs that have previously been given at intervals. These approaches are also considered to reduce the development of resistance as well as being more effective in providing microbiological cure. Some drugs have a post-antibiotic effect, defined as inhibition of bacterial growth after concentrations of an antibiotic reach zero. Inhibitors of protein and nucleic acid synthesis (e.g. aminoglycosides, quinolones, clindamycin and tetracyclines) have the longest post-antibiotic effects, suggesting that it is due to alteration of bacterial DNA synthesis.

Patients with burns, renal replacement therapy or extracorporeal membrane oxygenation present special situations that require dose alteration. There are excellent reviews in the further reading section.

Anti-viral drugs

The viral life cycle consists of four sections (entry, replication, shedding or latency). Most drugs act on the viral DNA polymerase enzyme during replication. Common viral infections encountered in ICU include meningoencephalitis (enterovirus or herpes simplex), pneumonitis (influenza viruses, or varicella in immunocompromised patients) or human immunodeficiency virus and acquired immunodeficiency syndrome. Cytomegalovirus (CMV) infection is relevant to immunosuppressed patients, particularly those after bone marrow or solid organ transplant, or with HIV infection.

Aciclovir and ganciclovir are phosphorylated within the virus into a triphosphate compound, which competitively inhibits viral DNA polymerase. Aciclovir is active against herpes simplex and zoster viruses, while ganciclovir is used against CMV. Resistance is due to the virus producing altered phosphorylation enzymes, or altered viral DNA polymerase.

Foscarnet binds to viral DNA polymerase, preventing DNA replication. It is inhibitory against most varicella zoster, and aciclovir-resistant herpes simplex and ganciclovir-resistant CMV strains. However CMV and HSV can develop resistance due to viral mutations in DNA polymerase. Renal toxicity, and metabolic derangements (hypocalcaemia, hypercalcaemia, hypomagnesaemia and hypophosphataemia) can develop.

Cidofivir also acts against viral DNA polymerase enzymes. It is active against herpes viruses (including acyclovir-resistant strains), ganciclovir-resistant CMV and papilloma, pox and adenoviruses.

Oseltamivir is used for prophylaxis and treatment of influenza A and B. It acts by inhibiting viral neuraminidase, an enzyme which enables release of the virus from the host cell. Early treatment of influenza infection can reduce the time to functional recovery by 1–3 days, and decrease the risk of lower respiratory tract complications requiring hospitalisation. It is generally well tolerated, but can be associated with headache, rash, hepatic inflammation and thrombocytopenia.

Anti-fungals

Risk factors for invasive fungal disease include neutropenia, stem cell transplantation, HIV infection/AIDS, total parenteral nutrition, fungal colonisation, renal replacement therapy, infection and sepsis, mechanical ventilation and diabetes. Fungal infection causes high mortality and morbidity. Common fungal infections include *Candida albicans* (cutaneous and invasive fungal disease), *Aspergillus* spp, *Cryptoccus* spp (in immunocompromised patients) and *Pneumocystis jirovecii* (previously *Pneumocystis carinii*), which is now classified as a fungal organism.

There are three groups of anti-fungal drugs:

1. Polyenes (e.g. amphotericin B): Binds to ergosterol in the fungal cell wall, leading to leakage and cell death. Ergosterol is not present in mammalian cell walls, hence giving fungal selectivity. It has a broad spectrum of activity against most fungi causing human disease, but is ineffective against some *Aspergillus* or *Candida* strains. Conventional amphotericin B causes reactions related directly to the infusion and is nephrotoxic. Lipid-based formulations enable higher doses to be used. Liposomal amphotericin B has fewest toxic effects, and is most widely used.

2. Azoles (e.g. fluconazole and itraconazole): These inhibit the fungal enzyme lanosterol demethylase, which synthesizes ergosterol, and thereby disrupts cell membrane synthesis. Fluconazole is active against *Candida albicans* as well as other fungi, but not *Candida glabrata* or *Aspergillus* spp. Fluconazole has an excellent safety profile and has 100% oral bioavailability. Itraconazole and voriconazole are active against all *Candida* spp and *Aspergillus*, but are more likely to cause drug interactions and side effects.

3. Echinocandins (e.g. caspofungin and micafungin): These drugs inhibit cell wall synthesis by non-competitive inhibition of 1,3-β-D-glucan synthase. They are fungicidal against *Candida* and fungistatic against *Aspergillus* spp (including strains resistant to fluconazole), but inactive against *Cryptococcus neoformans*. They are generally well tolerated, but risk renal and hepatic impairment. Oral bioavailability is very low requiring intravenous administration.

Further reading

Ulldemolins M, Roberts JA, Lipman J, Rello J. Antibiotic dosing in multiple organ dysfunction syndrome. Chest 2011; 139:1210–1220.

Jamal JA, Economou CJ, Lipman J, Roberts JA. Improving antibiotic dosing in special situations in the ICU. burns, renal replacement therapy and extracorporeal membrane oxygenation. Curr Opin Crit Care 2012; 18:460–471.

Pagani L, Afshari A, Harbarth S. Year in review 2012: Critical Care – infection. Crit Care 2011; 15:238.

Related topics of interest

Arterial blood gases – acid–base physiology

Key points

- The body's defence against an H⁺ load involves several compensatory mechanisms: dilution, buffers and compensation by the lungs, kidneys, liver and bone
- Stewart's approach to acid–base balance is conceptually simple and elegant but is operationally complicated and unwieldy

A biochemical milieu maintained within a narrow range is required for the normal function of enzymes within the cells of the body. The concentration of hydrogen ions (H^+) is low but crucial for normal enzyme function.

The following definitions are essential to the understanding of acid–base physiology:

Acid	Proton donor
Base	Proton acceptor
Strong acid	Fully dissociates in solution
Weak acid	Partially dissociates in solution
Buffer	A chemical substance that prevents large changes in H⁺ concentration when an acid or base is added to a solution
Acidaemia	Decrease in pH
Acidosis	Increase in H⁺ concentration

The normal plasma concentration of sodium is 140 mmol L^{-1} while that of H^+ is 0.00004 mmol L^{-1}. Thus, H^+ concentration is represented as pH, which is the negative Log_{10} of the H^+ concentration. The normal extracellular pH is 7.4, venous blood 7.35, red blood cells 7.2, muscle cells 6.8–7.0 (in anaerobic metabolism 6.40) and that of CSF 7.32

Aerobic metabolism produces 1400 mmols of carbon dioxide per day. This is termed volatile acid because it is excreted via the lungs. Amino acid metabolism produces approximately 80 mmol day^{-1} of non-volatile acid.

Anaerobic metabolism produces ATP, lactate, protons and water and the abnormal metabolism of fats produces keto-acids (e.g. diabetic ketoacidosis).

The body's defence against an H^+ load involves the following compensatory mechanisms.

Dilution

Acid produced in cells is diluted in total body water because it diffuses into the extracellular fluid and into other cells. Each 10-fold dilution increases the pH by 1 unit.

Buffers

An acid–base buffer is a solution of two or more chemical compounds that prevents marked changes in H⁺ concentration when an acid or a base is added. The pK of a buffer system defines the pH at which the ionised and unionised forms are in equilibrium. It is also the pH at which the buffer system is most efficient.

Important buffer systems are found in plasma and cells (including red blood cells).

The Henderson Hasselbalch equation considers the relationship of a buffer system to pH.

$$pH = pKa + Log_{10}\ base/acid$$

For the bicarbonate system: $pH = 6.1 + Log_{10}\ HCO_3^-/Paco_2$

Hence at plasma bicarbonate of 24 mmol L^{-1} and a $Paco_2$ of 5.3 kPa the equation becomes: $pH = 6.1 + Log_{10}\ 24/(2.3 \times 5.3)$

(2.3 = solubility coefficient of carbon dioxide, mmol kPa^{-1})

$$pH = 7.4$$

Respiratory compensation

The respiratory system is able to regulate pH. An increase in CO_2 concentration leads to a decrease in pH and a decrease in CO_2 leads to a rise in pH. If the metabolic production of CO_2 remains constant the only factor that affects CO_2 concentration is alveolar ventilation. The respiratory centre in the medulla oblongata is sensitive to H^+ concentration and changes alveolar ventilation accordingly. This affects H^+ concentration within minutes. Thus, the respiratory system is a 'physiological buffer'.

Renal control

The kidneys control acid–base balance by controlling the secretion of H^+ relative to the amount of filtered bicarbonate.

Tubular secretion of hydrogen ions

Hydrogen ions are secreted throughout most of the tubular system. There are two distinct methods of secretion:

- Secondary active transport of H^+ occurs in the proximal tubule, thick segment of the ascending loop of Henle and the distal tubule. Within the epithelial cell, carbon dioxide combines with water under the influence of carbonic anhydrase to form carbonic acid. This then dissociates into H^+ and bicarbonate. The H^+ is secreted into the tubular lumen by a mechanism of sodium/hydrogen counter-transport
- Primary active transport occurs in the latter part of the distal tubules all the way to the renal pelvis. This transport system accounts for less than 5% of the total H^+ secreted. However, it can concentrate H^+ 900-fold compared to fourfold for secondary active transport. The rate of H^+ secretion changes in response to changes in extracellular H^+ concentration

Interaction of bicarbonate and hydrogen ions in the tubules

The bicarbonate ion does not diffuse into the epithelial cells of the renal tubules readily because it is a large molecule and is electrically charged. However, it combines with a secreted H^+ to form carbon dioxide and water and is, effectively, 'reabsorbed'. The CO_2 diffuses into the epithelial cell and combines with water to form carbonic acid, which immediately dissociates to bicarbonate and H^+. The bicarbonate ion then diffuses into the extracellular fluid.

The rate of H^+ secretion is about 3.5 mmol min^{-1} and the rate of filtration of bicarbonate is 3.46 mmol min^{-1}. Normally, the H^+ and bicarbonate titrate themselves. The

mechanism by which the kidney corrects either acidosis or alkalosis is by incomplete titration. An excess of H^+ in the urine can be buffered by phosphate and ammonia.

The liver

The liver assists in acid–base balance by regulating ureagenesis. Amino acid metabolism leads to the generation of bicarbonate and ammonia. These combine to form urea, CO_2 and water:

$$2NH_4^+ + 2HCO_3^- \rightleftharpoons NH_2\text{-}CO\text{-}NH_2 + CO_2 + 3H_2O$$

The lungs remove the CO_2 and there is no net acid or base production. The liver is able to regulate the metabolism of ammonia and bicarbonate to urea. In alkalosis, ureagenesis increases, consuming bicarbonate. In acidosis, ureagenesis decreases, increasing available bicarbonate. The liver also affects acid–base balance by carbon dioxide production from complete oxidation of substrates (carbohydrates and fats), metabolism of organic acid anions (lactate, ketones and amino acids) and the production of plasma proteins especially albumin.

Bone

Extracellular H^+ can exchange with cations from bone and cells (e.g. sodium, potassium, magnesium and calcium). This is a slow process and may take hours or days.

The Stewart approach to acid–base balance

The concept of acid–base balance has historically been expressed in terms of the balance between respiratory and non-respiratory (metabolic) systems. Stewart's physico-chemical approach is similar to the traditional empirical approach in its classification and measurement of acid–base disturbances. The difference lies in the explanation and interpretation of acid–base disturbances and control mechanisms. Stewart's approach is conceptually simple and elegant but is operationally complicated and unwieldy.

The biochemistry of aqueous solutions is complex. All human solutions contain water, which is an inexhaustible supply of H^+. Hydrogen ion concentration is determined by the dissociation of water. The laws of physical chemistry, particularly electro neutrality and conservation of mass, determine the dissociation of water. In plasma, the determinants of H^+ concentration can be reduced to three: strong ion difference (SID), partial pressure of carbon dioxide (Pco_2) and total weak acid concentration (A_{TOT}). Neither H^+ concentration nor bicarbonate ion concentration can change unless there is a change in one or more of these variables. The principle of conservation of mass shows that strong ions can neither be destroyed nor created to satisfy electro neutrality, but H^+ are generated or consumed by changes in water dissociation.

Saline administration

$$SID = (Na^+ + K^+ + Ca^+ + Mg^+) - (Cl^- + lactate^-)$$

From the above equation, sodium and chloride are the principle tools in altering SID.

An increase in sodium with respect to chloride increases the SID and increases the pH. The reverse occurs with an increase in chloride relative to sodium leading to a decrease in SID.

An increase in SID leads to a reduction in water dissociation and hence a reduction in plasma H^+. As sodium is controlled to maintain tonicity it appears that chloride is the principle tool in altering SID and hence plasma pH. Loss of strong anions, e.g. in conditions associated with nasogastric aspirates, will cause an increase in SID.

A decrease in SID may be brought about by the addition of strong anions (lactate or chloride). When saline is given to a patient, the relative excess of chloride reduces the SID and increases the dissociation of water and, therefore, the plasma H^+.

Stewart's approach provides an alternative method for assessing acid-base abnormalities. In particular, it provides a useful explanation for the aetiology of hyperchloraemic acidosis, which is seen commonly in critical ill patients.

Further reading

Cowley NJ, Owen A, Bion JF. Interpreting arterial blood gas results. Br Med J 2013; 346:f16.

Hickish T, Farmery AD. Acid-base physiology: new concepts. Anaesth Intensive Care Med 2012; 13:567–572.

Badr A, Nightingale P. An alternative approach to acid-base abnormalities in critically ill patients. Contin Educat Anaesth Crit Care Pain 2007;7:107–111.

Sirker AA, Rhodes A, Grounds RM, Bennett ED. Acid-base physiology: the traditional and the modern approaches. Anaesthesia 2002; 57:348–356.

Related topics of interest

Arterial blood gases – analysis

Key points

- An understanding of arterial blood gases (ABGs) is fundamental to the management of critically ill patients
- Arterial blood gas data must be considered within the context of the wider clinical picture and can be interpreted systematically with a five-step approach

Having processed an arterial blood sample the blood gas analyser will display typically the following information:

Pao$_2$ – partial pressure of oxygen in arterial blood

This is measured directly. Its relationship with the fractional inspired oxygen concentration (Fio$_2$) is described by the alveolar gas equation:

$$P\text{AO}_2 = F\text{IO}_2\,(P_b - P_{H_2O}) - P\text{ACO}_2/RQ$$

    Pao$_2$ = Alveolar oxygen pressure
    Fio$_2$ = Inspired oxygen fraction
    P_b = Atmospheric pressure
    Paco$_2$ = Alveolar CO_2 pressure
    PA$_{H_2O}$ = Water vapour pressure [6.27 kPa (47 mmHg)]
    RQ = Respiratory quotient (0.8)

When breathing air at an atmospheric pressure of 100 kPa (760 mmHg), the partial pressure of inspired oxygen is 20.9 kPa (158 mmHg). Having become fully saturated with water in the upper respiratory tract the partial pressure of oxygen falls to 19.5 (148 mmHg). At the alveolus, oxygen is taken up and replaced by CO_2, which reduces the Pao$_2$ to 14 kPa (106 mmHg). Because of shunt, the arterial oxygen pressure is always slightly lower than that in the alveolus. Shunt increases with age. When breathing air, the normal Pao$_2$ is 12.5 kPa (92 mmHg) at the age of 20 years and 10.8 kPa (82 mmHg) at 65 years.

Paco$_2$ – partial pressure of carbon dioxide in arterial blood

This is measured directly and is normally 4.4–6.1 kPa (33–46 mmHg).

pH

This is the negative Log_{10} of the hydrogen ion concentration and is measured directly. The normal pH is 7.35–7.45.

Standard bicarbonate

This is calculated from the CO_2 and pH using the Henderson Hasselbach equation. It is the concentration of bicarbonate in a sample equilibrated to 37 °C and Paco$_2$ 5.3 kPa. Thus, the metabolic component of acid-base balance can be assessed. The normal value is 22–26 mmol L^{-1}.

Actual bicarbonate

This reflects the contribution of both the respiratory and metabolic components. The normal value in venous blood is 21–28 mmol L^{-1}.

Base excess and base deficit

This is a measure of the amount of acid or base that needs to be added to a sample, under standard conditions (37 °C and Paco$_2$ 5.3 kPa), to return the pH to 7.4. It is traditionally reported as 'base excess'. The normal range is +2 mmol L^{-1} to –2 mmol L^{-1}.

Interpretation of blood gas data

When evaluating respiratory and acid–base disorders arterial blood gas data must be considered within the context of the wider clinical picture. Having noted the Fio$_2$ and Pao$_2$, the ABG results should be assessed as follows:

1. Assess the hydrogen ion concentration.
   pH > 7.45 – alkalaemia
   pH < 7.35 – acidaemia
   7.35–7.45 no disturbance or mixed disturbance
2. Assess the metabolic component
   HCO$_3$ > 26 mmol L^{-1} – metabolic alkalosis
   HCO$_3$ < 22 mmol L^{-1} – metabolic acidosis
3. Assess the respiratory component

Pa_{CO_2} > 5.9 kPa – respiratory acidosis
Pa_{CO_2} < 4.6 kPa – respiratory alkalosis

4. Combine the information from 1, 2 and 3 and determine if there is any metabolic or respiratory compensation.
5. Consider the anion gap. This indicates the presence of non-volatile acids (lactic acid, keto-acids and exogenous acids). The normal anion gap is 10–18 mmol L^{-1} and can be estimated using the following equation:

$$([Na^+] + [K^+]) - ([Cl^-] + [HCO_3^-])$$

Disorders of acid–base balance are divided into acidosis and alkalosis and into those of metabolic and respiratory origin. They can be subdivided by the presence or absence of an abnormal anion gap.

Pre-analytical sources of error include air bubbles, time delays, heparin, leucocytosis, halothane and labelling. When blood is cooled CO_2 becomes more soluble, hence Pa_{CO_2} falls. With every degree centigrade fall in temperature, pH increases by 0.015. Haemoglobin accepts more hydrogen ions when cooled.

Disorders of acid–base balance
1. Metabolic acidosis (with a normal anion gap)
- Increased gastrointestinal bicarbonate loss (e.g. diarrhoea, ileostomy and ureterosigmoidostomy)
- Increased renal bicarbonate loss [e.g. acetazolamide, proximal renal tubular acidosis (type 2), hyperparathyroidism, tubular damage, e.g. drugs, heavy metals and paraproteins]
- Decreased renal hydrogen secretion [e.g. distal renal tubular acidosis (type 1) and type 4 renal tubular acidosis (aldosterone deficiency)]
- Increased HCl production (e.g. ammonium chloride ingestion and increased catabolism of lysine)
2. Metabolic acidosis with abnormal anion gap
Accumulation of organic acids. A useful memory aid is the acronym KUSMEL: Ketones, Uraemia, Salicylate, Methanol, Ethylene glycol and Lactate.
- Lactic acidosis
L-Lactic acid – Type A (anaerobic metabolism, hypotension/cardiac arrest, sepsis and poisoning – ethylene glycol and methanol). Type B (decreased hepatic lactate metabolism, insulin deficiency, metformin accumulation, haematological malignancies and rare inherited enzyme defects)
D-Lactic acid (fermentation of glucose in the bowel, e.g. in blind loops).
- Ketoacidosis (e.g. insulin deficiency, alcohol excess and starvation)
- Exogenous acids (e.g. salicylates)
3. Metabolic alkalosis
- Loss of acid (e.g. hydrogen ion loss from GI tract – vomiting, nasogastric suction, hydrogen loss from kidney – diuretics, hypokalaemia, excess mineralocorticoid and low chloride states – diuretic therapy)
- Addition of alkali [e.g. sodium bicarbonate (paradoxical intracellular acidosis], addition of substance converted to bicarbonate – citrate, lactate and acetate).
4. Respiratory acidosis
- Respiratory depression (e.g. drugs and cerebral injury)
- Muscle weakness (e.g. Guillain-Barré, myasthenia, polio and muscle relaxants)
- Trauma (e.g. flail chest and lung contusion)
- Pulmonary insufficiency (e.g. pulmonary oedema, pneumonia and ARDS)
- Airway obstruction (e.g. COPD)
- Artificial ventilation (e.g. inadequate minute volume and excessive PEEP)
5. Respiratory alkalosis
- Excessively high minute volume
- Hypoxaemia
- Pulmonary embolism
- Asthma (early)
- Impairment of cerebral function (e.g. head injury and meningo-encephalitis)
- Respiratory stimulants (e.g. salicylate overdose – early)
- Sepsis (early)
- Parenchymal pulmonary disorder (e.g. oedema)
6. Mixed disorders
- Metabolic acidosis and respiratory acidosis (e.g. cardiac arrest and respiratory failure with anoxia)
- Metabolic alkalosis and respiratory alkalosis (e.g. CCF and vomiting, diuretics

and hepatic failure and diuretic therapy and pneumonia)

- Metabolic alkalosis and respiratory acidosis (e.g. COPD and diuretics, COPD and vomiting)
- Metabolic acidosis and respiratory alkalosis (e.g. salicylate overdose, septic shock, sepsis and renal failure and CCF and renal failure)
- Metabolic alkalosis and metabolic acidosis (e.g. diuretics and ketoacidosis, vomiting and renal failure and vomiting and lactic acidosis)
- Pyloric stenosis – hypochloraemic alkalosis with paradoxical aciduria
- Urinary diversion, e.g. ileal conduit, sigmoid implantation, recto-vesical fistula – hyperchloraemic acidosis

Lactate

Anaerobic metabolism produces ATP, lactate and water. H^+ is generated from breakdown of ATP (36 ATP in aerobic metabolism and 2 ATP in anaerobic metabolism)

Hyperlactataemia = > 2 mmol/L

Lactic acidosis = > 5 mmol/L and pH < 7.35

The term lactic acidosis is not strictly correct; a better term is hyperlactataemia with an excess of protons, which are not used in the aerobic pathway to form $NADH_2$. There are two main mechanisms that can cause hyperlactataemia without acidosis:

1. Type A – Impaired oxygen delivery.
2. Type B – Normal oxygen delivery but with increased cellular production, reduced uptake/utilisation of oxygen or reduced lactate clearance.

Lactate increases with increased glycolysis (adrenergic stimulation); examination of the lactate:pyruvate (LP) ratio will distinguish tissue hypoxia (LP ratio > 10:1) from normoxic conditions (LP ratio ≤ 10:1).

Alpha-stat versus pH stat

The alpha-stat hypothesis recognises that the degree of ionisation (alpha) of imidazole groups of proteins remains constant in the face of different temperatures. The pK of imidazole structures on histidine changes with temperature. Hence, intracellular pH is maintained at different temperatures. The alpha-stat theory does not require physicians to alter patient parameters to maintain pH in the face of changes of temperature.

The pH-stat hypothesis relies on correction of blood gas results for temperature. All blood gas machines are compensated to 37 °C. The pH is corrected using the Rosenthal correction factor. Hence physiological parameters should be altered in the face of changing temperature to maintain a constant pH.

When using pH-stat, at lower temperatures a respiratory acidosis would be required to maintain a normal pH (7.4). The potential physiological effect of this is to increase cerebral blood flow. Differences in clinical outcomes using alpha-stat or pH-stat remain unclear; there may be some benefit to the pH-stat approach in children.

Simple arithmetic related to acid–base disorders

- If pH = 7.*ab* and [H^+] = *cd* nanomols/L, then *ab* + *cd* = 83
  e.g. pH = 7.23, [H^+] = 83 – 23 = 60
- For a 1.6 kPa (12 mmHg) change in PCO_2 there will be a 0.1 change in pH and a 6 mmol change in BE

Further reading

Cowley NJ, Owen A, Bion JF. Intepreting arterial blood gas results. Br Med J 2013; 346:f16.

Hickish T, Farmery AD. Acid-base physiology: new concepts. Anaesth Intensive Care Med 2012; 13:567–572.

Related topics of interest

Arterial cannulation

Key points

- Most patients on a critical care unit will have an arterial cannula to enable continuous blood pressure measurement and repeated blood sampling
- The radial artery is the most common site for arterial cannulation
- Several technologies enable fluid responsiveness and cardiac output to be estimated from the peripheral arterial waveform
- Serious complications from arterial cannulae occur in less than 1% of cases

Introduction

Peripheral arterial cannulation is a common procedure performed in critical care units. The radial artery at the wrist is the most popular site but there are a number of other suitable arteries: the ulnar, dorsalis pedis and posterior tibial arteries are, like the radial artery, relatively small distal vessels, but each has a collateral vessel. The brachial, femoral and axillary arteries do not have collaterals but are much larger and less likely to thrombose.

Indications

1. Continuous monitoring of arterial blood pressure:
   a. Where haemodynamic instability is anticipated:
      - Major surgical procedures, e.g. cardiac and vascular
      - Large fluid shifts, e.g. major trauma
      - Medical problems, e.g. heart valve disease
      - Drug therapy, e.g. inotropes and/or vasopressors
   b. For neurosurgical procedures.
   c. Where non-invasive blood pressure monitoring is not possible, e.g. burns and morbid obesity.
2. Sampling:
   - Blood gases
   - Repeated blood sampling (to prevent the need for multiple punctures)
3. To assess fluid responsiveness and to enable non-invasive measurement of cardiac output.

Contraindications

- Local infection
- Coagulopathy is a relative contraindication
- Inadequate circulation to the extremity

Technique

A modified Allen's test may be performed to assess the adequacy of collateral blood flow to the hand before cannulating the radial artery. However, ischaemia may occur despite a normal result and an abnormal result does not predict this complication reliably. Consequently, most clinicians have discarded the Allen's test; if there is any doubt about the perfusion of the hand after radial cannulation, remove the cannula immediately. Radial artery cannulation is made easier by hyperextending the patient's wrist to 30° using a fluid bag or rolled towel.

A 20 gauge arterial cannula may be inserted under local anaesthesia in the same way as a venous cannula, although on occasions it can be easier to transfix the vessel first. Alternatively, a Seldinger technique (the cannula is inserted over a guidewire) can be used. Ultrasound may be helpful in identifying a peripheral artery, particularly in the shocked patient.

Alternatives to radial artery cannulation

Ulnar artery

The ulnar artery can be cannulated using the position and technique described above. If multiple attempts at cannulation of the radial artery have been unsuccessful, do not attempt to cannulate the ipsilateral ulnar artery.

Brachial artery

The brachial artery may be cannulated just proximal to the skin crease of the antecubital fossa, medial to the biceps tendon and lateral to pronator teres.

Dorsalis pedis

If perfusion to the foot is satisfactory, the dorsalis pedis or posterior tibial arteries may be cannulated safely with a 20 gauge catheter.

Femoral artery

The femoral artery may be cannulated 1–2 cm distal to the inguinal ligament at the midpoint of a line drawn between the superior iliac spine and the symphysis pubis. Insert an 18 gauge central venous cannula into the artery using a Seldinger technique. A standard 20 gauge arterial cannula is too short for reliable femoral access. The anatomical relationship of the femoral artery and vein is variable – ultrasound is very helpful for identifying the artery and guiding cannulation.

Sources of error

An over damped trace will under read the systolic pressure and over read the diastolic pressure. Causes of over damping include a kinked cannula, partial obstruction of the cannula by blood clot or by the vessel wall, and air bubbles in the manometer line or transducer. An under damped trace will over-read the systolic and under-read the diastolic pressure. The usual cause of this is resonance in long manometer lines. The mean arterial pressure should remain accurate even in the presence of damping or resonance.

In the supine patient, the systolic pressure increases and diastolic pressure decreases (pulse pressure widens) the further from the aortic valve that the arterial pressure measurement is made. This reflects increasing stiffness of the arterial tree in the periphery. The mean arterial pressure should be consistent wherever it is measured. An exception to this principle occurs in the presence of very high doses of vasopressors when intense vasoconstriction can result in arterial pressure measured from the radial artery, for example, being substantially lower than a larger artery such as the femoral.

Estimating cardiac output and fluid responsiveness from an arterial catheter

In patients undergoing positive pressure ventilation the cyclical changes in the arterial waveform that occur with respiration [pulse pressure variation (PPV)] can be used to estimate fluid responsiveness – a PPV of more than 10% generally indicates that the cardiac output will increase in response to a fluid challenge. There are now several monitors that enable the measurement of PPV or a variant of this and they generally also provide a continuous estimate of cardiac output by using complex algorithms to analyse the arterial waveform.

Complications

The most significant complications are ischaemia and infection but, overall, the incidence of serious complications is less than 1% of cases. Thrombosis is more likely to occur when the cannula is large relative to the artery, particularly if it is left in place for longer than 72 h. The incidence of complications from radial, femoral and axillary artery cannulation is shown in **Table 7**. Thrombi at the catheter tip can embolise peripherally. Flushing the arterial catheter can cause retrograde emboli of thrombus or clot. Disconnection can cause extensive haemorrhage, and bleeding around the catheter site can cause haematomas, particularly in patients with a coagulopathy.

Infection is extremely rare in patients who have arterial catheters solely for intraoperative monitoring, but it may occur in the critical care unit, particularly after about 4 days. The rate is probably similar to that in concurrently placed central venous catheters. The site must be inspected regularly for signs of local inflammation and the arterial catheter removed immediately if any is identified. Accidental injection of drugs may cause distal gangrene. Aneurysms and pseudoaneurysms are rare, late complications.

Table 7 Complications following radial, femoral and axillary artery cannulation. Incidence given as n cases/n catheterisations (%).

Complication	Radial artery		Femoral artery		Axillary artery	
Permanent ischaemic injury	4/4217	(0.09)	3/1664	(0.18)	2/989	(0.20)
Temporary occlusion	831/4217	(19.7)	10/688	(1.45)	11/930	(1.18)
Sepsis	8/6245	(0.13)	13/2923	(0.44)	5/989	(0.51)
Local infection	45/6245	(0.72)	5/642	(0.78)	16/713	(2.24)
Pseudoaneurysm	14/15,623	(0.09)	6/2100	(0.3)	1/1000	(0.1)
Haematoma	418/2903	(14.4)	28/461	(6.1)	17/744	(2.28)
Bleeding	2/375	(0.53)	5/316	(1.58)	10/711	(1.41)

Data from Scheer BV et al. Crit Care 2002;6:198–204.

Further reading

Scheer BV, Perel A, Pfeiffer UJ. Clinical review: complications and risk factors of peripheral arterial catheters used for haemodynamic monitoring in anaesthesia and intensive care medicine. Crit Care 2002; 6:198–204.

Koh DB, Gowardman JR, Rickard CM, Robertson IK, Brown A. Prospective study of peripheral arterial catheter infection and comparison with concurrently sited central venous catheters. Crit Care Med 2008; 36:397–402.

Related topics of interest

- Arterial blood gases – analysis (p 41)
- Cardiac output measurement (p 83)
- Cardiac surgery – postoperative care (p 91)

Asthma

Key points

- The decision to initiate mechanical ventilation for acute severe asthma is based on clinical judgment and is undertaken cautiously
- Approximately 4% of patients hospitalised for acute asthma require mechanical ventilation
- Patients with status ashmaticus who require mechanical ventilation have increased in-hospital and long-term mortality

Epidemiology

Bronchial asthma affects more than 300 million people worldwide. In infants, males generally have more severe disease whilst in older children there is no sex predilection with regard to severity. Its incidence is higher among adult females.

Clinical features

Pathophysiology

Central to the pathogenesis of asthma is airway inflammation of the bronchi leading to smooth muscle constriction and excessive secretion.

This consists of:

- Mucosal and submucosal oedema
- Cellular infiltration of smooth muscles particularly by eosinophils and mast cells
- Increased airway secretions, capillary engorgement
- Deposition of excess collagen immediately beneath the basement membrane of the epithelium

Clinical features

Asthma is a diagnosis made on clinical, physiological and pathological characteristics. There is no standardised definition. It is a chronic disease. The presence of one or more of wheeze, breathlessness, cough and chest tightness along with the presence of variable but reversible airflow obstruction supports its diagnosis.

Severe asthma is diagnosed with any one of the following:

1. Peak expiratory flow (PEF) 33–50% best or predicted.
2. Unable to complete sentences in one breath.
3. Respiratory rate ≥ 25 breaths min^{-1}.
4. Pulse rate ≥ 110 beats min^{-1}.

Life-threatening asthma is diagnosed with any one of the following in a severe asthma patient:

1. PEF <33% best or predicted, Spo_2<92%, Pao_2 <8 kPa, normal $Paco_2$.
2. Silent chest, cyanosis or feeble respiratory effort.
3. Dysrhythmia or hypotension.
4. Exhaustion, confusion or coma.

Features of near-fatal asthma involve raised $Paco_2$ and/or the need for mechanical ventilation with raised pressures.

Differential diagnosis of acute severe asthma includes airway foreign body, bronchiolitis, congenstive heart failure, vocal cord dysfunction, gastro-oesophageal reflux and pulmonary fibrosis.

Investigations

Spirometry is increasingly available and is preferable to peak expiratory flow as it is less dependent on patient effort and gives a clearer indication of airway obstruction. Features of airflow obstruction with a forced expiratory volume (FEV)$_1$/ forced vital capacity (FVC) ratio <65%, or FEV$_1$ <70% predicted and features of reversibility with increase of FEV$_1$ >12% from baseline and at least 200 mL increase after an inhaled bronchodilator support the diagnosis of asthma.

Other investigations include eosinophil count, IgE levels and allergen testing.

Investigations in acute attacks should include an assessment of the level of the severity of the asthma, PEF or FEV$_1$, pulse oximetry and CXR. Where the arterial blood oxygen saturation is <92% or the patient has features of life-threatening asthma an arterial blood gas should be performed.

Treatment

The best strategy for management of acute exacerbations of asthma is early recognition and intervention, before attacks become severe and potentially life threatening. Detailed investigations into the circumstances surrounding fatal asthma have frequently revealed failures on the part of both patients and clinicians to recognize the severity of the disease and to intensify treatment appropriately.

The basic principles in the management of acute severe asthma include:

- Assessing the severity of the attack
- Correcting hypoxemia by administering supplemental oxygen
- Reversing airway obstruction with the use of β$_2$-agonist agents and early use of corticosteroids
- Preventing or treating complications
- Frequent objective assessments of the response to therapy until definite, sustained improvement is documented
- Transferring patient to a critical care unit if they do not improve after 4–6 h
- Once the patient is better, educating them about the principles of self-management for early recognition and treatment

Treatment – immediate

- Oxygen: aim for arterial blood oxygen saturation of 94–98%
- β$_2$-agonist via oxygen driven nebuliser (salbutamol 5 mg or terbutaline 10 mg – halve doses in very young children). Intravenous β$_2$-agonists should be reserved for those patients in whom inhaled therapy cannot be used reliably including while on mechanical ventilation
- Prednisolone 40–50 mg orally (daily) or 100 mg hydrocortisone i.v. every 6 h

- Chest X-ray to exclude a pneumothorax or consolidation

If acute severe or life-threatening asthma or in those with a poor initial response:

- Add ipratropium (0.5 mg 4–6 h) to nebulised β$_2$ agonist
- Intravenous magnesium sulphate (2 g infused over 20 min)
- Intravenous aminophylline is not likely to result in any additional bronchodilatation in acute asthma compared to treatment with β$_2$-agonists and steroids, unless the patient has life-threatening or near fatal asthma with a poor response to initial therapy, when it may be of benefit. Side effects such as palpitations, arrhythmias and vomiting are increased if i.v. aminophylline is used
- There is no evidence for the use of leukotriene receptor antagonists in acute severe asthma
- Antibiotics are not indicated routinely
- Hypokalaemia can be caused or exacerbated by β$_2$-agonist and/or steroid treatment and must be corrected

Repeat PEF measurements every 15–30 min from starting treatment. Measure blood gases and maintain arterial blood oxygen saturation above 92%.

Indications for admission to a critical care unit include worsening hypoxaemia and hypercapnea despite intervention, drowsiness or unconsciousness or respiratory arrest. Transfer the patient accompanied by a doctor prepared to intubate.

Mechanical ventilation in patients with acute severe asthma.

Consider mechanical ventilation when medical therapy is failing; do not leave this until it's too late. Intubation, ventilation and subsequent management on ICU should be performed by an experienced intensive care clinician. Ventilator settings are optimised for individual patients and will vary considerably over time.

The principles of mechanical ventilation in severe airflow obstruction are to reduce dynamic hyperinflation and achieve adequate oxygenation. This can be achieved by:

- Controlled hypoventilation
- Prolonging the expiratory time
- Unloading breathing effort
- Promoting synchrony between patient and ventilator

Do not overventilate or aim for normocarbia. Permissive hypercarbia is frequently well tolerated with a pH > 7.2. Permissive hypoventilation helps limit inspiratory pressures and reduce barotrauma and cardiovascular depression. Prolonging the expiratory phase is important as it helps reduce dynamic hyperinflation.

Reasonable initial ventilator settings include:
- Respiratory rate from 10 to 14 breaths/min
- Tidal volume less than 8 ml/kg
- Minute ventilation less than 115 ml/kg
- Inspiratory flow from 80 to 100 l/min and extrinsic positive end-expiratory pressure (PEEP) that is less than 80% of the intrinsic PEEP

Adjust the settings to minimise Pplat and intrinsic PEEP, preferably maintaining Pplat less than 30 cmH_2O and intrinsic PEEP less than 10 cmH_2O

Muscle relaxation using neuromuscular blocking drugs is frequently needed to achieve the above aims. Patients with severe asthma needing mechanical ventilation are also on high-dose steroids and therefore at an increased risk of critical illness neuropathy. Reduce this risk by minimising the duration of therapy with neuromuscular blocking drugs.

Continue maximal medical therapy throughout the period of ventilation.

Fluid therapy in severe asthma

Dehydration is common in the patient with severe asthma. Oral intake is often low and the patient has increased fluid losses caused by sweating and increased work of breathing. High positive intrathoracic pressures during mechanical ventilation reduce venous return and can lead to significant hypotension. Before induction of anaesthesia and intubation infuse fluids rapidly to avoid such complications.

Heliox

Heliox is a mixture of helium and oxygen (usually in a 70:30 ratio) and has a lower density than oxygen-enriched air; thus, enabling higher flows through the airways. It reduces dynamic hyperinflation, intrinsic PEEP and peak airway pressures. Heliox is easier to administer via a facemask and can be technically challenging when delivered whilst on mechanical ventilation. There is currently not enough evidence to support its use outside of a clinical trial.

Anaesthetics

Volatile anaesthetics can be added to the ventilator gas mixture to provide further bronchodilatation. This can be administered either as an intravenous infusion, i.e. ketamine or an inhalation agent, i.e. isoflurane.

Extracorporeal life support

Consider extracorporeal support in patients not responding to aggressive medical therapy and failing on mechanical ventilation, i.e. developing refractory status asthma.

Prognosis

Patients who survive to hospital discharge remain at high risk of death; this excess risk is only beginning to be recognised and may have a worse prognosis than some malignancies. Close medical follow-up is important for long-term survival. Survivors of near death due to asthma often deny the severity of their illness, and anxiety appears to be more common among close family members than the patients themselves. Depression is strongly associated with an increased risk of asthma mortality, and suspicion of depression in a survivor of a near-fatal asthma attack warrants formal evaluation and treatment.

Further reading

British Thoracic Society Scottish Intercollegiate Guidelines Network. British Guideline on the Management of Asthma, a national clinical guideline, Guideline 101. Edinburgh: SIGN, 2012.

Louie S, Morrissey BM, Kenyon NJ, et al. The critically ill asthmatic–from ICU to discharge. Clin Rev Allergy Immunol 2012; 43:30–44.

Related topics of interest

- Refractory hypoxaemia (p 295)
- Acute respiratory distress syndrome (ARDS) – diagnosis (p 8)
- Acute respiratory distress syndrome (ARDS) – treatment (p 11)
- Pulmonary function tests (p 280)

Blood and blood products

Key points

- The safety of blood is maintained by strict donor selection criteria and screening
- Blood is separated into components so that each component is available for specific clinical indications
- Perioperative cell salvage and autologous donation may avoid homologous transfusion

Screening

In England in 2009, 2.1 million blood donations were collected from 1.6 million donors. Donor selection guidelines are used to exclude donors at risk to themselves and recipients. Those with risk factors for HIV, Creutzfeldt–Jakob disease (CJD), variant CJD and intercurrent illnesses are excluded from donation. International blood screening varies, UK and Australia screen for:

- ABO and Rhesus (Rh) D blood groups
- Red cell antibodies
- Hepatitis B (surface antigen and DNA), HIV (antibody and RNA), HTLV (antibody), Hepatitis C (antibody and RNA) and Syphilis (antibody)
- Malaria antibodies, *T. cruzi* antibodies or West Nile virus RNA for donors at risk due to travel
- CMV antibody for blood for transplant recipients
- Platelets – screened at 24 h for bacterial contamination

Collection and storage

Approximately 450 mL (±10%) of whole blood is collected into a sterile pack containing CPD-A (citrate, phosphate and dextrose-adenine) anticoagulant. Red cells, platelets and plasma are separated by stepwise centrifugation. Components are resuspended in optimal additives to maximise their shelf life. Continuing metabolic activity causes storage lesion:

- Depletion of 2,3-diphosphoglycerate (2,3-DPG), adenosine triphosphate (ATP), PO_4^{2-}, platelets and factors V and VIII
- Accumulation of CO_2, H^+, K^+, activated clotting factors, denatured and activated proteins, microaggregates of platelets, white cells and fibrin
- The Hb-O_2 dissociation curve is shifted to the left by depletion of 2,3 DPG and hypothermia, but offset by a right shift due acidosis
- The P_{50} is less than 2.4 kPa (18 mmHg) after 1 week
- A reduction in red cell membrane integrity causes osmotic fragility, cell lysis and an increase in free haemoglobin

Leucodepletion, washing, irradiation and pathogen inactivation

Leucodepletion of blood products was introduced in 1999 in the UK. This reduces storage lesion, some immune and non-immune transfusion reactions, and viral and prion transmission. Other methods of reducing antigenicity include a triple saline wash (removes plasma proteins and antibodies), and irradiation [reduces T – cell proliferation and subsequent graft-versus-host-disease (GvHD), but reduces shelf-life of red cells]. Pathogen-inactivation methods used for FFP include photochemical inactivation with methylene blue (single units), and detergent methods (pooled donations).

Blood components

Whole blood

Few centres store whole blood. The shelf life is only 5 days and the risk of haemolysis and GVHD is higher because of larger amounts of plasma and white cells. Whole 'hot' blood < 24 h old can be provided only by special arrangement.

Red cells

In the UK, a standard unit of red cells contains only 20 mL of residual plasma; the rest of the plasma is replaced with an 'optimal additive' solution of saline, adenine, glucose and mannitol (SAGM). The final mean volume [standard deviation (SD)] of these red cell solutions is 282 mL ($\pm$ 32) and the haematocrit is 57% ($\pm$ 3). In the UK, these red cells have a shelf life of 35 days but elsewhere in the world it is 42 days. One unit should increase the patient Hb by 10 g L^{-1}. Red cells less than 5 days old are richer in clotting factors and platelets, however factors V and VIII decline over 24 h. Frozen red cells are used for rare blood groups, autologous storage or for combat field hospitals.

Platelets

An adult dose unit comprises the platelets from 4 to 6 whole blood donations. It will include about 250 mL of plasma and 60 mL of anticoagulant. Platelets are best stored at 22 °C and are agitated continuously (shelf life 5–7 days). This temperature is accompanied by the risk of bacterial contamination and platelets are now cultured before being issued. An adult dose unit will increase the platelet count by approximately 35×10^9 L^{-1}. If ABO-Rh incompatible platelets are transfused, donor red cells can cause Rhesus (Rh) sensitisation and low-grade haemolysis.

Fresh frozen plasma

A single pack of fresh frozen plasma (FFP) includes a mean of 220 mL of plasma and 60 mL of anticoagulant. The usual adult dose is 12–15 mL kg^{-1}, which is typically about four packs. FFP contains significant quantities of fibrinogen (20–50 g L^{-1}) and an adult dose will typically increase the fibrinogen concentration by about 1 g L^{-1} – this is the same as would result from an adult dose of cryoprecipitate. The risk of microbial infectivity with FFP can be reduced with treatment with either methylene blue (single donor units) or solvent and detergent (pools of 300–5000 plasma donations). It carries infection risks, and donor plasma leucocyte antibodies can cause transfusion-related acute lung injury.

Cryoprecipitate

Cryoprecipitate is prepared from FFP. It is high in fibrinogen and contains factors VIII (FVIII:C), XIII, von Willebrand's factor and fibronectin. It is indicated in fibrinogen deficiency/depletion, particularly in disseminated intramuscular coagulation and massive transfusion. A typical adult therapeutic dose is equivalent to 10 single donor units – this contains 3–6 g fibrinogen in a volume of 200–500 mL. Fibrinogen concentrate from pooled donors has recently become available and may provide an alternative to cryoprecipitate.

Other plasma products

All plasma products are derived from large plasma pools. Recipients are exposed to multiple donors. The sterilisation processes are thought to inactivate enveloped viruses but may not be sufficient to inactivate non-enveloped viruses or prions. The factor concentrates are freeze dried powders for reconstitution, and due to further processing, also inactivate non-enveloped viruses.

Albumin is made by cold fractionation followed by heating to 60 °C for 10 h. It is supplied as 4–5% or 20% albumin solutions.

Prothrombin complex concentrate contains factors IX, II, X and a small amount of VII. It is used for bleeding in patients with single or multiple congenital deficiencies of these factors, and for reversal of Vitamin-K inhibitors, where FFP thawing is delayed or a large FFP volume is undesirable.

Factors VIII and activated FactorVIIa (rFVIIa) are available in recombinant form and used in haemophilia. rFVIIa has been used off label for severe bleeding in trauma, surgical and obstetric haemorrhage. If used, it should be according to accepted guidelines after expert assessment. There may be increased risks of thrombosis, and it is expensive.

Alternatives to homologous blood

Autologous donation

Patients can pre-donate their own blood. This autologous blood is subject to the same screening tests as the homologous supply. The process is expensive with significant wastage. The risk of administrative errors is the same as for homologous blood. It is very rarely used in the UK.

Perioperative red cell salvage

This includes pre-operative normovolaemic haemodilution, intraoperative cell saver, and surgical drain reinfusion. Cell saver blood consists of washed red cells without platelets or clotting factors with risks of traumatic haemolysis, air/micro emboli, infusion of irrigants and hyperkalaemia.

Red cell substitutes

Haemoglobin based oxygen carriers (HBOCs) – from human, animal or recombinant Hb are either polymerised or linked to larger molecules to improve their half-life. Most of the first generation HBOCs caused vasoconstriction due to nitric oxide uptake.

They lack 2, 3-DPG and thus have a low P_{50}. A glutaraldehyde polymerised bovine HBOC Hemopure, is licensed for clinical use only in South Africa. The P_{50} is 4.9 kPa (30 mmHg). Newer products, Hemospan and PHP (pyridoxylated Hb polyoxyethylene), both conjugated human Hb, are in clinical trials.

Perfluorocarbons (PFCs) – are hydrocarbons with F^- ions replacing H^+ ions. This increases the solubility for oxygen. They are chemically inert and immiscible in water, but can be emulsified with surfactant. They have linear oxygen kinetics and require a high FIO_2. Newer generation agents have higher O_2 carrying capacity but remain investigational.

Further reading

Retter A, Wyncoll D, Pearse R, et al. Guidelines on the management of anaemia and red cell transfusion on adult critically ill patients. Br J Haematol 2013; 160:445–464.

McClelland DBL. United Kingdom Blood Services Handbook of Transfusion Medicine 4th Edition. Norwich; The Stationary Office, 2007 www. transfusionguidelines.org.uk
www.transfusion.com.au

Related topics of interest

- Blood coagulopathies (p 54)
- Blood transfusion and complications (p 58)

Blood coagulopathies

Key points

- Coagulation failure is common in critically ill patients and increases morbidity and mortality
- Delays associated with current laboratory testing may be improved with point of care testing
- Early expert haematological advice should be sought

Epidemiology

Coagulation failure occurs because of loss of normal haemostasis which requires equilibrium between the fibrinolytic and the clotting systems, the vascular endothelium and platelets. Twenty-five percent of major trauma patients have a coagulopathy by the time they reach hospital and it is an independent predictor of increased mortality. Abnormalities of coagulation are seen in 80% of patients with severe sepsis.

Pathophysiology

There are many reasons for coagulation failure in the critically ill:
- Surgical and non-surgical vessel trauma
- Acquired deficiencies of clotting factors and excessive fibrinolysis [e.g. major trauma with shock, massive transfusion, disseminated intravascular coagulation (DIC), extracorporeal circuits and liver disease]
- Thrombocytopenia: [e.g. drug-induced, anti-platelet antibodies (idiopathic thrombocytopenic purpura (ITP), heparin-induced thrombotic thrombocytopenic syndrome (HITTS) and sepsis]
- Hypothermia, which impairs clotting factor activity
- Anticoagulants (e.g. heparin, warfarin, aspirin and thrombolytics)
- Congenital coagulation factor deficiency

Clinical features

Coagulopathy should be suspected in any patient with abnormal bruising or signs of petechiae and purpura (including purpura fulminans seen in menigococcal sepsis), bleeding from mucous membranes and the GI tract, or continued bleeding from puncture sites, vascular access sites and wounds.

Investigations

Coagulation tests

Traditional laboratory coagulation tests [Prothrombin time (PT), Activated partial thromboplastin time (APTT), and Thrombin time (TT) take significant time to perform and do not assess all components involved in in vivo coagulation, e.g. vascular integrity and platelet function. Point of care testing has the potential for more rapid results and when combined with transfusion management algorithms may result in better outcomes. Available devices can test platelet function, clot viscoelasticity, heparin activity, PT and APTT.

PT tests the extrinsic pathway, with vitamin K-dependent factors (II, VII and X). Factor VII is the first to decrease with warfarin therapy. A normal time is 12–14 s for clot formation; the test sample should clot within 3 s of the control. Prolonged PT occurs in factor VII deficiency, liver disease, vitamin K deficiency or oral anticoagulant therapy.

APTT tests the intrinsic pathway (factors XII, XI, IX, VIII and X) activated by kaolin or cephaloplastin. The normal time is 30–45 s (method dependent) and samples that clot more than 6 s beyond the control are abnormal. APPT is prolonged in the presence of heparin, the haemophilias, von Willebrand's disease, severe fibrinolysis and DIC.

Activated clotting time is measured after whole blood is activated with diatomaceous earth. Clot formation normally occurs 90–130 s later. It tests predominantly the intrinsic pathway and is used as a bedside test for the action of heparin, but is also prolonged by thrombocytopenia, hypothermia, fibrinolysis and high-dose aprotinin.

TT: both the PT and the APTT include the final common pathway in their tests. This is tested specifically by the addition of thrombin to plasma (TT). A normal time is 9–15 s. Unlike a reptilase test, it is affected by heparin and fibrin degradation products (FDPs).

Bleeding time (normal range: 3–9 min) tests primary haemostasis of platelets and vessels. A blood pressure cuff is inflated to 40 mmHg and a standardised skin incision is made distal to it. If bleeding stops within 9 min, this is considered normal. Platelet count (normal range: $150–400 \times 10^9 \ L^{-1}$): Thromboelastography allows some functional assessment and point of care testing of platelet function is increasingly available.

All factors can be assayed, but factor VII components and fibrinogen are the ones most commonly measured. Normal fibrinogen level is $2–4.5 \ gL^{-1}$. Factor Xa assays are used to monitor the anticoagulant effect of low molecular weight heparins that do not affect APTT.

D-dimers and FDPs released by plasminolysis can be assayed and are often measured to confirm DIC. Minor elevations in levels of $20–40 \ \mu g \ mL^{-1}$ occur following surgery and trauma and may also accompany sepsis, DVT and renal failure. Assay of the D-dimer fragments is more specific but less sensitive for fibrinolysis. High D-dimer levels suggest excessive fibrinolysis (e.g. DIC). Euglobulin lysis time (ELT): ELT reflects the presence of plasminogen activators. With fibrinolytic activation the ELT time is shortened (normal range >90 min).

Specific problems

Haemophilias

Haemophilia A (classical haemophilia) is a sex-linked deficiency of factor VIII. Haemophilia B or Christmas disease is due to factor IX deficiency, and is less common than haemophilia A. Treatment is with factor VIII and IX respectively or rFVIIa for those with inhibitors.

Von Willebrand's disease

Autosomal dominant and the commonest hereditary coagulation disorder. Prophylactic infusion of DDAVP $0.3 \ \mu g \ kg^{-1}$ augments release of factor VIII and von Willebrand's factor and reduces the risk of haemorrhage.

Cryoprecipitate and fresh frozen plasma (FFP) will also correct the defects.

Haemostatic failure associated with liver disease

Cholestasis is associated with deficiencies of the vitamin K-dependent coagulation factors (II, VII, IX and X). This is reversed rapidly with vitamin K therapy. In the presence of extensive hepatocellular damage, vitamin K may be ineffective. Liver disease is also associated with thrombocytopenia secondary to splenomegaly.

Oral anticoagulant agents

These agents cause deficiencies of vitamin K-dependent clotting factors (II, VII, IX and X). Prothrombin complex concentrate (a mixture of human Factor II, IX, X and antithrombin III) will rapidly reverse warfarin in cases of life-threatening bleeding. FFP will also provide short-term reversal of anticoagulation (factor VII has a half-life of around 7 h) while vitamin K provides long-term antagonism of warfarin.

New oral anticoagulant agents, e.g. rivaroxaban (Xa inhibitor) and dabigatran (thrombin inhibitor) offer some advantages over warfarin but cannot be reversed by current usual therapies, specific antidotes are in development. Bleeding will require expert haematology input.

Heparin

Heparin potentiates the action of antithrombin III, and can be measured by prolongation of APTT. Protamine sulphate is a direct antagonist and 1 mg protamine will neutralise 100 units of heparin. In overdose, protamine is anticoagulant and it must be given slowly to avoid hypotension caused by pulmonary vasoconstriction. The low molecular weight heparins do not affect APPT; anti-Xa levels can be used for monitoring; their effect may not be fully reversed by protamine.

Anti-platelet agents

Aspirin and other non-steroidal anti-inflammatory drugs (NSAIDs) have Platelet inhibitory effects. Platelet function effects are largely irreversible, lasting up to 10 days after administration. Platelet transfusion may be required despite a normal platelet count.

Disseminated intravascular coagulopathy

Disseminated intravascular coagulopathy occurs when a powerful or persisting trigger activates haemostasis. The release of free thrombin leads to widespread deposition of fibrin and a secondary fibrinolytic response.

The major problem and presenting feature of acute disseminated intravascular coagulopathy (DIC) is bleeding. Thrombotic, haemorrhagic or mixed manifestations in various organ systems may also coexist. DIC is associated with numerous underlying problems:

- Sepsis (bacterial, especially Gram-negative organisms, viral, protozoal, especially malaria)
- Burns, snake bite and heat stroke
- Eclampsia, placental abruption, amniotic fluid embolism, retained products of conception and puerperal sepsis
- Hepatic failure and autoimmune diseases
- Malignancy (promyelocyte leukaemia and mucin-secreting adenocarcinomas)
- Surgery (cardiac, vascular neurosurgery and prostatic)
- Incompatible blood transfusion
- Extensive intravascular haemolysis
- Extracorporeal circuits

Diagnosis of DIC is usually based on the clinical picture with a supportive pattern of laboratory tests. A PT >15 s, a prolonged APPT, fibrinogen level <160 mg dL^{-1} and platelet count < 150×10^9 L^{-1} with high levels of FDPs (D-dimers) are confirmatory although they may not be present in all cases. The blood film may show fragmentation of the red cells (microangiopathic haemolytic anaemia), which is more commonly seen in chronic DIC associated with malignancy.

Treatment is aimed at the precipitating cause while replacing clotting factors and platelets.

Thrombocytopenia

Thrombocytopenia results from decreased production, increased consumption or extracorporeal loss of platelets. All of these factors play a role in the thrombocytopenia associated with sepsis.

1. Decreased production. Leukaemias, drug-induced thrombocytopenia (thiazides, quinine, anti-tuberculis drugs, carbamazepine, chloroquine, chlorpropamide, gold salts, methyldopa, chloramphenicol, high-dose penicillin and chemotherapy agents), marrow depression or infiltration by malignancy.
2. Increased consumption. Sepsis. ITP due to antiplatelet IgG autoantibodies, thrombotic thrombocytopenic purpura, haemolytic uraemic syndrome, shock, DIC, hypersplenism due to splenomegaly and HITTS.
3. Extracorporeal loss. Due to haemorrhage and haemodilution. Extracorporeal circuits (cardiopulmonary bypass, renal replacement therapy and plasmapheresis).

Treatment is directed at the underlying cause. Platelet transfusion if count is <10–20 $\times$ 10^9 L^{-1}. Prophylactic platelets are given prior to surgery or an invasive procedure.

Bleeding related to thrombolysis

With increasing use of thrombolytic agents, haemorrhagic complications are more common. The majority of haemorrhage occurs from cannula sites or the urinary or gastrointestinal tract. Less than 1% of bleeding complications are intracranial but the mortality rate is high. The risk of bleeding increases with dose and is increased if heparin is also administered. In the presence of serious bleeding, stop the infusion of thrombolytic agents and correct clotting by giving FFP and platelets.

Tranexamic acid

The CRASH-2 study demonstrated improved mortality in trauma patients if this anti-fibrinolytic agent is given within 3 hours of injury. It is cheap and appears safe. CRASH-3 will investigate its use in brain trauma.

Recombinant factor VIIa (rFVIIa)

rVIIa is licenced for haemophiliacs with inhibitors to factors VIII or IX, but has also been used in non-haemophiliacs when conventional therapy has failed to stop severe bleeding. Clinical trials failed to demonstrate mortality benefits, it is expensive and may be associated with increased thrombotic complications.

General management principles for abnormal bleeding

- Prevent hypoxia, and correct hypothermia and acidosis
- Give tranexamic acid to trauma patients at risk of significant bleeding within 3 h of injury
- Exclude surgical bleeding: provide surgical and non-surgical haemostasis (e.g. fracture immobilisation and angio-embolisation) where appropriate
- Give vitamin K and FFP in liver failure and to reverse the effects of warfarin. Urgent reversal of warfarin may be achieved with prothrombin complex concentrate

- Give protamine to reverse heparin
- Take blood samples for coagulation studies and platelet count/function
- Activate massive transfusion protocol as needed and give blood to maintain adequate circulating haemoglobin
- Give FFP to replace lost coagulation factors
- Give platelets to maintain a platelet count of $>50-100 \times 10^9 \, L^{-1}$ in the presence of active bleeding. Ratio approaching 1:1:1 for RBCs:FFP:platelets may have better outcomes in massive transfusion
- Give platelets to those patients who are bleeding with known recent aspirin or NSAID use
- Give cryoprecipitate or fibrinogen concentrate to replace fibrinogen
- Give other specific clotting factors as indicated (e.g. VIII, IX for the haemophilias) and seek expert advice

Further reading

Enriquez LJ, Shore-Lesserson L. Point-of-care coagulation testing and transfusion algorithms. Br J Anaesth 2009; 103:i14–i22.

Rossaint R, Bouillon B, Cerny V, et al. Management of bleeding following major trauma: an updated European guideline. Crit Care 2010; 14:R52.

National Blood Authority: Blood management guidelines. http://www.nba.gov.au/guidelines/review.html

Brohi K, Cohen MJ, Davenport RA. Acute coagulopathy of trauma: mechanism, identification and effect. Curr Opin Crit Care 2007; 13:680–685.

McClelland DBL. United Kingdom Blood Services Handbook of Transfusion Medicine 4th Edition. Norwich, The Stationary Office, 2007.

www.transfusionguidelines.org.uk

www.transfusion.com.au

Related topics of interest

- Blood transfusion and complications (p 58)
- Blood and blood products (p 51)

Blood transfusion and complications

Key points

- Blood products are indicated to improve oxygen delivery, provide volume support and improve haemostasis
- Blood transfusion remains an independent risk factor for mortality. Complications include clerical errors, infection transmission, immune reactions, immune suppression and inflammatory responses
- Transfusion guidelines aim to minimise unnecessary transfusion and manage this resource; they include restrictive transfusion triggers, blood salvage techniques, use of local and systemic haemostatic agents and erythropoiesis optimisation

Anaemia in the critically ill

Anaemia is a risk factor for renal failure, myocardial infarction stroke and mortality. The causes of anaemia include pre-existing anaemia, overt or occult bleeding, frequent blood sampling and anaemia of critical illness. Anaemia of critical illness is characterized by:

- Bone marrow suppression
- Reduced erythropoietin (EPO) production by impaired kidneys
- Poor marrow response to EPO
- Altered iron metabolism

Strategies to reduce anaemia and blood transfusion in the ICU include vigilance for bleeding, tolerance of anaemia in low risk patients, scrutiny of indications for antiplatelet and anticoagulant drugs, postoperative cell salvage and restricted sampling. Erythropoiesis can be optimised with the use of iron supplementation, folic acid, vitamin B_{12}, vitamin C, EPO and adequate nutrition.

Blood transfusion triggers

Most patients tolerate normovolaemic anaemia down to a haemoglobin value of 70 g L^{-1}. Transfusion is usually appropriate when the Hb concentration is less than 70 g L^{-1}. At Hb concentrations of more than 100 g L^{-1}, RBC transfusion is usually unnecessary and potentially harmful.

A target Hb value of around 90 g L^{-1} may be appropriate for patients with cerebrovascular disease or acute coronary syndromes (ACS). Do not transfuse ACS patients with Hb concentration > 100 g L^{-1}, because this is associated with increased mortality. These triggers are assessed for each patient based on haemodynamic state, evidence of impaired tissue oxygenation, haemostasis and cardiopulmonary reserve. The safe lower limit for unstable patients with ongoing bleeding is uncertain.

Haemorrhage and massive transfusion

Control of haemorrhage may require surgical or radiological intervention, reversal of anticoagulation, correction of clotting abnormalities and thrombocytopenia and/or systemic haemostatic agents. Patients who receive multiple units of blood within 24 h are at risk of coagulopathy, thrombocytopenia, hypothermia and acidosis. Ensure a massive transfusion protocol is in place to trigger the rapid provision of red cells, fresh frozen plasma (FFP), platelets and other clotting factors, e.g. cryoprecipitate.

Compatibility testing

There are more than 30 common antigens and hundreds more rare antigens. The risks of immunological reactions are small if ABO-compatible blood is used.

- Group – recipient blood is typed for ABO and Rhesus antigens. This takes less than 5 min
- Screen – recipient blood is screened for red cell antibody, by adding the serum to Group O red cells expressing known

antigens. This enables an urgent directed immediate spin cross-match later on

- Immediate spin cross-match – involves the addition of recipient sera to donor cells and observing for immediate agglutination. It confirms ABO compatibility and takes about 5 min. It will not reliably detect unexpected antibodies
- Full cross-match – requires incubation of donor cells and recipient sera for at least 15 min with an enhancing agent, and observing for agglutination. A Coombs test is then performed to detect antibody on donor red cells. The full cross-match test takes about 45 min

The risk of a major incompatible reaction varies with the extent of compatibility testing undertaken:

- Randomly selected (untyped donor and recipient)   35.6%
- Group O   0.8%
- ABO-compatible   0.6%
- ABO and Rhesus compatible   0.2%
- ABO, Rhesus and negative antibody screen   0.06%
- Complete compatibility testing   0.05%

Group O red cells can be used safely in an emergency. Rh negative cells are used for premenopausal females, while Rh positive is suitable for others. Patients who are group O are most at risk for an incompatible transfusion reaction because of the presence of anti-A and anti-B in their plasma. Group AB FFP is also safe, as it has no anti-A or anti-B antibodies.

Complications of blood transfusions

Immediate immune reactions:

- Acute haemolytic transfusion reaction – due to ABO, Lewis, Kell or Duffy incompatible donor cells causing complement-mediated cytotoxicity and/or lysis of red cells. There may be fevers, rigors, chest pain, back pain, dyspnoea, headache, urticaria, cyanosis, bronchospasm, pulmonary oedema, acute renal failure and cardiovascular collapse
- Febrile non-haemolytic transfusion reactions – occur in 1–5% of all

transfusions and are caused by recipient antibody to donor leucocyte/platelet HLA. The incidence has halved with leucocyte-depleted red cells

- Allergy – reactions are usually mild but anaphylaxis can occur
- Transfusion-related acute lung injury (TRALI) – non-cardiogenic pulmonary oedema caused by recipient antibody to donor leucocyte HLA. It happens within 6 h and can occur with minimal volumes. FFP is the commonest cause of TRALI

Delayed immune reactions (4–14 days post transfusion): these are due to undetected antibody. Alloimmunisation – to cellular or protein antigens is common, and causes problems with subsequent blood transfusion.

- Graft-versus-host disease – due to donor lymphocytes in blood products that react against host tissue. It is more likely in immunocompromised individuals, or those with some shared HLA (family member donors)

Non-immune immediate reactions:

- Transfusion-associated circulatory overload – occurs in up to 5% of patients and is the commonest adverse blood event
- Microbial contamination – risk increases with storage length. The most common organism is Yersinia enterocolitica
- Immune suppression – increases the risk of infection that is independent of bacterial contamination and impairs wound healing. Whether blood transfusion increases the risk of recurrence of cancer is controversial
- Infammatory response – can be induced by microaggregates of proteins and cells and may cause SIRS and/or ARDS
- Storage lesion-related metabolic disturbances – occur with rapid administration or massive transfusion. Hyperkalaemia, metabolic acidosis and metabolic alkalosis (citrate metabolism) may occur. Citrate toxicity, resulting in hypocalcaemia, is rare and is caused usually by FFP (blood in optimal additive includes very little residual citrate)

Non-immune delayed reactions:

- Viral infections – estimated infection risks (per unit transfused) associated with voluntary donor programmes are approximately: HIV 1:5,000,000, hepatitis B 1: 740,000: hepatitis C 1: 2,700,000

- Iron overload – complicates multiple transfusions over a long period of time. It results in haemosiderin deposition with myocardial and hepatic damage

Further reading

www.transfusionguidelines.org.uk
www.shotuk.org
www.transfusion.com.au
Retter A, Wyncoll D, Pearse R, et al. Guidelines on the management of anaemia and red cell transfusion in adult critically ill patients. Br J Haematol 2013; 160:445–464

Murphy MF, Waters JH, Wood EM, et al. Clinical Review: Transfusing blood safely and appropriately. Br Med J 2013; 347:f4303.
Vlaar AP, Juffermans NP. Transfusion-related acute lung injury: a clinical review. Lancet 2013; 382:984–994.

Related topics of interest

Brain death and organ donation

Key points

- Diagnosis of death includes cardiorespiratory and neurological criteria
- Consider organ donation in all dying patients
- Donation after circulatory death is becoming increasingly common
- This topic represents UK guidance and will differ in other countries

Death constitutes the irreversible loss of the capacity to breathe and the capacity for consciousness.

Determination of death

Cardiorespiratory criteria

Diagnosing death by cardiorespiratory criteria is the commonest method. Absence of cardiac function is confirmed by the absence of central pulse on palpation and the absence of heart sounds on auscultation along with asystole on continuous ECG, absence of flow on an arterial trace or absence of contractility on echocardiography, should these methods be available. Following 5 min of observation to confirm cardiorespiratory arrest, neurological assessment is performed to confirm absence of pupillary response to light, absence of corneal reflex and absence of motor response to supra-orbital pressure. Once these criteria are met, the patient's death is confirmed. Observation times vary internationally.

Neurological criteria

In the UK, brainstem death is equivalent to whole brain death. There are three stages to diagnosis: fulfilment of preconditions; exclusion of reversible factors; demonstration of coma, absent brainstem reflexes and apnoea. Some countries require demonstration of whole brain death, which can be achieved clinically or require ancillary testing.

Diagnosis of death by neurological criteria

Preconditions

Prior to considering brainstem testing:
- The patient should be in a coma, apnoeic and requiring mechanical ventilation
- A diagnosis of irreversible brain damage of known aetiology is required

When the cause of the irreversible brain damage cannot be fully established, such as in cases of hypoxic brain injury, brainstem testing can be performed only if the possibility of a reversible or treatable cause has been excluded.

Exclusion of reversible causes

Prior to brainstem testing, the following criteria must be met to ensure that there are no endocrine, metabolic, drug induced or circulatory reversible causes to the patient's apnoea and coma.

Medications

Drugs can artificially maintain apnoea or coma – mainly sedative, analgesic and neuromuscular blocking agents. The time needed between discontinuation of the drug and brainstem testing needs careful consideration and varies according to the drug given, total dose given, duration of administration, use of other medications that may influence metabolism, any underlying hypothermia, hepatic or renal failure, and the age of the patient.
Exclusion of their effects can include:
- Waiting for a period exceeding four times the drug's elimination half-life (care required in hepatorenal dysfunction)
- Use of specific antagonists such as naloxone or flumazenil
- Serum testing for drug concentrations

If there are any concerns about residual effects of drugs, ancillary investigations of cerebral function will be necessary.

Cardiorespiratory parameters

Adequate mean arterial pressure (MAP), oxygenation, carbon dioxide and pH control are required prior to testing with the following parameters met:

MAP	> 60 mmHg (consistently)
pH	7.35–7.45
P_{CO_2}	<6.0 kPa
P_{O_2}	>10 kPa

Temperature

Core temperature must be >34 °C.

Biochemistry

Correct gross biochemical abnormalities to achieve the following values before testing:

Na^+	115–160 mmol L^{-1}
K^+	>2 mmol L^{-1}
Mg^{2+}	0.5–3 mmol L^{-1}
Phosphate	0.5–3 mmol L^{-1}
Glucose	3–20 mmol L^{-1}

Other causes of apnoea

Exclude cervical spine injury or severe neuromuscular weakness.

Testing

Brainstem function tests are carried out by two clinicians with at least 5 years registration, of which one must be a consultant. Testing must occur on two separate occasions, but time of death is recorded as the time of the first test.

Brainstem reflexes

To confirm irreversible loss of brainstem reflexes the following should be absent:

a. Pupillary response to light direct and consensual (cranial nerves [CNs] II, III; midbrain)
b. Corneal reflex to light touch (CNs V, VII; pons)
c. Oculo-vestibular reflex with absence of eye movements during or after the injection of 50 mL cold saline into each auditory canal over 60 s (CNs III, IV, VI, VIII; pons)
d. Response to supra-orbital painful stimulus (CNs V, VII; pons)
e. Gag reflex to posterior pharynx stimulus (CNs IX, X; medulla)
f. Cough reflex with stimulus of the carina (CN X; medulla)

Apnoea testing

This is the last brainstem reflex to be tested.

- Increase F_{IO_2} to 1.0
- Reduce minute ventilation until Pa_{CO_2} >6.0 kPa and pH <7.4 (in chronic hypercapnia, increase Pa_{CO_2} until >6.5 kPa and pH <7.4)
- If cardiovascularly stable, disconnect from ventilator and attach 5 L/min of oxygen via a tracheal catheter. Apply CPAP if arterial blood oxygenation is not maintained.
- Observe for respiratory effort for 5 min
- Confirm increase in Pa_{CO_2} by at least 0.5 kPa
- Reconnect ventilator

Other tests

Sometimes preconditions cannot be met, or full neurological examination is not possible. Here, ancillary tests of brainstem function aim to detect electrical activity (EEG; evoked potentials) or cerebral perfusion (angiography; CT/MRI angiography; Doppler; PET).

Organ donation and transplantation

Success rates of organ donation and transplantation have greatly improved since the first attempted renal transplant (1906). Reasons for this include better surgical techniques, tissue-matching, improved retrieval and storage, and immunosuppressive therapy. The limiting factor continues to be organ availability; donation after brain death (DBD) is reducing and demand is increasing. This gap has yet to be filled by increases in live donation (e.g. renal and hepatic) and donation after circulatory death (DCD).

Donor identification

Consider organ donation should be considered in all patients expected to die in ICU, but any decision to withdraw treatment must be completely divorced from the consideration of organ donation. Likewise, quality of care must not be altered by decisions made about organ donation.

Consent

If the patient is suitable for DBD or DCD, the local specialist nurse in organ donation

(SNOD) is contacted and the Organ Donation Pathway is commenced. Initial stages include checking the organ donor register and discussing with the Coroner (or Procurator Fiscal).

The patient's family is approached to discuss the options. If the family objects to donation, even with evidence of the patient's wish to donate, donation cannot proceed. With agreement to continue, the patient's organs are offered to transplant centres.

Donation after circulatory death

Controlled DCD is planned before death, usually with those patients who are to have active treatment withdrawn (although patients awaiting DBD may arrest and become DCD donors). Uncontrolled DCD involves patients who are dead on hospital arrival or who have undergone unsuccessful resuscitation and is therefore uncommon, requiring rapid decisions and prompt attendance of retrieval teams.

Contraindications to potential organ donation within the United Kingdom include:
- Age > 80 for DCD
- Age >85 for DBD
- Known or suspected CJD disease
- Known HIV disease but not infection alone
- Disseminated active cancer

If consent is obtained and organs accepted, treatment is continued until an appropriate time for withdrawal (considering family, ICU staff and the retrieval team). Treatment is withdrawn in accordance with the unit's procedure, unaltered by the consideration of donation. Relatives can stop the donation process at any time.

After cardiorespiratory arrest, death is confirmed by a doctor independent of the retrieval team after 5 min of observation of apnoea and mechanical asystole. The family is given time with the patient before transfer to theatre.

Maximum warm ischaemic times are organ specific:
- Liver <30 min
- Pancreas <30 min
- Lung <60 min
- Kidney <2 h

Donation after brain death

If consent is obtained and organs accepted, then appropriate treatment is continued. The aim is to optimise the condition of the organs until retrieval teams are in theatre. Organ donation pathway and bundles provide guidance as to what physiological parameters should be maintained and how.

Further reading

Murphy PG, Bodenham AR, Thompson JP. Diagnosis of death and organ donation in 2012. Br J Anaesth 2012; 108:i1–2.

Oram J, Murphy P. Diagnosis of Death. Contin Educ. Anaesth Crit Care Pain 2011; 11:77–81.

NHS Blood & Transplant website: www. organdonation.nhs.uk.

UK Donation Ethics Committee. An ethical framework for controlled donation after circulatory death. London: Academy of Medical Royal Colleges, 2011.

Academy of Medical Royal Colleges. A code of practice for the diagnosis and confirmation of death. London: Academy of Medical Royal Colleges, 2008.

National Institute for Health and Clinical Excellence (NICE). Organ donation for transplantation: improving donor identification and consent rates for deceased organ donation, Clinical Guidelines CG135. London: NICE, 2011.

Related topics of interest

Burns

Key points

- Major burns are associated with a significant inflammatory and hypermetabolic state
- Initial assessment should follow the principles of trauma management; consider early tracheal intubation in those with signs of inhalational injury
- Initial fluid resuscitation should follow the Parkland formula

Epidemiology

Each year approximately 140,000 new burn injuries present to the emergency department in England and Wales, 5–10% of these patients will require hospitalisation. Mortality rates for all burn inpatients are approximately 14%.

Pathophysiology

Systemic changes

Major burns cause the systemic inflammatory response syndrome (SIRS), with immediate activation of the inflammatory cascade. Vascular permeability increases dramatically leading to generalised oedema in patients with burns >30% of total body surface area (TBSA).

The first 24–48 h following a severe burn are associated with a decrease in cardiac output by up to 50% and an increase in systemic vascular resistance. Subsequently, with adequate fluid resuscitation, cardiac output increases and systemic vascular resistance decreases.

Metabolic

Major burns are associated with a profound hypermetabolic state; the metabolic rate may reach values two to three times greater than normal. There is an increase in catabolic hormones with catabolic protein loss, increased gluconeogenesis and decreased synthesis of new proteins.

Pulmonary

Upper airway injury results in oedema to the supraglottic structures potentially progressing to airway obstruction. Lower airway injury usually results from inhaled noxious gases damaging the mucosal epithelium causing increased mucus secretion, ciliary dysfunction, epithelial sloughing, inflammation and atelectasis.

Multiple noxious gases maybe inhaled in smoke – carbon monoxide and cyanide the two best described. Carbon monoxide binds to haemoglobin with an affinity approximately 250 times greater than oxygen; it shifts the oxyhaemoglobin dissociation curve to the left and interferes with the cytochrome oxidase system. Hydrogen cyanide inhibits the cytochrome oxidase system causing cellular hypoxia and forcing ATP generation via anaerobic metabolism producing lactate.

Immune system

The burn injury results in loss of the protective dermal barrier; in addition, the major burn patient frequently requires multiple invasive procedures including line placements which increase the risk of septic complications.

Clinical features

Lund and Browder charts provide an accurate assessment of burn injury as % of TBSA in adults and children (**Figure 3**). The degree of tissue damage is defined by the burn depth. In superficial burns only the epidermal layer is affected. It is erythematous, painful and dry, blisters are absent. Partial-thickness burns involve both the epidermal and dermal layers and may be superficial or deep depending on the degree of dermal damage. There is erythema, blisters, oedema and pain. Full thickness burns destroy all skin layers and if complex will involve subcutaneous structures. The burn is white and painless and there is no capillary return.

Clinical signs of inhalational injury include stridor, hoarse voice, oro-pharyngeal oedema, cyanosis, cough, wheeze and copious secretions which maybe carbonaceous and singeing of facial or nasal hair. The clinical

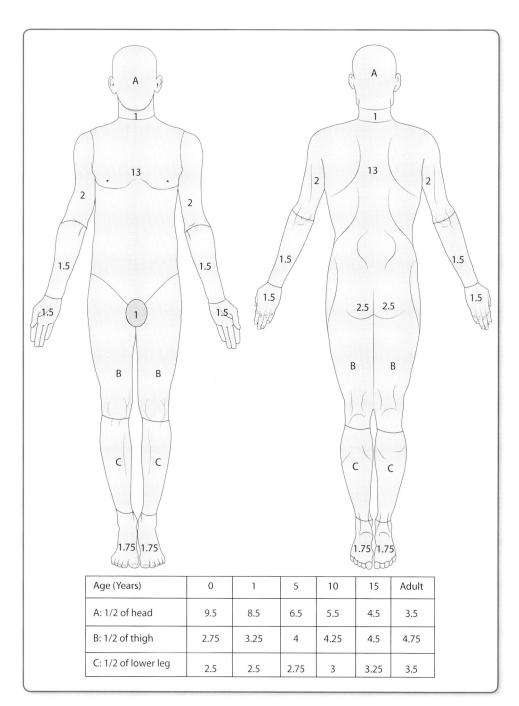

Age (Years)	0	1	5	10	15	Adult
A: 1/2 of head	9.5	8.5	6.5	5.5	4.5	3.5
B: 1/2 of thigh	2.75	3.25	4	4.25	4.5	4.75
C: 1/2 of lower leg	2.5	2.5	2.75	3	3.25	3.5

Figure 3 Lund and Browder chart. Numbers are % of total body surface area (TBSA). Letters are dependent on age and read from the table.

signs of carbon monoxide poisoning include headache, nausea and vomiting, hypotension, seizures and coma.

Investigations

Arterial blood gases with co-oximetry (essential) allow assessment of the proportion of carboxyhaemoglobin in inhalational injury. A persisting lactic acidosis should alert to the possibility of cyanide poisoning.

Fibreoptic bronchoscopy can aid in the diagnosis and management of inhalation injury, changes can take several days to develop.

Diagnosis

The nature and severity of a burn is defined by the causative agent (thermal, electric, chemical or radiation), the proportion of TBSA and anatomical locality involved, depth, associated inhalational injury, co-morbidities and age. Referral to a specialist burn centre should follow national guidelines.

Treatment

The principles of severe trauma management should be followed when assessing a burns patient – airway with cervical spine control, breathing, circulation and neurological disability. Burns patients may sustain other serious trauma which should be treated in a timely manner.

Airway and inhalational injury

Early tracheal intubation should be performed in the presence of stridor, respiratory failure, decreased conscious level, facial or neck burns or oro-pharyngeal oedema. Use an uncut tracheal tube to allow for evolving facial swelling. Suxamethonium is safe in the first 24 h after the burn, after this it is contraindicated up to 1 year because it may cause hyperkalaemia.

Treatment of carbon monoxide poisoning is with 100% oxygen, which reduces the half-life of HbCO from 4 h to 1 h. Consider invasive ventilation in those with HbCO levels >25%. Hyperbaric oxygen therapy at 3 atm will further reduce the half-life to under 30 min and should be considered in pregnant or comatose patients, those with HbCO levels >40% and patients who are failing to respond to standard treatment.

Fluid resuscitation

Intravenous fluid resuscitation is needed in any adult with burns involving >15% TBSA or >10% TBSA if associated with an inhalational injury. The Parkland formula is the most commonly used method to calculate resuscitative fluid volume, the volume of fluid infused in the first 24 h from the time of the burn is 4 mL × weight (kg) × %TBSA burnt; half is given in the first 8 h, the other half given over the remaining 16 h. Warmed Hartmann's solution is the most commonly used fluid. The Parkland formula acts as a guide and other endpoints of resuscitation should be monitored including urine output. Use invasive haemodynamic monitoring in the more severely burnt patient.

Ventilation

Use lung protective ventilator techniques. Specific treatments for inhalational injury include pulmonary toilet, regular bronchodilator therapy and bronchoscopic lavage.

Analgesia

Initial analgesia comprises titrated intravenous morphine, followed by regular paracetamol and oral opiates. Post-surgical analgesia can be managed with an opiate-based patient controlled analgesic system, operation maybe difficult if both hands are injured. Dressing changes require short acting analgesia – intravenous opiates, ketamine or Entonox are valuable solutions.

Nutrition and metabolism

Early enteral nutrition is associated with improved survival. Gastrointestinal mucosal protection is best achieved with early enteral nutrition and either a proton pump inhibitor or H_2-receptor antagonist.

Control the environmental temperature at 28–32 °C with high humidity to decrease evaporative heat and fluid losses. Emerging evidence suggests the hypermetabolic state can be attenuated with insulin, synthetic testosterone or beta-blockers.

Infection

Infective complications are common and a significant source of morbidity and mortality. The identification of sepsis is complicated because the burns patient will already have signs of SIRS. The avoidance of infection by meticulous asepsis and hand hygiene is vital.

Surgical management

Early excision, debridement and burn closure are important in reducing the hypermetabolic state, infection, pain, length of stay and mortality. Circumferential full thickness burns of the thorax, limb(s) or neck may necessitate urgent escharotomies.

Complications

Generalised oedema from over resuscitation can lead to abdominal compartment syndrome and pulmonary oedema. Infective complications are common, including wound and indwelling device sepsis and pneumonia. Early complications include venous thromboembolism, gastro-duodenal ulceration and renal failure. Late complications include pulmonary fibrosis, contractures, chronic pain and post-traumatic stress disorder.

Further reading

McClure J, Moore EC. Burns and inhalational injury. Anaesthesia and Intensive Care 2011; 12:393–398.

National Network for Burn Care (NNBC). National Burn Care Referral Guidance, Version 1. London: NBBC, 2012.

Greenhalgh DG, Saffle JR, Holmes JH, et al. American Burn Association consensus conference to define sepsis and infection in burns. J Burn Care Res 2007; 28:776–790.

Related topics of interest

- Abdominal compartment syndrome (p 1)
- Infection acquired in hospital (p 192)
- Nutrition (p 230)

Calcium, magnesium and phosphate

Key points

- Measurement of ionised calcium is necessary for the accurate diagnosis of hypocalcaemia
- Severe hypocalcaemia may follow parathyroidectomy
- Initial treatment of hypercalcaemia involves rehydration, whatever the cause

Calcium

Over 99% of body calcium is in bone, and about 1% is freely exchangeable with extracellular fluid (ECF). Ionised calcium is crucial to many processes, including nerve and neuromuscular conduction/contraction and coagulation. Normal daily intake is 10–20 mmol and normal total serum calcium is in the range 2.25–2.7 mmol L^{-1}. Intestinal calcium absorption is enhanced by 1,25-dihydroxy-vitamin D_3 (1, 25 $(OH)_2$ D_3). Around 40% is bound to albumin and total serum calcium decreases 0.02 mmol L^{-1} for each 1 g L^{-1} decrease in albumin. Ionised calcium is the physiologically important form and the normal level is 1.15 mmol L^{-1}.

Hypocalcaemia

Hypocalcaemia occurs when calcium is lost from the ECF (most commonly through renal mechanisms) in greater quantities than can be replaced by bone or the intestine. As a result of reduced absorption or poor dietary intake, hypocalcaemia and hypomagnesaemia often coexist. Common causes of hypocalcaemia are:

- Renal failure
- Hypoparathyroidism (including post-parathyroidectomy)
- Sepsis
- Burns
- Hypomagnesaemia
- Pancreatitis
- Malnutrition
- Osteomalacia
- Alkalosis (reduced ionised calcium)
- Citrate toxicity (e.g. large volumes of fresh frozen plasma during massive transfusion)

Clinical features

Symptoms of hypocalcaemia correlate with the magnitude and rate of the decrease in serum calcium. Main features include neuromuscular irritability evidenced by extremity and circumoral paraesthesiae, Chvostek and Trousseau signs, muscle cramps, tetany, laryngospasm and seizures. A prolonged QT is seen on ECG and may progress to VT/VF.

Treatment

Therapy depends on the severity of the hypocalcaemia and its cause. Check and correct serum magnesium and phosphate. Chronic asymptomatic mild hypocalcaemia can be treated with oral calcium supplements. If metabolic acidosis accompanies hypocalcaemia, correct the calcium concentration before the acidosis. Calcium and hydrogen ions compete for protein-binding sites, so an increase in pH will lead to a rapid decrease in ionised calcium. In the presence of acute symptomatic hypocalcaemia, give an intravenous bolus of calcium (100–200 mg or 2.5–5 mmol) over 5 min. This can be followed by a maintenance infusion of 1–2 mg $kg^{-1}h^{-1}$. Calcium chloride 10% contains 27.2 mg Ca mL^{-1} (0.68 mmol mL^{-1}) and calcium gluconate 10% contains 9 mg mL^{-1} (0.225 mmol L^{-1}). Calcium gluconate causes less venous irritation than calcium chloride.

Calcium management following parathyroidectomy

In chronic renal failure the glomerular filtration rate decreases and phosphate (PO_4) is not excreted. Phosphate levels in the blood rise and this decreases the level of the active metabolite of 1, 25$(OH)_2D_3$. As a result, patients have hypocalcaemia and defective bone mineralisation. The low calcium stimulates the parathyroid gland to increase production of parathyroid hormone, PTH (secondary hyperparathyroidism). If the secondary hyperparathyroidism is prolonged, the secretion of PTH becomes autonomous – tertiary hyperparathyroidism. This leads to high calcium values. High calcium and high PO_4 values cause precipitation of calcium in tissues and organs. After total or partial parathyroidectomy the calcium value can fall rapidly, particularly in patients who have evidence of 'hungry bone syndrome' (high alkaline phosphatase). These patients may need large quantities of i.v. calcium replacement. Some patients have hypercalcaemia with calcification of small and medium blood vessels, leading to skin necrosis and ulcers particularly on their legs. This is called calciphylaxis and these patients' calcium levels should be kept at the lower limit of normal.

Calcium infusion after parathyroidectomy

Calcium infusions are best given through a central venous catheter because peripheral i.v. calcium may cause necrosis. Check calcium values 4 h until stable, then 6 h. Check the patient's alkaline phosphatase concentration preoperatively: the higher the value, the more likely that symptomatic hypocalcaemia will occur postoperatively. Prescribe oral calcium medications. If the corrected calcium value is <2.4 mmol L^{-1}, commence a calcium infusion.

Dilute 20 mL 10% calcium chloride in 100 mL 0.9% sodium chloride (**Table 8**). Check corrected calcium 4 h, and adjust rate (**Table 9**). If the patient has tertiary hyperparathyroidism or calciphylaxis, choose the lower infusion rate; if they have alkaline phosphatase > 300 units L^{-1}, choose the higher infusion rate. All patients require oral calcium, 1 g, 8-hourly, and calcitriol, 0.5–1.0 µg daily in two divided doses, as soon as they are able to drink.

Hypercalcaemia

Hypercalcaemia occurs generally when the influx of calcium from bone or the intestine exceeds renal calcium excretory capacity. Common causes include:

- Hyperparathyroidism (accounts for > 50% of cases)
- Neoplasms (primary with ectopic PTH secretion, secondary with bone metastases)
- Sarcoidosis (increased production of $1,25(OH)_2D_3$ by granulomatous tissue)
- Drugs (thiazides and lithium)
- Immobilisation of any cause

Table 8 Starting rate of calcium infusion	
Preoperative alkaline phosphatase (ALP) level (unit L^{-1})	Calcium chloride infusion rate (mL h^{-1})*
200–100	5
400–800	10
>800	15
*20 mL 10% calcium chloride in 100 mL 0.9% sodium chloride.	

Table 9 Adjusted rate of calcium infusion	
Plasma corrected calcium (mmol L^{-1})	Calcium chloride infusion rate (mL h^{-1})*
2.0–2.4	5–10
1.8–2.0	10–15
1.7–1.8	25–30
<1.7	35–40
*20 mL 10% calcium chloride in 100 mL 0.9% sodium chloride.	

- Vitamin D intoxication
- Thyrotoxicosis
- Milk-alkali syndrome (consumption of calcium-containing antacids)

Clinical features

Symptoms depend on the rate of rise as well as the absolute value of calcium. Mild hypercalcaemia is usually asymptomatic. Severe hypercalcaemia causes neurological, gastrointestinal and renal symptoms. Features range from mild weakness, depression, psychosis and drowsiness to coma. Gastrointestinal effects include nausea, vomiting, abdominal pain, constipation, peptic ulceration and pancreatitis. Nephrogenic diabetes insipidus, renal stones, nephrocalcinosis and ectopic calcification may occur.

Treatment

Treat the underlying cause of hypercalcaemia. Most cases of mild hypercalcaemia are caused by primary hyperparathyroidism and many will require parathyroidectomy. Patients with symptomatic moderate (serum calcium >3.0 mmol L^{-1}) or severe (>3.4 mmol L^{-1}) hypercalcaemia require intravenous saline to restore intravascular volume and enhance renal calcium excretion. Avoid thiazide diuretics but furosemide (frusemide) will enhance calcium excretion. Patients with severe hypercalcaemia associated with raised PTH should be referred for urgent parathyroidectomy. Bisphosphonates (e.g. etidronate and sodium pamidronate) have become the main therapy for the management of hypercalcaemia caused by enhanced osteoclastic bone reabsorption. Steroids are effective in hypercalcaemia associated with haematological malignancies and in diseases related to $1,25(OH)_2D_3$ excess (e.g. sarcoidosis and vitamin D toxicity).

Magnesium

Magnesium is essential for cellular and enzyme function. Total body magnesium store is about 1000 mmol, of which 50–60% is in bone. The normal plasma range is 0.7–1.0 mmol L^{-1}. The normal daily intake is 10–20 mmol, which is balanced by urine and faecal losses. The kidney is the primary organ involved in magnesium regulation.

Hypomagnesaemia

Hypomagnesaemia occurs in up to 65% of critically ill patients and is often associated with hypokalemia. Usually follows loss of magnesium from the gastrointestinal tract or kidney.

- Gastrointestinal causes include prolonged nasogastric suction or vomiting, diarrhoea, extensive bowel resection, severe malnutrition and acute pancreatitis
- Renal losses occur with volume expanded states, hypercalcaemia, diuretic therapy, alcohol, aminoglycosides and cisplatin exposure and the polyuric phase of acute kidney injury
- Other causes include phosphate depletion, hyperparathyroidism and diabetes mellitus

Clinical features

Most symptoms are non-specific. The accompanying ion abnormalities such as hypocalcaemia, hypokalaemia and metabolic alkalosis account for many of the clinical features. Neurological signs include confusion, weakness, ataxia, tremors, carpopedal spasm and seizures. A wide QRS, long PR, inverted T, and U wave may be seen on ECG. Arrhythmias may occur, including severe ventricular arrhythmias (torsades de pointes), and there is increased potential for cardiac glycoside toxicity.

Treatment

Treat the underlying cause. Treat moderate-to-severe hypomagnesaemia, especially if associated with acute arrhythmia or seizure, with 8–10 mmol of magnesium sulphate i.v. over 5 min followed by additional doses titrated against serum levels. Replace potassium at the same time. Oral magnesium sulphate is a laxative and may cause diarrhoea.

Hypermagnesaemia

Hypermagnesaemia is usually caused by excess IV administration. High magnesium concentrations antagonise the entry of calcium and prevent excitation.

Clinical features

Include hypotension, bradycardia, drowsiness and hyporeflexia (knee jerk is a useful clinical test and is lost above 4 mmol L^{-1}). Values >6 mmol L^{-1} cause coma and respiratory depression.

Treatment

Stop giving magnesium. Give calcium chloride to antagonise the effect of magnesium. Diuretics increase renal loss. In severe cases dialysis may be required.

Phosphate

Total body phosphate in adults is about 700 g: approximately 85% is in bone and 15% is in ECF and soft tissue. Phosphate is found in adenosine triphosphate (ATP), 2,3-diphosphoglycerate (2, 3-DPG) in red blood cells, phospholipids and phosphoproteins. Phosphate is essential in many cellular functions and also acts as a buffer. The normal serum value is 0.85–1.4 mmol L^{-1}.

Hypophosphataemia

Hypophosphataemia results from internal redistribution, increased urinary excretion and decreased intestinal absorption.

- Internal redistribution of phosphate may result from respiratory alkalosis, re-feeding after malnutrition, recovery from diabetic ketoacidosis and the effects of hormones and other agents [insulin, glucagon, adrenaline (epinephrine), Cortisol and glucose]
- Increased urinary excretion of phosphate occurs in hyperparathyroidism, vitamin D deficiency, malabsorption, volume expansion, renal tubular acidosis and alcoholism
- Decreased intestinal absorption of phosphate occurs in antacid abuse, vitamin D deficiency and chronic diarrhoea

Clinical features

Clinical features are usually seen when the phosphate value has decreased below 0.3 mmol L^{-1}. They may include weakness (which may contribute to respiratory failure and problems with weaning from mechanical ventilation), cardiac dysfunction, paraesthesia, coma and seizures.

Treatment

Correct the underlying cause. Ten mmol phosphate (as potassium dihydrogen phosphate) can be given i.v. over 60 min and repeated depending on measured values (a sodium phosphate preparation is also available). There is a risk of hypocalcaemia associated with i.v. replacement and serum calcium must be maintained. Oral phosphate can be given in doses of 2–3 g daily.

Hyperphosphataemia

Renal failure is the most common cause.

- Reduced renal excretion: renal failure, hypoparathyroidism, acromegaly, bisphosphonate therapy and magnesium deficiency
- Increased exogenous load: i.v. infusion, excess oral therapy, phosphate-containing enemas
- Increased endogenous load: tumour lysis syndrome, rhabdomyolysis, bowel infarction, malignant hyperthermia, haemolysis and acidosis
- Pseudo-hyperphosphataemia: multiple myeloma

Clinical features

Hypocalcaemia and tetany may occur with a rapid rise in phosphate concentration. A large rise in calcium × phosphate product causes ectopic calcification in tissues, nephrocalcinosis and renal stones.

Treatment

Aluminium hydroxide is used as a binding agent. Magnesium and calcium salts are also effective and aluminium accumulation is a risk. Dialysis may be required.

Further reading

Marcocci C, Cetani F. Clinical practice. Primary hyperparathyroidism. N Engl J Med 2011; 365:2389–2397.

Aguilera IM, Vaughan RS. Calcium and the anaesthetist. Anaesthesia 2000; 55:779–790.
Weisinger JR, Bellorin-Font E. Magnesium and phosphorus. Lancet 1998; 352:391–396.

Related topics of interest

Cancer patients and critical care

Key points

- Advances in cancer treatment have resulted in improved patient survival and more cancer patients are being considered for admission to critical care units
- Duration of stay, mechanical ventilation and number of organs involved are important predictors of survival of cancer patients
- The outcomes of cancer patients admitted to critical care units have improved over time

Introduction

Recent advances in cancer treatment have improved life expectancy in patients with haematological and solid malignancies. The outcomes of cancer patients in critical care units have also been improving. Admission may be precipitated for the management of complications associated with the disease and its treatment, administration of specific cancer therapy or post-operative care. Factors that predict critical care mortality in cancer patients include the duration of stay, mechanical ventilation and number of organ system failures rather than specific cancer characteristics. The following discussion highlights conditions affecting cancer patients that may precipitate their admission to a critical care unit.

Oncological and haematological emergencies

Direct tumour involvement

Superior vena cava syndrome

Superior vena cava obstruction is most commonly caused by compression from a malignant mediastinal mass and can be life-threatening if associated with tracheal obstruction. Treatment includes corticosteroids, chemotherapy or radiotherapy for sensitive tumours or surgical resection. Anticoagulation is administered as thrombus formation is frequently observed.

Neurological complications

Spinal cord compression is seen more commonly in patients with prostate, lung and breast cancer. Prompt management is critical to alleviate pain and preserve neurological function. Magnetic Resonance Imaging (MRI) of the spine is the investigation of choice (**Figure 4**).

Treatment consists of high-dose corticosteroids, radiotherapy and/or surgery. Indications for surgery include spinal instability, a radio-resistant or undiagnosed tumour or a single level of cord compression.

Brain tumours, either primary or metastatic, can result in a number of neurological emergencies including cerebral herniation, haemorrhage and seizures.

Malignant pericardial effusion

Malignant pericardial disease can be caused by direct invasion from thoracic tumours or haematogenous spread. It can be complicated by life-threatening tamponade. Echocardiography is the diagnostic imaging of choice and can guide pericardiocentesis in haemodynamically unstable patients. Given fluid re-accumulates in approximately half of cases, consideration should be given to definitive therapy such as the creation of a pericardial window.

Metabolic complications

Malignant hypercalcaemia

Hypercalcaemia of malignancy is predominantly due to humoral factors but can also be caused by local osteolysis from bony metastases. The severity of symptoms and signs correlates with the rate of serum calcium rise rather than the absolute value. Management consists of rehydration, diuresis and bisphosphonate administration. Haemodialysis is reserved for cases with

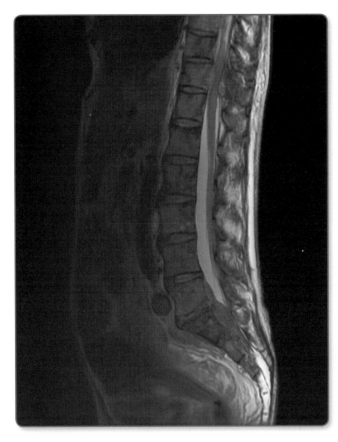

Figure 4 Sagittal T2-weighted MRI showing malignant spinal cord compression at T11 with associated cord oedema at T10-T12. There is also an epidural mass extending between L5 and S3, resulting in obliteration of the spinal canal at S1. This patient had a history of prostate cancer and presented with progressive bilateral leg weakness.

concurrent congestive cardiac failure, severe renal injury or clinically significant neurological findings.

Syndrome of inappropriate secretion of anti-diuretic hormone

Syndrome of inappropriate secretion of anti-diuretic hormone (SIADH) causing hyponatraemia is most frequently associated with small cell lung cancer, however can occur in cancer patients due to non-malignant causes such as infections, drugs and central nervous system and respiratory processes. Mild cases can be treated with fluid restriction, while symptomatic cases may require intravenous hypertonic saline.

Complications of treatment

Treatment-related toxicities involve a complex interplay between individual cytotoxic agents, their dose and schedule, and host and tumour factors. Some complications are dose-dependent and predictable, while others are idiopathic.

Respiratory complications

Acute respiratory distress syndrome is the most common reason for patients receiving chemotherapy to be admitted to ICU. Infection and pneumonitis are common underlying causes, which can be difficult to differentiate on clinical grounds. Other causes of respiratory failure in cancer patients include alveolar haemorrhage, pulmonary embolism and airway obstruction by tumour. Confirmatory tests include CT scan, bronchoalveolar lavage, bronchial brushings and biopsies. Initial management is empirical and supportive until a diagnosis is reached and specific treatment can be instituted. In the setting of infection, antimicrobial therapy often requires multiple drugs and close microbiological collaboration. In cases of drug-induced pneumonitis, the offending agent is ceased and corticosteroids instituted.

There is evidence that in haematology/oncology patients with respiratory failure management with non-invasive ventilation is beneficial.

Febrile neutropaenia

Neutropaenia is defined as a neutrophil count $< 1.0 \times 10^9$ cells. The risk of infection is related to the nadir neutrophil count and duration of neutropaenia. The classic signs of infection are commonly absent and sepsis should be assumed in any neutropenic patient presenting with a temperature >38 °C. Commonly observed pathogens include Gram-negative bacilli and gram-positive cocci; however, the possibility of multi-drug resistant bacteria or fungi should be considered. In the majority of cases, an underlying aetiology is not identified.

Prompt management is essential and a septic screen should not delay the commencement of empirical broad-spectrum IV antibiotics. Recommended treatment regimens include a β-lactam penicillin (or third generation cephalosporin) with anti-pseudomonal activity combined with an aminoglycoside. Vancomycin should be considered if the patient is in shock or if there is a high probability of a staphylococcal infection. Anti-fungal treatment should be added if fever and neutropaenia persist for >5 days. Ongoing treatment should be refined on the basis of culture results.

Gastrointestinal toxicities

Mucositis   Mucositis may affect the whole gastrointestinal tract. Oral mucositis occurs frequently during treatment with 5-fluorouracil, methotrexate and anthracyclines (daunorubicin, doxorubicin, epirubicin and idarubicin). It increases the risk of infection, may compromise nutritional intake and is painful. Supportive treatment is essential and wherever possible, enteral nutrition is preferred.

Diarrhoea   Diarrhoea can be a major cause of morbidity in patients undergoing chemotherapy with agents such as irinotecan

and 5-fluorouracil. It can be complicated by dehydration, renal failure, thrombo-embolic events and gram-negative sepsis. Management includes aggressive rehydration and measures to reduce diarrhoeal volume with loperamide, codeine or octreotide in severe refractory cases.

Constipation   Constipation is frequently seen in cancer patients and can be due to chemotherapy or supportive agents such as 5-HT3 antagonists and opioid analgesia. Vinca alkaloids can rarely cause a paralytic ileus. Prevention with the use of aperients is important.

Cardiac toxicities

Anthracyclines are implicated as causative agents in cardiomyopathy and the HER2-monoclonal antibody trastuzumab, used in the management of HER2-positive breast cancer, can also cause a cardiomyopathy which is typically reversible on treatment cessation. 5-fluorouracil can rarely cause coronary artery spasm.

Neurological complications

The incidence of chemotherapy-induced neurotoxicity is increasing due to use of higher doses and novel mechanism chemotherapy agents (e.g . tyrosine kinase inhibitors). Complications observed include peripheral and autonomic neuropathies (platinum drugs, taxanes and vinca alkaloids), cerebellar toxicity (5FU), myeloradiculopathies and encephalopathy.

The diagnosis is one of exclusion and management is limited. Hence, close monitoring, early recognition and treatment modification is essential.

Tumour lysis syndrome

Tumour lysis syndrome results from the destruction of tumour cells and release of intra-cellular components into the circulation. It is most commonly observed in haematological malignancies following chemotherapy. It is characterised by a number of metabolic abnormalities (hyperkalaemia, hyperphosphataemia, hypocalcaemia, hyperuricaemia and lactic acidosis) and can result in renal failure, seizures and arrhythmias. Prophylactic measures employed in high risk patients include hydration to maintain urine output and administration of hypouricaemic agents. Haemodialysis may reverse toxicity in severe cases.

Graft versus host disease

Graft versus host disease (GVHD) is a common, potentially fatal complication of allogeneic bone marrow transplantation. It is caused by an immunological reaction of donor lymphocytes reacting to antigens present on the surface of host cells. Clinical manifestations frequently include a rash associated with variable degrees of hepatic abnormalities and gastrointestinal failure. Histocompatibility matching and post-transplant immunosuppression are important measures to reduce its incidence.

Toxicities of targeted therapies

Recent advances in the molecular characterisation of tumours have led to the development of agents that target cancer cell-specific attributes that are essential for growth and survival. They can be classified into two broad categories – monoclonal antibodies and tyrosine kinase inhibitors (e.g. bortezomib). These targeted agents differ from conventional chemotherapy in their mechanisms of action and toxicity profiles. Furthermore, their side-effect profiles are, to an extent, specific to the pathways inhibited and hence specific to each agent. Adverse events common to the class of agents include acute infusion reactions to monoclonal antibodies and skin rash and diarrhoea with small molecular inhibitors.

The dilemma of admission

The decision to admit a patient with an oncological emergency is complicated and should be made by experienced doctors in oncology and critical care. Despite advances in treatment mortality often remains high. There is widespread adoption of a trial of intensive care where full treatment is instituted for 5 days to see if there is likely to be a benefit. This practice has been widely adopted in France with improvement in survival.

Further reading

McCurdy MT, Shanholtz CB. Oncologic emergencies. Crit Care Med 2012; 40:2212–2222.

Soares M, Caruso P, Silva E, et al. Characteristics and outcomes of patients with cancer requiring admission to intensive care units: a prospective multicenter study. Crit Care Med 2010; 38:9–15.

Azoulay E, Alberti C, Bornstain C, et al. Improved survival in cancer patients requiring mechanical ventilatory support: impact of noninvasive mechanical ventilatory support. Crit Care Med 2001; 29:519–525.

Azoulay E, Soares M, Darmon M, et al. Intensive care of the cancer patient: recent achievements and remaining challenges. Ann Intensive Care 2011:1–5.

Related topics of interest

Cardiac arrhythmias

wKey points

- Arrhythmias occur in about 12% of general ICU patients
- The presence or absence of adverse signs or symptoms will dictate the appropriate treatment for most arrhythmias
- The options for the immediate treatment of arrhythmias are: electrical cardioversion, antiarrhythmic drugs and cardiac pacing
- In general, if a patient has a life-threatening tachyarrhythmia other than sinus tachycardia, prompt electrical cardioversion is indicated

Epidemiology

Arrhythmias occur in about 12% of general ICU patients with atrial fibrillation being most common.

Pathophysiology

Arrhythmias can be caused by a primary cardiac abnormality such as myocardial ischaemia or infarction, or secondary to a variety of toxic and metabolic disturbances in patients with a systemic inflammatory response syndrome or multiple organ failure. Arrhythmias result from disturbances in automaticity or conduction through myocardial tissue. Risk factors include increasing age, cardiac disease, illness severity, mechanical ventilation and vasopressor infusion. Arrhythmias are most common in the first 48 h after ICU admission. Tachyarrhythmias can be classified as supraventricular or ventricular. Supraventricular arrhythmias include:

- Sinus tachycardia
- Atrial flutter and fibrillation
- Ectopic atrial tachycardia
- Multifocal atrial tachycardia
- Junctional tachycardia
- Atrioventricular (A-V) nodal re-entrant tachycardias
- Accessory pathway reciprocating tachycardias

Ventricular arrhythmias include:
- Premature ventricular beats
- Torsade de pointes
- Ventricular tachycardia
- Ventricular fibrillation

Assessment

Answering the following questions will help determine the correct treatment of all arrhythmias:

1. How is the patient?
2. What is the arrhythmia?

The presence or absence of certain adverse signs or symptoms will dictate the appropriate treatment for most arrhythmias:

- Evidence of low cardiac output includes sweating, cold and clammy extremities (increased sympathetic activity), impaired consciousness (reduced cerebral blood flow) and hypotension
- Excessive tachycardia (> 150 beats min^{-1}) reduces cardiac output and causes myocardial ischaemia as diastole is shortened to a greater degree than systole
- Excessive bradycardia is defined as a heart rate of < 40 beats min^{-1}. Patients with a poor stroke volume may need much higher rates to maintain an adequate cardiac output
- Pulmonary oedema (failure of the left ventricle) or raised jugular venous pressure, and hepatic engorgement (failure of the right ventricle)

Treatment options

First, attempt to correct any precipitants for the arrhythmia. These can include:

- Myocardial ischaemia
- Respiratory compromise (hypoxia and hypercarbia)
- Circulatory compromise (hypovolaemia, hypotension, hypertension, low haemoglobin and reduced cardiac output)
- Electrolyte abnormalities (especially of potassium, magnesium and calcium)

- Metabolic abnormalities (acidosis and alkalosis)
- Presence of drugs (tricyclics, monoamine oxidase inhibitors, quetiapine, cocaine, amphetamine, antiarrhythmic overdose/toxicity)
- Excessive endogenous catecholamines (inadequate sedation, pain and phaeochromocytoma)
- Exogenous catecholamines (catecholamine infusions, direct and indirect vasopressors and theophylline toxicity)
- Mechanical stimulation (pacing wire, CVP line and pulmonary artery catheter)
- Mechanical cardiac abnormalities (cardiomyopathy, valvular heart disease, pulmonary embolism and tamponade)
- Raised intracranial pressure
- Hypo- or hyperthermia
- Hyper- and hypothyroidism
- Sepsis-related myocardial dysfunction

The options for the immediate treatment of arrhythmias are:

1. Electrical cardioversion
2. Antiarrhythmic (and other) drugs
3. Cardiac pacing

In general, if a patient has a life-threatening tachyarrhythmia other than sinus tachycardia, prompt electrical cardioversion is indicated. If the patient is stable, there is more time to establish the diagnosis and decide on the most appropriate course of treatment. Whenever possible, record a 12-lead ECG to help identify the precise rhythm and later expert review if needed.

1. Electrical cardioversion with a synchronised shock can convert a tachycardia to sinus rhythm. The shock is synchronised to occur with the R wave of the electrocardiogram rather than the T wave to avoid the relative refractory period. This reduces the risk of precipitating ventricular fibrillation. Serial shocks are not appropriate for recurrent (within hours or days) paroxysms (self-terminating episodes) of atrial fibrillation. This is relatively common in critically ill patients, who may have ongoing precipitating factors for their arrhythmia (e.g. metabolic disturbance or sepsis). Conscious patients will require sedation or anaesthesia for cardioversion. Cardioversion does not prevent subsequent arrhythmias. If there are recurrent episodes, drug therapy is needed. For a broad complex tachycardia or atrial fibrillation start with a 120–150 Joule biphasic shock and increase if this fails. Atrial flutter and regular narrow complex tachycardias can usually be terminated with lower energy shocks (start with 70–120 J biphasic). When feasible, antero-posterior pads should be used for cardioversion of atrial fibrillation or atrial flutter.

2. Antiarrhythmic drugs tend to be reserved for patients without adverse signs. All drugs that are used to treat arrhythmias can cause arrhythmias. Ideally, the aim of arrhythmia treatment is to achieve sinus rhythm. In elderly patients with atrial fibrillation, ventricular rate control can be equally good in terms of haemodynamic stability and prognosis. Antiarrhythmic drug therapy should be reviewed once the arrhythmia has resolved. This avoids continuing drugs unnecessarily in patients where the arrhythmia was precipitated by non-cardiac problems that have been corrected (e.g. sepsis and metabolic disturbance).

3. Cardiac pacing using external transcutaneous pacing is simple and reliable for treating symptomatic bradycardias resistant to atropine or adrenaline/isoprenaline infusion. It also buys time for transvenous pacing to be initiated.

Further reading

http://www.resus.org.uk/pages/guide.htm
Resuscitation Council (UK) Guidelines 2010. Website with more information on the peri-arrest arrhythmia.

Annane D, Sébille V, Duboc D, et al. Incidence and prognosis of sustained arrhythmias in critically ill patients. Am J Respir Crit Care Med 2008; 178:20–25.

Lip GYH, Tse HF, Lane DA. Atrial fibrillation. Lancet 2012; 379:648–661.

Link MS. Clinical practice. Evaluation and initial treatment of supraventricular tachycardia. N Engl J Med 2012; 367:1438–1448.

Related topics of interest

Cardiac failure – acute

Key points

- Acute heart failure is associated with high morbidity and mortality
- Treatment is aimed at improving haemodynamics and symptoms while avoiding myocardial ischaemia and organ hypoperfusion
- Pharmacological treatment is based on vasodilators and careful use of diuretics while reserving inotropes for patients with shock and hypoperfusion

Epidemiology

Acute heart failure is defined as the rapid or gradual onset or worsening of signs and symptoms of heart failure leading to unplanned hospitalisation or emergency room attendance. AHF commonly presents as acute decompensation of chronic heart failure (65–85% of cases), less frequently as new acute heart failure in a patient with a previously mildly impaired or normally functioning heart (e.g. acute myocardial infarction, fulminant myocarditis or hypertensive crisis) and rarely as cardiogenic shock (<2% of cases).

Acute decompensated heart failure (ADHF) is the most frequent cause for hospital admission in people older than 65 years. In-hospital mortality is approximately 10%. There is a high risk of readmission to hospital (20%) and mortality (5–10%) at 6 months following hospital discharge. Hospitalisation for AHF doubles the 4-year mortality rate (60%) compared with stable CHF (25%). Most patients are hypertensive on presentation and 50% have preserved systolic function. Coronary artery disease exists in most patients and myocardial ischaemia is associated with worse outcomes.

Pathophysiology

Congestive heart failure (CHF) is characterised by reduced myocardial contractility followed by neurohormonal compensatory mechanisms leading to fluid retention, increased venous return and restoration of cardiac output (CO) at a higher end diastolic volume/pressure. Further impairment of contractility or fluid accumulation in patients with stable CHF will cause acute decompensation leading to symptoms and signs of pulmonary congestion and decreased CO. Hypovolaemia (excessive diuretic use, poor fluid intake or GI losses) can lead to non-congestive, low output ADHF. Some patients with AHF have preserved systolic function and hypertension on presentation, and diastolic dysfunction is commonly present. Increased vascular resistance creates an afterload mismatch and fluid redistribution (more than overload) into the pulmonary circulation causing pulmonary congestion. This mechanism of AHF is called vascular failure. Treatment non-compliance, myocardial ischaemia, arrhythmias, renal dysfunction, infection and inflammation can initiate or amplify the pathophysiology.

Clinical features

Clinical assessment helps to establish the diagnosis, guide treatment and monitor response. Findings relate to increased ventricular filling pressures and/or decreased CO. Most patients with AHF present with hypertension or normotension and tachycardia may be blunted by chronic beta-blocker use. The main symptoms associated with left-sided failure are dyspnoea, orthopnoea, paroxysmal nocturnal dyspnoea (PND) due to pulmonary congestion and fatigue (due to low CO). Right-sided failure causes abdominal discomfort, ankle swelling, fatigue, nausea, vomiting and early satiety. The main signs are caused by:

- Sympathetic stimulation: tachycardia, sweating and peripheral vasoconstriction
- Myocardial dysfunction: cardiomegaly, added heart sounds (gallop rhythm), functional tricuspid and mitral regurgitation
- Sodium and water retention: elevated venous pressure, pulmonary and peripheral oedema, pleural effusions, hepatomegaly and ascites

Sudden deterioration in well-compensated chronic cardiac failure may be caused by ischaemia/infarct, arrhythmias, pulmonary embolism, hypertension, and increased cardiac work, e.g. due to asthma, infection and poor compliance with medical therapy. In patients difficult to wean from ventilation, consider occult cardiac failure.

Investigations

Investigations aim to confirm/exclude AHF diagnosis, assess organ perfusion, identify treatable and reversible causes, and assist in prognosis. They include:

- FBC, platelets, creatinine, urea, electrolytes, LFTs, glucose and thyroid function tests to assess organ function and identify triggers
- ABG, lactate, and central venous oximetry ($ScvO_2$) help determine the degree of respiratory insufficiency and perfusion status
- Brain natriuretic peptide (BNP) or pro-BNP. Over-distended ventricles release BNP. Low BNP values help to exclude a cardiac origin of dyspnoea and increased values are associated with a worse prognosis
- Echocardiography to determine ventricular systolic and diastolic function, valve abnormalities, estimation of ventricular filling pressures, and signs of myocardial ischaemia
- ECG for rhythm analysis and identification of myocardial ischaemia and myocarditis
- Chest X-ray to identify pulmonary pathology, pre-existing cardiac conditions, pulmonary congestion and may help to follow response to treatment, but may be normal despite LV dysfunction and pulmonary congestion
- Troponins (Tn) are released in the presence of myocyte necrosis. Acute coronary syndromes (ACS) can trigger AHF but Tn values can also be elevated in AHF without ACS. Elevated Tn values are associated with worse outcomes

Diagnosis

The diagnosis of AHF relies on history and clinical examination accompanied by complementary tests. Clinical diagnosis can be challenging in the absence of previous history of cardiac disease and the presence of co-morbidities such as chronic obstructive pulmonary disease. Insertion of a pulmonary artery catheter (PAC) may be useful when the patient remains unstable despite adequate treatment or in the presence of hypoperfusion and unclear diagnosis. The PAC helps guide fluid, inotropic and vasopressor therapy and enables assessment of perfusion by determining $ScvO_2$. Search for reversible triggering conditions (e.g. ACS, arrhythmias, electrolyte abnormalities, thyroid function abnormalities and infection) which must be treated simultaneously.

Treatment

Treatment objectives are to:
- Improve haemodynamics
- Relieve symptoms
- Avoid myocardial injury and end-organ hypoperfusion

Drugs used during the initial stabilisation phase may effectively improve haemodynamics and relieve symptoms but do not improve long-term outcome; inotropes may even increase mortality. Start disease and prognosis modifying CHF medication (angiotensin converting enzyme inhibitors, β-blockers, angiotensin receptor blockers and spironolactone) soon after stability is achieved.

Use supplemental oxygen to correct hypoxia and maximise oxygen delivery, but avoid hyperoxia.

Positive pressure ventilation (PPV) improves oxygenation by increasing functional residual capacity and alveolar recruitment. It also decreases the work of breathing and, thus, oxygen consumption, and can help the failing heart by reducing preload and afterload. PPV can be provided noninvasively (CPAP or BIPAP) and invasively (mechanical ventilation via a tracheal tube). Whenever possible, perform a trial of non-invasive ventilation before intubation and mechanical ventilation. Consider invasive ventilation if NIV fails to improve hypoxaemia, and to treat severe shock or acute pulmonary oedema, or for procedures requiring the patient to be supine (angiography).

Base the initial treatment on clinical profile. 'Wet and warm' patients are treated initially with vasodilators and diuretics are added as needed. 'Wet and cold' patients are treated initially with vasodilators; diuretics are used cautiously and inotropes considered if unresponsive. AHF can be difficult to diagnose in 'dry and cold' patients. Attempt to optimise preload with small boluses of fluid before starting vasodilators and inotropes.

Vasodilators are the first line of treatment if blood pressure is normal. Venous and arterial vasodilations reduce preload and afterload, improving CO and organ blood flow. Nitroglycerin is preferable in AHF associated with ACS, and sodium nitroprusside in AHF and hypertensive crisis. Morphine is a vasodilator and is useful when anxiety and restlessness are present. Use diuretics cautiously in patients with evidence of fluid overload because they may further activate the renin-angiotensin-aldosterone system and worsen renal function.

Dobutamine, dopamine and milrinone are the most used inotropes. Reserve inotropes for patients with low CO and signs of hypoperfusion. Although effective in improving haemodynamics and symptoms, inotropes are associated with increased mortality, possibly by increasing myocardial oxygen consumption and ischaemia. Levosimendan is a calcium sensitiser with inodilator properties. It improves contractility without increasing myocardial work and oxygen consumption, but may cause hypotension requiring a vasopressor (e.g. noradrenaline). Levosimendan reduces mortality in AHF associated with ACS, especially in those patients already on beta-blockers.

Vasopressors (e.g. noradrenaline) are used to ensure end-organ perfusion if hypotension persists after optimisation of volume, but vasoconstriction can worsen heart failure.

Consider mechanical assist devices in patients with AHF not responsive to conventional treatment with potential for recovery or as a bridge to transplantation. Intra-aortic balloon counterpulsation (IABP) is indicated in cardiogenic shock unresponsive to conventional treatment and associated with severe mitral regurgitation, interventricular septal rupture or myocardial ischaemia. IABP works through synchronised inflation and deflation of a balloon advanced through the femoral artery and positioned in the thoracic aorta. Aortic diastolic pressure and coronary perfusion are augmented during inflation and afterload decreased and LV emptying facilitated during balloon deflation. Left ventricular assist devices decrease myocardial work and improve organ perfusion by unloading the ventricle and ensuring adequate blood flow into the arterial circulation. They are used as a bridge to recovery or transplantation in specialist centres. Treatment of the underlying cause is essential and commonly involves the management of arrhythmias and reperfusion strategies for ACS.

Further reading

Nieminen MS, Böhm M, Cowie MR, et al. Executive summary of the guidelines on the diagnosis and treatment of acute heart failure: the Task Force on Acute Heart Failure of the European Society of Cardiology. Eur Heart J 2005; 26:384–416.

Summers RL, Sterling S. Early emergency management of acute decompensated heart failure. Curr Opin Crit Care 2012; 18:301–307.

Cotter G, Felker GM, Adams KF, Milo-Cotter O, O'Connor CM. The pathophysiology of acute heart failure – Is it all about fluid overload? Am Heart J 2008;155:9–18.

Krum H, Abraham WT. Heart failure. Lancet 2009; 373:941–955.

Related topics of interest

Cardiac output measurement

Key points

- Cardiac output is the major determinant of oxygen delivery
- In most general intensive care units, the pulmonary artery floatation catheter (PAC) has been largely replaced by non-invasive cardiac monitors
- Non-invasive options include the oesophageal Doppler, the LiDCO plus and LiDCO rapid systems, the FloTrac / Vigileo system, the PiCCOPlus System and echocardiography (**Table 10**)

Introduction

The maintenance of adequate tissue perfusion is one of the primary goals in the management of the critically ill patient. Cardiac output (CO) is the major determinant of oxygen delivery and the variable that can be most effectively manipulated therapeutically. Preload, after-load, cardiac contractility and compliance affect CO. The monitoring and manipulation of cardiac filling and CO form the basis of much of critical care practice.

Clinical features

Clinical assessment, vital signs, urine output and core/peripheral temperature gradients can provide valuable information about the cardiac output and circulation. In all forms of shock there is evidence of poor end organ perfusion (oliguria, altered mental state and lactic acidosis). In low CO states, the peripheries are cool and the pulse volume low, whereas in septic shock the peripheries are warm and the pulse volume high. However, in critically ill patients with multisystem failure, clinical assessment alone may be inadequate and the accuracy of estimation of volume status compared to invasive techniques may be as low as 30%.

Pulmonary artery floatation catheter

The PAC enables catheterisation of the right heart and pulmonary artery without the need for X-ray, through a percutaneous sheath placed in a central vein. The waveform and pressure are monitored continually, allowing the catheter to be floated through the tricuspid valve into the right ventricle and finally wedged in the pulmonary artery. It allows direct measurement of central venous pressure, pulmonary artery pressure and pulmonary artery occlusion pressure, which gives an indication of the preload of the left ventricle. The addition of a thermistor near the tip enables determination of CO by the thermodilution technique. A known volume of liquid at a known temperature is injected as a bolus into the atrium. This mixes with and cools the blood, causing a drop in temperature at the thermistor in the pulmonary artery. The area under the dilution curve is analysed by computer to calculate the CO using the Stewart Hamilton equation.

The PAC has been widely used to guide haemodynamic management since its introduction in the 1970s but concerns were raised about the evidence base for its widespread use. In recent years, several well-designed studies have demonstrated no evidence of increased harm but also have failed to show that use of the PAC improves patient outcome.

The PAC is the considered the gold standard device for measuring cardiac output at the bedside; however, several new devices are less invasive and have replaced the PAC for the measurement of cardiac output in a variety of clinical settings.

Oesophageal Doppler

When a sound wave is reflected off a moving object the frequency is shifted by an amount proportional to the relative velocity of the object – this is the Doppler effect. Reflected signals from a flexible probe placed in the oesophagus are analysed to produce a velocity-time curve for blood flow in the aorta. The area under this curve, known as the stroke distance, represents the distance travelled by the blood during systole. This is multiplied by the cross section diameter of the aorta (derived from a built-in nomogram) to enable stroke volume (SV) to be calculated. The device also provides peak velocity (an indication of ventricular contractility) and corrected flow time (the duration of flow during systole – an indicator of preload and after-load). The accuracy of the measurements depends on the assumption that the cross-sectional area of the aorta is constant throughout the cardiac cycle, that the angle of the probe to the direction of blood flow is constant, and that there is laminar flow within the aorta. Additionally, since flow is measured in the descending aorta, which represents only 70% of the total cardiac output, the displayed cardiac output has to be adjusted accordingly. Since probe position is crucial to obtaining an accurate measurement of aortic blood flow, this device is significantly operator-dependent.

The major advantage of this technique is that the probes are relatively noninvasive and easy to place, although in some patients, signal strength can be poor. Despite some limitations of oesophageal Doppler devices, their utility appears to be confirmed by several perioperative haemodynamic optimisation studies that have consistently demonstrated a reduction in complication rates and hospital length of stay. In the United Kingdom, NICE (National Institute for Health and Care Excellence) advises that the oesophageal Doppler should be considered for use in patients undergoing major or high-risk surgery.

LiDCO plus and LiDCO rapid systems

The LiDCO plus and LiDCO rapid systems use the same pulse power analysis algorithm (PulseCO) to track continuous changes in SV.

This algorithm is based on the assumption that fluctuations of arterial pressure around the mean, termed the pulsatility, are proportional to SV. The accuracy of the system is complicated by the non-linear compliance of the arterial wall, wave reflection and damping. The system uses a proprietary autocorrelation algorithm to resolve these problems.

The LiDCO *plus* requires calibration using the transpulmonary lithium indicator dilution technique every 8 h. Lithium is not toxic in small doses and can be easily measured in vivo using a lithium sensitive electrode. A small bolus dose of lithium is injected into a peripheral or central vein, and the cardiac output is derived from the area under the dilution curve generated by a sensor attached to a standard radial arterial line. The LiDCO plus has been used widely within the critical care environment and studies have generally demonstrated its ability to track reliably cardiac output after changes in volume status, inotropes and systemic vascular resistance, but recalibration is recommended after major haemodynamic changes. The complexity of requiring calibration by lithium thermodilution and concerns about the calibration being adversely affected by concomitant use of muscle relaxants, have limited the adoption of the system within the operating theatre.

The LiDCO *rapid* uses nomograms for cardiac output estimation rather than calibration, and therefore displays nominal CO and SV. It has a simpler display and analysis of the changes in nominal SV are utilised to optimise haemodynamics during the preoperative period. The system can be calibrated with an externally validated CO from other devices.

FloTrac/Vigileo system

The FloTrac/Vigileo system is a pulse contour device which provides continuous CO measurement from a proprietary FloTrac transducer, attached to a standard radial or femoral arterial catheter, which is connected to the Vigileo monitor. The system analyses the arterial waveform over 20 s and along with the patients demographics calculates the standard deviation of the arterial pressure (σAP). The σAP is proportional to pulse pressure, whilst resistance and compliance is estimated from further waveform analysis and demographics to generate a non-calibrated SV and CO. After conflicting results of early validation studies, the cardiac output algorithm has been repeatedly modified since its launch in 2005. Although studies using the Flotrac/Vigileo system for intra-operative optimisation have demonstrated a decreased complication rate and reduced length of hospital stay, there remain concerns about the accuracy of the device during periods of rapid haemodynamic change.

PiCCOPlus System

The PiCCOPlus system uses a dedicated thermistor-tipped catheter (typically placed in the femoral artery) to assess beat-by-beat SV along with CO and SV variation. The system uses pulse contour analysis and assumes that the area under the systolic portion of the arterial waveform is proportional to SV. Calibration via transpulmonary thermodilution requires the insertion of a central venous catheter and is typically repeated every 6 hours or up to hourly during periods of major haemodynamic instability. The PiCCOPlus system has been validated in different patient populations. Although the accuracy of transpulmonary thermodilution may be affected by the long transit time, errors from airway pressure variation are minimised. The major advantage of the PiCCOPlus system is that it provides key information about preload and alveolar oedema, as well as the SV. Further analysis of the dilution curve enables determination of global end diastolic volume (GEDV) and extravascular lung water (EVLW). GEDV is considered an effective and reliable preload indicator, and hence predictor of fluid responsiveness, while EVLW is a measure of pulmonary oedema and can be used as a limit on further fluid resuscitation.

Reduction of EVLW after the acute phase of critical illness can reduce ventilator days.

Echocardiography

Echocardiography utilises an ultrasound beam to generate intermittent real-time images of the heart. It has been traditionally performed via the transthoracic approach, but up to 30% of mechanically ventilated patients have poor transthoracic windows, particularly those who have undergone cardiothoracic surgery. Transoesphageal echocardiography (TOE) uses a transducer mounted on the tip of an endoscope. The image obtained is more refined since the transducer within the oesophagus is juxtaposed against the heart and it is easier to maintain a stable transducer position. TOE can be used to assess preload either qualitatively (signs of hypovolaemia include left ventricular outflow tract turbulence and systolic cavity obliteration) or by measurement of the volume of the ventricle. Cardiac performance can be estimated by the calculation of ejection fractions and from Doppler velocity traces of aortic flow. Echocardiography can provide only an intermittent assessment of cardiac filling and its chief advantage is its ability to detect other cardiac pathologies. TOE is sensitive enough to detect ischaemia by regional wall motion abnormalities prior to any ECG changes. Other diagnostic uses include the detection of aortic dissection or trauma, cardiac tamponade, valvular lesions and intracardiac thrombus.

Bioimpedance and bioreactance

Newer devices measure cardiac output from changes in electrical current produced by fluid shifts in the thorax and measured by skin electrodes. They have the potential to be very accurate and non-invasive but relatively few data are available to confirm their precision and accuracy.

Haemodynamic optimisation

The optimal SV and cardiac output has yet to be defined. The evidence for haemodynamic optimisation comes mainly from small perioperative studies and the findings are inconsistent.

1. In the perioperative setting, repeated fluid challenges until SV is maximised, measured by several devices (particularly oesophageal Doppler), may produce better outcomes (e.g. reduced length of stay and faster recovery of gastrointestinal function).

2. During mechanical ventilation in a fluid depleted patient, the increase in intra-thoracic pressure during inspiration causes a decrease in SV due to reduced venous return to the heart. As the patient is fluid resuscitated the effect on venous return is reduced and variation in SV with mechanical ventilation also decreases. SV variation (SVV) and pulse pressure variation (PPV) are good predictors of fluid responsiveness: the patient is considered fluid optimised when the SVV is 5–10%.

3. The oxygen saturation of blood returning to the heart from the peripheries is determined predominantly by oxygen delivery to the peripheries (DO_2), which itself is dependent on cardiac output. Hence, when the cardiac output is low, the central venous arterial saturation ($ScvO_2$) will also be low. $ScvO_2$ optimisation to a target of 70% has been associated with improved outcome in the early treatment of sepsis.

4. DO_2 can be derived from CO, haemoglobin concentration and haemoglobin saturation; studies have demonstrated targeting a $DO_2 > 600$ mL min^{-1} m^{-2} improves outcome.

System	Variables	Requirements	Advantages	Limitations
LIDCO plus	Intermittent CO Continuous SV CO SVV	Arterial line Peripheral or central venous line	Directly calibrated CO	Requires high fidelity arterial waveform Requires calibration with transpulmonary lithium dilution
LIDCO rapid	Continuous SV CO SVV	Arterial line	Easy to setup Simple interface	Non-calibrated Caution after rapid changes in vascular tone
PiCCO plus	Intermittent CO, GEDV, EVLW Continuous SV CO SVV	Arterial line Central venous line	Directly calibrated CO Additional measured GEDV and EVLW	Requires high fidelity arterial waveform Requires calibration with transpulmonary thermodilution
FloTrac	Continuous SV CO SVV	Proprietary FloTrac arterial sensor	Easy to setup, simple interface	Non-calibrated Reliability uncertain especially after rapid changes in vascular tone
CardioQODM	SV, FTc, PV	Oesophageal probe	Non-invasive Easy to setup Simple interface	Operator dependent Only really suitable in intubated patients

Table 10 Minimal invasive cardiac output techniques

Cardiac Output (CO), Stroke Volume (SV), Stroke Volume Variation (SVV), Global End Diastolic Volume (GEDV), Extravascular Lung Water (EVLW), Flow Time Corrected (FTc) and Peak Velocity (PV).

Further reading

Allsager CM, Swanevelder J. Measuring cardiac output. Br J Anaesth 2003; 3:15–19.

Alhashemi JA, Cecconi M, Hofer CK. Cardiac output monitoring: an integrative perspective. Crit Care 2011; 15:214.

Related topics of interest

- Cardiac failure – acute (p 80)
- Inotropes and vasopressors (p 200)
- Post-resuscitation care (p 269)

Cardiac pacing

Key points

- Cardiac pacemakers can be temporary or permanent
- Temporary pacing includes transvenous, transcutaneous, epicardial, transoesophageal and percussion pacing
- Assessment of a patient with a permanent pacemaker should include why the pacemaker was inserted and what type it is
- Implantable cardioverter-defibrillators are encountered increasingly frequently

Introduction

Cardiac pacing devices can be either temporary or permanent. Cardiac pacing is necessary when normal impulse formation fails (bradyarrhythmias) or conduction fails (heart block) and there is a decrease in cardiac output with associated hypotension or syncope. Pacing can be used to override tachyarrhythmias. Antiarrhythmia devices enable cardioversion and defibrillation, and biventricular pacing can be used for cardiac resynchronisation to treat chronic heart failure.

Permanent pacemakers

Assessment of a patient with a permanent pacemaker should include the following key points

1. *Why was the patient's heart paced?*
   Indications include symptomatic heart block, sinus node disease, carotid sinus or malignant vasovagal syndromes. The underlying cause may be idiopathic or include congenital abnormalities, ischaemic heart disease, valve disorders, connective tissue diseases and problems associated with antiarrhythmic drug therapy. An ECG rhythm strip will indicate the underlying rhythm or if the patient is pacemaker dependent.
2. *What type of pacemaker is fitted?*
   Pacemakers are classified using the North American Society of Pacing and Electrophysiology/British Pacing and Electrophysiology Group (NASPE/BPEG) five-letter code (NBG code). The first letter refers to the paced chamber and the second to the sensed chamber. The chamber codes are A (atrium), V (ventricle), D (dual), O (none) or S (single-atrium or ventricle). The third letter refers to the sensing mode and may be T (triggering), I (inhibition), D (dual, inhibition and triggering) or O (none, pacemaker in asynchronous mode). The fourth letter indicates rate response to activity (e.g. mechanical vibration, acceleration or changes in minute ventilation) and may be O (none) or R (rate modulation). The fifth letter refers to multi-site pacing (i.e. more than one stimulation site in any single cardiac chamber or a combination) and may be A (atrium), V (ventricle), D (dual) and O (none). There is a separate NASPE/BPEG coding system (NBD code) for implantable cardioverter-defibrillators (ICDs).

Temporary pacemakers

1. Indications include
   - Life threatening bradyarrhythmia until a permanent pacemaker is implanted
   - Temporary bradyarrhythmia. Transient atrioventricular block may occur after myocardial infarction, cardiac surgery, especially valve surgery, or with drug therapy, e.g. amiodarone toxicity
   - Pacemaker-dependent patients who develop pacemaker malfunction. Temporary pacing allows the permanent pacemaker to be changed
   - Patients undergoing surgical procedures at risk of life threatening bradyarrhythmia
   - Temporary overdrive pacing may be used to control tachyarrhythmias
2. Pacing is at a fixed rate (asynchronous or non-demand) or on demand. Fixed rate systems produce electrical stimuli at the selected rate regardless of any intrinsic cardiac activity. If the pacing stimulus falls on the apex of a T wave ventricular tachycardia or ventricular fibrillation can

occur. Demand pacing is preferable as it senses intrinsic QRS complexes and only delivers electrical stimuli when needed.

- Transvenous pacing is the commonest temporary mode. A single bipolar right ventricular lead is placed with fluoroscopy. Temporary dual chamber pacing is also possible. The lead is connected to a pacing box. The commonest modes are VOO or VVI. Leads can stay in place for 1–2 weeks although puncture site infection and septicaemia is a risk
- Transcutaneous pacing is rapid, safe and easy to initiate. Adhesive electrodes with a large surface area are used. The negative electrode is placed anteriorly (cardiac apex) and the second electrode posteriorly (below the tip of the scapula). Multifunction electrodes (pacing and defibrillation) are placed in the usual positions for defibrillation. The electrical stimulus causes skeletal muscle contraction. Patients often require analgesia and sedation to tolerate transcutaneous pacing. In an emergency, transcutaneous pacing buys time for transvenous pacing to be initiated
- Epicardial pacing is used after cardiac surgery. Wires are positioned on the atrial and ventricular surfaces at the end of surgery and passed out through the chest wall
- Transoesophageal pacing. The posterior left atrium comes into close proximity with the oesophagus. Ventricular capture is difficult to achieve and use of this method is limited
- Percussion pacing by gentle blows over the precordium lateral to the lower sternal edge may produce a cardiac output in patients with ventricular standstill where P waves are seen. This temporising manoeuvre may buy time to institute other therapies and avoid the need for CPR

Pacemaker problems

It is important to ensure that a palpable pulse accompanies electrical activity on the ECG.

A CXR will show position of leads and may indicate misplacement, dislodgement or damage.

1. Failure to capture. The ECG shows pacing spikes with no following P or QRS waves. Myocardial ischaemia at the site of electrode attachment or of conducting pathways can cause loss of capture of the pacemaker impulse by the heart. There may be scarring at the contact site. Increasing the generator output may correct this. Potassium abnormalities also cause failure to capture. These affects are amplified in critically ill patients who may have hypoxia, acidosis, and other metabolic abnormalities. Antiarrhythmic drug therapy may also alter the threshold for pacing.
2. Failure to pace. There are no pacing spikes when they should occur. Exclude battery failure, loose connections and lead damage.
3. Failure to sense. Pacing spikes occur inappropriately. May precipitate ventricular arrhythmias. Exclude inappropriate sensitivity setting, battery depletion and lead damage.
4. Oversensing. Pacemaker is inhibited by non-cardiac stimuli. Electro-magnetic interference from diathermy, MRI scanners and mobile phones (in close proximity) can interfere with pacemakers. Patient shivering can also interfere with pacemaker function.
5. Defibrillation. Place paddles at least 12–15 cm from the pacing unit.

Some permanent pacemakers can be converted to a VOO (asynchronous) mode by placing a magnet over the pacemaker box but it is preferable to use the programming transceiver for adjustment as a magnet may result in an unpredictable resetting.

Implantable cardioverter-defibrillators

Critical care staff are increasingly likely to encounter patients with ICDs. The list of indications for which they are beneficial is growing. These include idiopathic ventricular fibrillation (VF) or ventricular tachycardia (VT), hereditary long QT syndromes and hypertrophic cardiomyopathy. These devices deliver a programmed number of low energy shocks (up to 41 J). Once the device has delivered all programmed shocks, therapy is discontinued even if the patient remains in VT or VF.

ICDs can also be classified by a four-letter code (NBD code). The first letter refers to the chamber shocked and the second to the anti-tachycardia pacing chamber (O= none, A= atrium, V=ventricle and D=dual). The third letter refers to the mode of tachycardia detection (E= electrical and H= haemodynamic). The fourth letter refers to the anti-bradycardia pacing chamber (O,A,V,D).

Early intervention can be life saving in ICD-related emergencies. These include lack of response to ventricular tachyarrhythmias, pacing failure and multiple shocks. A magnet placed on top of all ICD models will temporarily disable the tachyarrhythmia function. Different models of ICD will respond slightly differently. The pacing function should continue whilst the magnet is in place. If there is time it is preferable to contact the ICD programmer to change the settings.

Diathermy during surgery can be used safely if the ICD is deactivated before the procedure and reactivated and reassessed immediately afterwards. Peripheral nerve stimulators used to assess neuromuscular blockade may interfere with pacemakers and ICDs. The 2-Hz frequency (120 beats/min) used for 'train-of-four' assessment is unlikely to trigger the ICD unless the detection rate is very low (in patients with slow ventricular tachycardia). Transcutaneous electrical nerve stimulation should be avoided it can trigger spurious shocks.

The ICD patient in cardiac arrest should receive standard cardiopulmonary resuscitation (including prompt external defibrillation). The ICD should be deactivated if resuscitative efforts are unsuccessful to avoid inadvertent shocks during post mortem examination or removal of the ICD.

Multiple ICD discharges in a short period of time constitute a serious situation. Causes include ventricular electrical storm, inefficient defibrillation, nonsustained ventricular tachycardia and inappropriate shocks caused by supraventricular tachyarrhythmias or oversensing of signals. Antiarrhythmic drugs may increase defibrillation energy requirements.

Deactivation of an ICD with the consent of the patient or relatives should be considered when withdrawing treatment or instituting a do not attempt cardiopulmonary resuscitation order.

Further reading

Bernstein AD, Daubert JC, Fletcher RD, et al. The revised NASPE/BPEG generic code for antibradycardia, adaptive-rate and multisite pacing. North American Society of Pacing and Electrophysiology/British Pacing and Electrophysiology Group. Pacing Clin Electrophysiol 2002; 25:260–264.

National Institute of Health and Clinical Excellence (NICE). Implantable cardioverter defibrillators for arrhythmias, review of technology appraisal 11. London: NICE, 2007.

Epstein AE, DiMarco JP, Ellenbogen KA, et al. ACC/AHA/HRS 2008 Guidelines for Device-Based Therapy of Cardiac Rhythm Abnormalities: a report of the American College of Cardiology/American Heart Association Task Force on Practice Guidelines (Writing Committee to Revise the ACC/AHA/NASPE 2002 Guideline Update for Implantation of Cardiac Pacemakers and Antiarrhythmia Devices) developed in collaboration with the American Association for Thoracic Surgery and Society of Thoracic Surgeons. J Am Coll Cardiol 2008; 51:e1–62.

Resuscitation Council (UK). Adult advance life support, 6th edn. London: Resuscitation Council UK, 2010.

Related topics of interest

Cardiac surgery – postoperative care

Key points

- The pattern of injury following cardiac surgery is predictable and many patients are suitable for protocol driven care
- Mild derangements of organ function are extremely common and often resolve spontaneously. Organ failure is much less common and associated with high mortality and morbidity
- Negative echocardiography should not prevent return to theatre in the case of suspected tamponade

Although cardiac surgery encompasses many procedures, the pattern of injury and many of the goals in the post-operative period are common to all. This makes many patients suitable for protocol driven care by nursing staff, with only fine-tuning by the medical team. Indications for medical referral must be clearly understood by both nurses and doctors.

A normal cardiac surgery time-course:
- admit to the intensive care unit (ICU)
- within 3 h – warm to 36.5 °C
- within 6 h – extubate
- overnight – wean vasoactive/inotropic drugs and ensure adequate analgesia
- the following morning – multidisciplinary ward round, remove drains, arterial lines and pulmonary artery catheter (if used)
- by the afternoon – transfer to ward or high-dependency unit

As with all intensive care, cardiac intensive care lends itself to an ABCDE approach to acute problems and a systems-based approach to longer term care.

Cardiovascular issues

The approach to all cardiovascular issues is that of optimising organ perfusion, particularly the heart and brain.

Heart rate

In most cases, the optimal heart rate is 80 bpm. This provides the ideal balance between a high heart rate (to achieve maximal cardiac output) and enough diastolic time to allow coronary perfusion and ventricular filling. In some patients with a poor cardiac output and a paced rhythm, a higher rate may improve cardiac output.

Pacing

Epicardial pacing wires are placed in many cardiac surgical patients. Some surgeons place them for all cases and some only when specifically indicated, e.g. valve surgery, where there is often transient injury to the AV-node or conducting system. Temporary epicardial pacing wires are removed at day 4. Patients who still require pacing on day 5 should be considered for a permanent pacemaker. There is a risk of tamponade on removing the wires and patients should be closely observed for 4 h after removal.

Pre-load

Most patients are in a state of moderate sodium and water overload after cardiopulmonary bypass, but may also be hypovolaemic. Small boluses of fluid are given to achieve optimum filling.

Contractility

Temporary decline in ventricular function is common after cardiac surgery. In patients with normal preoperative left ventricular (LV) function undergoing routine surgery, the decline reaches a nadir 24 h post-operatively and returns to pre-operative values by one week. In those starting with impaired LV function, or having long or complicated surgery, the nadir is deeper and tends to occur later; furthermore, ventricular function may never recover to pre-operative values.

Inotropes are often required if pre-operative ventricular function is impaired, aortic cross-clamp times are long (>2 h) or surgery is complicated. There is limited evidence that inotropes improve outcome after cardiac surgery and no evidence supporting any specific inotrope over another.

Afterload

Afterload is the work done by the LV after the aortic valve has opened – it is not merely a function of systemic vascular resistance (SVR). Other factors that influence afterload around the time of cardiac surgery are:

- Aortic stenosis
- A prosthetic aortic valve that is too small
- A previously incompetent mitral valve that is repaired/replaced
- Systolic anterior motion of the anterior mitral valve leaflet (AMVL). After mitral valve repair, the AMVL can be 'sucked' into the left ventricular outflow tract (LVOT) during systole – effectively obstructing the LVOT and impairing cardiac output, a situation akin to hypertrophic obstructive cardiomyopathy (HOCM). Treatment is volume loading and beta-blockers; adrenaline will make the situation worse

Right ventricular dysfunction

Right ventricular (RV) dysfunction accounts for 20% of circulatory failure after cardiac surgery. This presents a complex problem because the RV is:

- Relatively tolerant of volume loading – this can result from excess fluid administration, regurgitation of the pulmonary or tricuspid valves, or an atrial septal defect
- Intolerant of pressure loading – this can be caused by hypoxia, hypercarbia, acidosis, excess positive end-expiratory pressure (PEEP) and lung disease – chronic obstructive pulmonary disease (COPD), acute respiratory distress syndrome (ARDS) and pulmonary embolism (PE)
- Affected by LV size, shape and compliance (ventricular interdependence)

Treatment is aimed at:

- Removal of precipitating factors
- Maintaining sinus rhythm at optimal rate
- Maintaining RV perfusion pressure
- Limiting preload
- Improving contractility
  - Inodilators such as enoximone, milrinone and dobutamine will improve RV perfusion pressure and reduce pulmonary vascular resistance.

Noradrenaline may be added to manipulate the blood pressure

- Reducing RV afterload
  - Simple measures such as avoiding hypoxia, hypercapnia, acidosis and optimising PEEP are often extremely helpful
  - Other treatments include sildenafil, nitric oxide and nebulised prostacyclin

Tamponade

The characteristic triad of decreasing blood pressure and cardiac output in the context of a rising central venous pressure is indicative of tamponade. It may be immediate or subacute after cardiac surgery. The treatment is to return to theatre for drainage/exploration. Emergency opening of the sternotomy wound on the ICU is required for patients that are arrested or in extremis. Serious tamponade can be caused by a small amount of blood.

Cardiac arrest after cardiac surgery

Cardiac arrest after cardiac surgery essentially follows similar guidelines to those who have not had cardiac surgery. The essential difference is to ensure rapid re-opening of the sternotomy – equipment and personnel experienced to do this should be immediately available. Early institution of pacing using the *in situ* epicardial wires is also an option in those patients with asystolic cardiac arrest.

Mechanical support

Intra-aortic balloon pump

The intra-aortic balloon pump (IABP) is placed in the descending aorta distal to the left subclavian artery and proximal to the renal arteries. The inflated balloon should occupy around 80–90% of the diameter of the aorta; it is triggered by the invasive blood pressure or the ECG. Low viscosity helium is rapidly injected into the balloon during cardiac diastole and withdrawn during cardiac systole. This increases diastolic perfusion pressure in the coronary arteries and cerebral circulation; the reduction in LV afterload during systole increases stroke volume by approximately 40 ml per beat.

This should improve cardiac output and mean blood pressure, decrease the heart rate and improve renal and other organ blood flow. It improves RV function as well as LV function because of ventricular interdependence and improved right coronary perfusion.

Indications for inserting an IABP are:
- Cardiogenic shock, particularly if caused by ischaemia
  - Papillary muscle rupture and mitral regurgitation (MR)
  - Post-myocardial infarction (MI) ventricular septal defect
- Unstable angina
- High-risk cardiothoracic surgery
  - Unstable angina
  - Poor ejection fraction
  - Difficulty weaning from cardiopulmonary bypass (CPB)

Contraindications to insertion of an IABP are:
Absolute
- Moderate or severe aortic regurgitation
- Aortic aneurysm and dissection
- Patent ductus arteriosus

Relative
- Severe bilateral peripheral arterial disease
- Major bleeding disorders
- HOCM with dynamic LVOT obstruction

Complications of IABP include:
- Stroke
- Bleeding
- Limb ischaemia
- Pseudoaneurysm
- Haemolysis/thrombocytopaenia
- Renal ischaemia – balloon obstructs renal arteries
- Balloon rupture

Left ventricular assist devices

Left ventricular assist devices (LVADs) are a mechanical therapeutic option in severe heart failure. They are used as a bridge to transplantation and to decision-making, and as a treatment in their own right.
Complications of LVADs include:
- Infection – bacterial, viral and fungal
- Immunosuppression
- Bleeding – because of anticoagulation (INR 1.5 – 2.5)
- Strokes – caused by emboli

Respiratory issues
Ventilation

Virtually all cardiac surgical patients will develop some lung inflammation. This may be caused by direct injury (surgical touch) or indirect injury associated with systemic inflammation. There is now good evidence that mechanical ventilation impacts outcome after cardiac surgery and a protective ventilation strategy with tidal volumes of 6 mL kg^{-1}, high PEEP and permissive hypercapnia should be used. This should be balanced against the risk of RV dysfunction associated with hypoxia, hypercapnia and high PEEP.

Post-operative pulmonary function

Forced vital capacity and forced expiratory volume in 1 s (FEV_1) may be reduced by 50% immediately after surgery and may take months to recover. Respiratory complications include:
- Altered chest wall dynamics from median sternotomy
- Pulmonary oedema
- Acute respiratory distress syndrome
- Pneumonia
- Atelectasis – present in >70% of patients
- Pleural effusion
- Pneumothorax
- Phrenic nerve damage (rare)

Renal issues

Virtually all patients having cardiac surgery will develop renal injury. This generally follows a predictable course with the creatinine peaking on day 3. In those with pre-existing renal impairment, the peak occurs later and is higher.

Only 1% of patients will require renal replacement therapy (RRT) after cardiac surgery but the mortality rate among these is 60%. Preventing renal failure is an important focus of perioperative cardiac surgery care. Numerous strategies have been tried to prevent acute kidney injury, but with little evidence of success. The risk factors for renal dysfunction after cardiac surgery are outlined in **Table 11**.

Table 11 Risk factors for impaired renal function after cardiac surgery		
Patient factors	Operative factors	Pharmacological factors
Increasing age	Redo/emergency surgery	Contrast media
Diabetes	Valve and combined surgery	NSAIDs
Systemic hypertension	Hyperglycaemia	Aminoglycosides
Pre-op MI	Haemorrhage	Ciclosporin
Low CO state	Infection / sepsis	Amphotericin
Pre-op creatinine > 130 mmol l^{-1}		
Raised intra-abdominal pressure		

Maintaining cardiac output with volume loading and inotropes is the mainstay of both prevention and treatment. Maintain the mean arterial pressure at pre-operative values. Use loop diuretics to achieve fluid balance. There is rarely a need for renal replacement therapy (RRT) in the first 24 h after cardiac surgery. The anticoagulation required for RRT added to the post-operative coagulopathy can cause catastrophic bleeding requiring re-operation and complications such as tamponade.

Gastrointestinal issues

The incidence of gastrointestinal (GI) complications after cardiac surgery is around 1–3% but is associated with a high mortality of > 60%. The most common complication is GI tract ischaemia and infarction caused by low cardiac output, excessive vasoconstriction, altered gut flow during bypass and thromboembolism.

Pancreatitis

Pancreatitis is uncommon after cardiac surgery, although there may be transient increases in amylase values caused by low cardiac output, hypothermia and/or excessive calcium administration.

Cholecystitis

Acalculous cholecystitis occurring after cardiac surgery is associated with a mortality of > 75%. Exclude this diagnosis with abdominal ultrasound in anyone with persistent abdominal pain or clinical deterioration.

Hepatic dysfunction

Mild derangements in hepatic function and hyperbilirubinaemia are common after cardiac surgery. Clinical jaundice is uncommon and frank hepatic failure is extremely rare and associated with a poor outcome.

Feeding

Early enteral feeding of post cardiac-surgical patients is encouraged. Those who need prolonged intensive care will likely require nutritional assessment and supplementation.

Neurological issues

Delirium occurs in more than 50% of cases; transient personality change occurs in up to 40% and fatal brain injury in <1%. Risk factors for neurological damage after cardiac surgery are:
- Increasing age
- Unstable angina
- Diabetes mellitus
- Pre-existing neurological disease
- Prior CABG
- Vascular disease
- Pulmonary disease
- Post-operative AF

Cerebral oxygen saturation monitoring is being used to direct blood transfusion, use of inotropes, manipulation of cardiopulmonary bypass (CPB) cannulae and reperfusion during deep hypothermic circulatory arrest.

Haematological issues

Excessive postoperative bleeding is an important and frequent complication of cardiac surgery; causes include:

- Surgical bleeding – usually from the sternal wires and anastomoses
- CPB related coagulopathy – platelet destruction and fibrinolysis
- Drug related coagulopathy – either preoperative drugs such as clopidogrel, prasugrel and tirofiban or peri-operative residual heparinisation

Chest tube drainage is measured hourly after cardiac surgery. Acceptable blood loss is defined by the '3, 2, 1' approach (**Table 12**).

Management of the bleeding patient:

- Clotting tests: FBC, APTT, PT, Fibrinogen
- Red cell transfusion to maintain haemoglobin > 100 g L^{-1}
- Transfusion of blood components is guided by:
  - Coagulation screen
  - Thromboelastograph (TEG) – clopidogrel and aspirin do not affect the TEG, therefore empiric treatment with platelets may be required

Platelets are commonly required after CPB. FFP is useful in those with pre-existing coagulopathy (warfarin and liver disease) and in those who have had long bypass times. Cryoprecipitate is given if fibrinogen is <1.5 g L^{-1}. Activated Factor VII has been used off licence for patients with life-threatening bleeding refractory to other treatments.

- Drugs affecting bleeding
  - Protamine: The half-life of heparin is significantly longer than that of protamine; there is often residual heparinisation, particularly if the 'pump blood' (blood salvaged from the CPB circuit) is given back to the patient

Table 12 Acceptable blood loss according to the 3, 2, 1 approach	
Post-op hours	Acceptable bleeding (mL $kg^{-1} h^{-1}$)
1	3
2–4	2
4–12	1

- Many cardiac surgical units routinely give tranexamic acid; aprotinin is no longer used

Other factors to consider include maintaining a SBP of 100–120 mmHg; restoration of normothermia; addition of PEEP (may reduce bleeding by increasing mechanical intrathoracic pressure); obtaining a chest X-ray or transoesophageal echo (TOE) (large pleural or pericardial collections will necessitate immediate return to theatre regardless of coagulation status). Approximately 2–5% of patients need re-exploration for bleeding and this is associated with a significant increase in morbidity and mortality.

Infective issues

An increase in white blood cell count and C-reactive protein after surgery (peaking at day 3) is common and caused by the inflammatory response. It can be difficult to distinguish infection from inflammation. Sternal wound infections occur in about 10% of cardiac operations; however, only about 4% are severe.

Predisposing factors are diabetes mellitus, long operations, internal mammary artery grafts and obesity. The usual infective organisms are *Staphylococcus aureus* (>20%), *Staphylococcus epidermidis* and coliforms. Simple infections can be managed with wound dressing and antibiotics. More severe infections require surgical debridement and reconstruction. Mediastinitis is the most severe form with a mortality of up to 25%.

Re-introduction of medicines

Cardiovascular

- Beta-blockers are usually re-introduced on the first post-operative day (at half-dose). This prevents tachycardia and acts as prophylaxis against atrial fibrillation
- Rapid withdrawal of calcium channel blockers can cause coronary artery spasm after CABG surgery. They should be re-introduced early in the post-operative period

- Re-introduction of angiotensin converting enzyme inhibitors, angiotensin receptor blockers and spironolactone should be delayed until all inotropic drugs have been weaned and renal function is satisfactory
- Digoxin can be re-introduced on the first post-operative day

Diabetes

Insulin infusion is used throughout the perioperative period. Subcutaneous insulin and oral anti-hyperglycaemics are re-introduced when the patient is eating a normal diet. Metformin can cause fatal lactic acidosis in those with elevated creatinine; it should be restarted only when the creatinine is < 150 mmol L^{-1}.

Central nervous system

Psychiatric medicines may be introduced on the first post-operative day but may prolong the QT interval.

Long-term steroids

Those on long-term steroids require the intravenous equivalent to cover the surgery and immediate post-operative period.

Further reading

Tubaro M (Editor in Chief), Danchin N, Filippatos G et al (Co-Ed). The ESC Textbook of Intensive and Acute Cardiac Care. Oxford; Oxford University Press, 2011.

Klein A, Vuylsteke A, Nashef SAM (Eds). Core Topics in Cardiothoracic Critical Care. Cambridge; Cambridge University Press, 2008.

Related topics of interest

Cardiac valve disease

Key points

- Degenerative valvular heart disease has replaced rheumatic heart disease as the reason for valve replacement in developed nations and transthoracic echocardiography is the investigation of choice
- Mitral regurgitation is commonly associated with cardiomyopathy and myocardial infarction
- Cardiac surgery may be lifesaving in acute valvular failure

Epidemiology

Life expectancy of patients with valvular heart lesions has improved dramatically over the past 20 years. This coincides with a reduction in rheumatic fever in the developed world but degenerative valve disease requiring management is common in the elderly. Improved imaging by echocardiography, multi-detector CT and MRI and improved prostheses and surgical techniques, including less invasive procedures are now frequently available. Surgery is performed for symptoms or prognostic reasons. Surgery is generally indicated when the valve pathology is severe (usually graded on echocardiography), and the patients either have symptoms or signs of ventricular dysfunction or dilatation on imaging. Conservation of the native valve structure is preferable to mechanical replacement where possible.

Aortic stenosis

Aortic stenosis may be congenital (bicuspid valve) or acquired (calcification and rheumatic fever). Symptoms include dyspnoea, angina and syncope. Signs include a slow rising anacrotic pulse and an ejection-systolic murmur that is loudest at the second right intercostal space and radiating to the neck. There may be an associated thrill if there is severe stenosis, when the murmur occurs late. The S_2 is soft and there may be reversed splitting of the second sound.

Investigations

- ECG may show left ventricular hypertrophy
- CXR: heart is normal size unless there is left ventricular dilatation. There may be aortic calcification or post-stenotic dilatation of the aorta
- Echocardiographyestimation of the valve area, the transvalvular gradient, ventricular hypertrophy and ejection fraction
- Cardiac catheterisation will add to the echocardiographic findings as well as define the anatomy of the coronary arteries

Management

The cardiac output is 'fixed'; the blood pressure is thus directly related to SVR. Tachycardia will reduce time for diastolic myocardial perfusion and should be avoided. The presence of symptoms and a documented stenotic valve should prompt immediate valve replacement. 75% of patients with symptomatic aortic stenosis die within 3 years of the onset of symptoms unless the valve is replaced. A gradient of >50 mmHg or a valve area <0.8 cm^2 represents severe stenosis. Balloon aortic valvotomy was initially introduced in the early 1990s but it is associated with serious complications (death, stroke, aortic rupture and aortic regurgitation in 10% of cases) and long term mortality similar to no treatment led to discontinuation. More recently balloon valvotomy as part of transcatheter aortic valve implantation is increasingly popular, especially for patients who are considered high risk for conventional valve replacement. A transapical aortic valve implantation technique is another new strategy where the valve is placed antegradely through an incision in the tip of the left ventricle after a mini-thoracotomy.

Aortic regurgitation

Chronic aortic regurgitation is due to disease of the aortic leaflets (infective endocarditis, rheumatic fever or the seronegative arthropathies) or disease affecting the aortic root (Marfan's syndrome, aortic dissection, syphilis or idiopathic associated with ageing and hypertension). Symptoms include fatigue, dyspnoea, orthopnoea (signs of left heart failure) or angina. The increased stroke volume produces a large pulse pressure with a Waterhammer (collapsing) pulse. Corrigan's sign (visible carotid pulses) and head nodding may be apparent. Quincke's sign (nail bed capillary pulsation) and pistol-shot femoral pulses are also a feature. The apex beat is displaced. The murmur of aortic regurgitation is typically high-pitched and early in diastole. The Austin Flint murmur (due to the aortic jet impinging on the mitral valve apparatus) may contribute to a physiological mitral stenosis (due to early closure of the mitral valve).

Investigations

- ECG may show left ventricular hypertrophy with or without strain.
- The CXR shows cardiomegaly.
- Echocardiography or cardiac catheterisation enables measurement of the aortic valve gradient and the extent of regurgitation. Left ventricular size and function may also be assessed.

Management

Vasodilators, e.g. ACE inhibitors are used to reduce afterload but may not slow the need for surgery. Surgery should be performed on the valve before the LV end-systolic dimension exceeds 55 mm or the ejection fraction is seriously compromised. Acute aortic regurgitation (or mitral regurgitation) is a surgical emergency. The left ventricle does not have time to adapt in the face of increased volume load, which causes cardiogenic shock and pulmonary oedema. The coronary blood vessels are affected both by the reduction in perfusion and the increase in left ventricular end-diastolic pressure, thus making myocardial ischaemia worse. Infective endocarditis is the usual cause. Concerns of valve replacement in infected patients are offset by the life-threatening nature of the insult; the risk of prosthetic valve infection is 10%.

Mitral regurgitation

Primary abnormality of the valve is usually degenerative (includes mitral valve prolapse and myxomatous disease), infective endocarditis, collagen vascular disease, rheumatic fever and spontaneous rupture of the chordae. Secondary mitral regurgitation results from left ventricular distortion or dilatation usually following infarction or associated with hypertrophic cardiomyopathy. In acute mitral regurgitation there is sudden volume overload on the left atrium and pulmonary veins leading to pulmonary oedema. In chronic mitral regurgitation the volume overload is compensated for by the development of cardiac hypertrophy. Symptoms are those of left and right heart failure. There is cardiac enlargement; the apex beat is displaced and there may be a parasternal heave. The S_1 is followed by a pansystolic murmur which radiates to the axilla. A third heart sound signifies reduced compliance.

Investigations

- ECG signs include left ventricular hypertrophy, P mitrale and possibly atrial fibrillation
- Echocardiography or cardiac catheterisation may show the enlarged cardiac chambers and permit estimation of the severity of regurgitation

Management

The amount of blood regurgitated depends on the gradient across the valve, the heart rate, and the SVR (a slow heart rate and raised SVR favour regurgitation). Vasodilators and a mild tachycardia will reduce regurgitation. Mitral valve repair is preferred to mitral valve replacement when possible and a minimally invasive technique involving femoralcardio-pulmonary bypass and a right mini-thoracotomy has been introduced that avoids sternotomy and its complications and may result in more rapid recovery. A transcatheter mitral valve repair is also possible placing a clip device on the mitral valve leaflets.

Mitral stenosis

Most cases of mitral stenosis are due to rheumatic fever which is now uncommon but other causes include left atrial myxoma, calcification of the annulus and SLE. Symptoms include dyspnoea, recurrent bronchitis, palpitations (atrial fibrillation), haemoptysis (due to pulmonary oedema) and acute neurological events (due to embolism). Signs are mitral facies, small volume pulse (+/− atrial fibrillation), tapping apex beat (palpable S_1), parasternal heave (RVH), loud S_1 and opening snap (if non-calcified). A diastolic murmur with or without presystolic accentuation may be present if the patient is in sinus rhythm.

Investigations

- The ECG may show P mitrale, atrial fibrillation or right ventricular hypertrophy

- CXR: may show an enlarged left atrium, calcification of the valve and pulmonary venous congestion
- Echocardiography enables an accurate calculation of the valve area (mitral stenosis is severe if the area is <1 cm^2)

Management

Digoxin or beta-blockers will increase diastolic filling time and reduce the heart rate. If atrial fibrillation is present, anticoagulation is needed to prevent neurological complications. Antibiotic prophylaxis is required to prevent infective endocarditis. Preload should be optimised and tachycardia avoided. Hypoxia will increase pulmonary vasoconstriction, putting further strain on the right ventricle. The high left atrial pressure associated with mitral stenosis eventually causes pulmonary hypertension. Balloon valvotomy, open valvotomy or valve replacement should be performed before irreversible pulmonary hypertension results.

Further reading

Vahanian A, Baumgartner H, Bax J, et al. Guidelines on the management of valvular heart disease: The Task Force on the Management of Valvular Heart Disease of the European Society of Cardiology. Eur Heart J 2007; 28:230–368.

Chen RS, Bivens MJ, Grossman SA. Diagnosis and management of valvular heart disease in emergency medicine. Emerg Med Clin North Am 2011; 29:801–810.

Rue M, Labinaz M. Transcatheter aortic-valve replacement: a cardiac surgeon and cardiologist team perspective. Curr Opin Cardiol 2010; 25:107–113.

Ray S. Changing epidemiology and natural history of valvular heart disease. Clin Med 2010;10:168–171.

Related topics of interest

- Acute coronary syndrome (p 4)
- Cardiac arrhythmias (p 77)
- Cardiac failure – acute (p 80)
- Cardiac output measurement (p 83)
- Venous thromboembolism (p 409)

Cardiopulmonary resuscitation

Key points

- The rate of survival to hospital discharge after treated out-of-hospital cardiac arrest is 6–10%; after in-hospital cardiac arrest it is approximately 20%
- Earlier identification of the deteriorating patient and effective implementation of a do-not-attempt cardiopulmonary resuscitation (CPR) policy should increase survival after in-hospital cardiac arrest
- National guidelines define the optimal approach to CPR

Epidemiology

In Europe, the annual incidence of emergency medical system-treated out-of-hospital cardiopulmonary arrest (OHCA) for all rhythms is 40 per 100,000 population. Ventricular fibrillation (VF) arrest accounts for about a quarter of these. Survival to hospital discharge is 6–10% for all-rhythm and around 25% for VF cardiac arrest.

The incidence of in-hospital cardiac arrest (IHCA) is influenced by factors such as the criteria for hospital admission and implementation of a do-not-attempt-cardiopulmonary resuscitation (DNACPR) policy. Data from the UK National Cardiac Arrest Audit indicate a treated cardiac arrest rate of 1.5 per 1000 admissions with 19.7% surviving to hospital discharge. The initial rhythm is VF or pulseless ventricular tachycardia (VT) in 17% of cases and, of these, 48% survive to leave hospital; after pulseless electrical activity (PEA) or asystole, 7% survive to hospital discharge. Many patients sustaining an in-hospital cardiac arrest have significant co-morbidity, which influences the initial rhythm; thus, strategies to prevent cardiac arrest are particularly important. In the United Kingdom, post cardiac arrest patients account for almost 6% of the intensive care unit bed days.

Pathophysiology

Approximately 80% of all OHCAs are caused by coronary heart disease – these are typically sudden, unpredicted events. In contrast, the majority of IHCAs are predictable events not caused by primary cardiac disease. In this group, cardiac arrest often follows a period of physiological deterioration involving unrecognised or inadequately treated hypoxaemia and hypotension. Many of these IHCAs could be prevented by implementing a rapid response system.

Resuscitation decisions

Cardiopulmonary resuscitation is not going to be successful if cardiac arrest occurs as the final stage of a progressive and irreversible decline in the patient's health. In these cases, a DNACPR decision should be made in advance of cardiac arrest. In this way, terminally ill patients will be allowed to die with dignity and the resources of the resuscitation team can be available for those with acute, reversible illness. The decision-making process should be based on current guidance from the British Medical Association, Resuscitation Council (UK) (RC (UK)) and Royal College of Nursing . A standardised form is used to record and communicate DNAR decisions. A DNACPR decision refers specifically to CPR and not to other treatment. Increasingly, DNACPR decisions are being incorporated into wider 'treatment limitation' decisions that focus more on what will be done for the patient rather than what will be withheld.

Basic life support

Basic life support refers to maintaining airway patency, and supporting breathing and circulation without the use of equipment. In hospital, resuscitation equipment should always be immediately available. Having confirmed cardiac arrest, the resuscitation team is called and someone sent to a fetch a defibrillator. Chest compressions are started using a rate of 100–120 min^{-1} and a depth of 5–6 cm, allowing full release after each compression. After 30 compressions, two ventilations are given with either a pocket mask or a bag-mask device. The emphasis is on high-quality CPR with minimal interruptions to chest compressions. The compression-ventilation (CV) ratio is 30:2 until an advanced airway is inserted; chest compressions are then continued without pausing during ventilation. To reduce fatigue, the individual undertaking compressions is switched every 2 min or earlier if necessary.

Feedback systems

There are now several defibrillator models that incorporate CPR feedback systems. These comprise either a puck that is placed on the sternum, or modified defibrillator patches, both of which incorporate an accelerometer that enables measurement of chest compression rate and depth. Measurement of the changes in chest impedance enable ventilation rate to be recorded. These modified defibrillators can provide audio feedback in real-time and downloaded data can be used for team debriefing after the event.

Advanced life support

The universal adult ALS treatment algorithm outlines the treatment of all cardiac arrest rhythms. After the initial assessment it divides into two pathways: arrest in VF/VT (shockable rhythms that require defibrillation) and other rhythms that are not treated with defibrillation (non-shockable) (**Tables 13** and **14**). During the treatment of cardiac arrest, emphasis is placed on good quality chest compressions between defibrillation attempts, recognising and treating reversible causes (4 Hs and 4 Ts), obtaining a secure airway, and vascular access. If return of spontaneous circulation is achieved, post-resuscitation care interventions are started.

Mechanical devices

It is difficult to maintain high quality chest compressions if CPR is prolonged or during transport to hospital. Under these circumstances mechanical chest-compression devices can provide high quality CPR for long periods. There are two mechanical chest compressions devices in clinical use: the AutoPulse (ZOLL Medical Corporation, Chelmsford, MA, USA), which comprises a backboard and battery powered band that tightens around the patient's chest at 80 min^{-1}, and the LUCAS (Physio-Control Inc./Jolife AB, Lund, Sweden) comprising a battery-powered suction cup that pushes down and pulls up (active compression-decompression) on the patient's sternum. Occasionally, an acute coronary occlusion will result in intractable VF, which is unresponsive despite repeated attempts at defibrillation. Under these circumstances, these mechanical devices have been used to provide CPR to enable patients in cardiac arrest to undergo percutaneous coronary intervention, revascularisation, followed by successful defibrillation.

Airway management

In the hands of skilled intubators, such as anaesthetists, tracheal intubation is the optimal method for securing the airway during CPR. In the absence of personnel skilled in tracheal intubation, a bag-mask, or preferably, a supraglottic airway device (SAD) should be used. Both the i-gel and the LMA Supreme have characteristics (ease of insertion and relatively high laryngeal seal pressures) that might make them suitable for use during CPR. Once a SAD has been inserted, attempt to deliver continuous chest compressions, uninterrupted during ventilation. Ventilate the lungs at 10 breaths min^{-1}; do not hyperventilate the lungs. If excessive gas leakage causes inadequate ventilation of the patient's lungs, chest compressions will have to be interrupted to enable ventilation (using a CV ratio of 30:2).

The risk of unrecognised oesophageal intubation can be minimised by using a reliable technique for detecting oesophageal placement of the tracheal tube. When tracheal intubation is undertaken less than 30 min after onset of cardiac arrest, waveform capnography has 100% sensitivity and 100% specificity for verifying placement of the tube in a major airway. During CPR, capnography also provides feedback on quality of chest compressions (better chest

Table 13 Treatment of shockable rhythms

Treatment of shockable rhythms

1. Confirm cardiac arrest – check for signs of life, breathing and pulse simultaneously.
2. Call the resuscitation team.
3. Perform uninterrupted chest compressions while applying self-adhesive defibrillation pads.
4. Plan actions before pausing CPR for rhythm analysis and communicate these to the team.
5. Stop chest compressions; confirm VF from the ECG.
6. Resume chest compressions immediately; another person charges the defibrillator (150-200 J biphasic for the first shock and 150–360 J biphasic for subsequent shocks).
7. While the defibrillator is charging, warn all rescuers other than the individual performing the chest compressions to 'stand clear'.
8. Once the defibrillator is charged, the 'stand clear' warning is given, a quick safety check undertaken, and the shock delivered when everyone is clear of the patient.
9. Without reassessing the rhythm or feeling for a pulse, restart CPR using a ratio of 30:2, starting with chest compressions.
10. Continue CPR for 2 min and ask the person delivering chest compressions to count down through the last set of compressions before pausing for rhythm assessment.
11. Pause briefly to check the monitor.
12. If VF/VT, repeat steps 6–11 above and deliver a second shock.
13. If VF/VT persists repeat steps 6–8 above and deliver a third shock. Resume chest compressions immediately and then give adrenaline 1 mg IV and amiodarone 300 mg IV while performing a further 2 min of CPR.
14. Repeat this 2 min of CPR-rhythm/pulse check – defibrillation sequence if VF/VT persists.
15. Give further adrenaline 1 mg IV after alternate shocks (i.e. approximately every 3–5 min).

If organised electrical activity compatible with a cardiac output is seen during a rhythm check, seek evidence of ROSC.

- Check a central pulse and capnograph if available (ROSC is typically accompanied by a sudden increase in the end tidal carbon dioxide (ET_{CO_2}).
- If there is evidence of ROSC, start post-resuscitation care (see below).
- If no signs of ROSC, continue CPR and switch to the non-shockable side of the algorithm.

If asystole is seen, continue CPR and switch to the non-shockable side of the algorithm.

The interval between stopping compressions and delivering a shock (the pre-shock pause) ideally should not exceed 5 s. Longer interruptions to chest compressions reduce the chance of a shock restoring a spontaneous circulation.

[Adapted, with permission, from Advanced Life Support 6th Edition, the Resuscitation Council (UK)]

Table 14 Treatment for PEA and asystole

Treatment for PEA and asystole

- Start CPR 30:2. Consider and treat reversible causes.
- Give adrenaline 1 mg IV/IO as soon as intravascular access is achieved.
- Continue CPR 30:2 until the airway is secured – then continue chest compressions without pausing during ventilation.
- Recheck the rhythm after 2 min:
– If organised electrical activity is seen, check for a pulse and/or signs of life:
  - If a pulse and/or signs of life are present, start post-resuscitation care.
  - If no pulse and/or no signs of life are present (PEA):
    – Continue CPR.
    – Recheck the rhythm after 2 min and proceed accordingly.
    – Give further adrenaline 1 mg IV every 3–5 min (during alternate 2 min loops of CPR).

– If VF/VT at rhythm check, change to shockable side of algorithm.

– If asystole or an agonal rhythm is seen at rhythm check:
  - Continue CPR.
  - Recheck the rhythm after 2 min and proceed accordingly.
  - Give further adrenaline 1 mg IV every 3–5 min (during alternate 2 min loops of CPR).

[Adapted, with permission, from Advanced Life Support 6th Edition, the Resuscitation Council (UK)] compressions will generate higher end-tidal (ET) CO_2 values) and provides an early indication of ROSC (the $ETco_2$ increases suddenly).

Vascular access

Although peak drug concentrations are higher and circulation times are shorter when drugs are injected into a central venous catheter compared with a peripheral cannula, insertion of a central venous catheter interrupts CPR and is associated with several potential complications. Peripheral venous cannulation is quicker, easier, and safer. Drugs injected peripherally must be followed by a flush of at least 20 ml of fluid and elevation of the extremity for 10–20 s to facilitate drug delivery to the central circulation. If intravenous access cannot be established within the first 2 min of resuscitation, insert an intraosseous (IO) device. Drugs injected via the IO route will achieve adequate plasma concentrations and fluid resuscitation can also be achieved effectively via an IO device.

Use of ultrasound during advanced life support

In the presence of PEA, in skilled hands, ultrasound can be useful for the detection of potentially reversible causes of cardiac arrest [e.g. cardiac tamponade, pulmonary embolism, ischaemia (regional wall motion abnormality), aortic dissection, hypovolaemia and pneumothorax]. Ultrasound examination must not cause prolonged interruptions to chest compressions and a sub-xiphoid probe position is recommended. By placing the probe just before chest compressions are paused for a planned rhythm assessment, a well-trained operator can obtain views within 10 s. PseudoPEA describes the echocardiographic detection of cardiac motion in the presence of a clinical diagnosis of PEA. The diagnosis of pseudoPEA is important because it carries a better prognosis than true PEA and will influence treatment (e.g. consider thrombolysis).

Extracorporeal life support

Several observational studies document the successful use of extracorporeal life support (ECLS) in selected cases of cardiac arrest refractory to standard ALS techniques. It has been generally used for IHCA or for patients admitted in refractory cardiac arrest following OHCA. Patients are selected for ECLS on the basis of having a potentially reversible cause of cardiac arrest, for example, an occluded coronary artery. The technique involves arteriovenous cannulation during CPR and rapid establishment of the patient on extracorporeal membrane oxygenation. The patient can also be rapidly cooled using the extracorporeal circuit, which will provide some neuroprotection.

Further reading

Nolan JP, Soar J, Perkins GD. Cardiopulmonary resuscitation. Br Med J 2012; 345:34–40.

Nolan JP, Hazinski MF, Billi JE, et al. Part 1. Executive Summary. 2010 International Consensus on Cardiopulmonary Resuscitation and Emergency Cardiovascular Care Science with Treatment Recommendations. Resuscitation 2010; 81:e1–25.

Nolan JP, Soar J, Zideman DA, et al. European Resuscitation Council Guidelines for Resuscitation 2010 Section 1. Executive summary. Resuscitation 2010; 81:1219–1276.

Related topics of interest

Care bundles

Key points

- A care bundle is a small set of evidence-based interventions for a defined patient segment/population and care setting that, when implemented together, will result in significantly better outcomes than when implemented individually
- Compliance with the elements of a care bundle must be easily measurable and all bundles are implemented with a target of 95% all-or-none compliance, i.e. all elements must be implemented every day unless clinically contraindicated
- High compliance with the individual elements of a care bundle requires a redesign of work processes, communication and the promotion of team work. This change in care process is likely to lead to improved outcomes

Background

The publication of the landmark report 'To err is human: Building a safer health system', by the Institute of Medicine in 1999 characterised preventable injury as an important and largely ignored cause of increased mortality and cost. The saving 100,000 lives campaign of the Institute of Healthcare Improvement (IHI) galvanised efforts to reduce preventable injury and advocated the use of care bundles. Care bundles now form a key part of a wider quality improvement movement which aims to change the way medicine is practised in order to provide more reliable, evidence based and safer patient care. The aim is to reduce unwanted variation, implement evidence based practice at the bedside and audit this with easily measurable interventions in order to deliver a minimum standard of care.

Care bundles are not intended to represent comprehensive care. They were developed to test a theory – that is, when compliance is measured for a core set of accepted elements of care for a clinical process, the necessary teamwork and cooperation required will result in high levels of sustained performance not observed when working to improve individual elements. There is a strong focus on performance management and it is hoped that the challenge to perform well provokes sustained institutional change.

Each care bundle is not set in stone but can be continuously developed as new evidence becomes available. For instance, chlorhexidine mouth wash was added to the IHI ventilator care bundle in 2010 as more evidence for its benefit became available. Each element of the bundle must have strong clinician agreement for it to be a success and the development of a care bundle must be a multidisciplinary effort. This promotes the team work which is such a key ingredient for success. Each element of a care bundle is descriptive rather than prescriptive, enabling local customisation of the bundle. Measurement of compliance with a care bundle is fundamental to its impact and is most often done with paper based tick box charts. The method of measurement is developed locally and performance should be benchmarked within individual organisations rather than compared between organisations.

Ventilator care bundle

The ventilator care bundle was developed by the IHI to reduce preventable harm in patients receiving mechanical ventilation. It has five elements.
- Elevation of the head of the bed to between 30° and 45°
- Daily 'sedation vacations' and assessment of readiness to extubate
- Peptic ulcer disease prophylaxis
- Deep venous thrombosis prophylaxis
- Daily oral care with chlorhexidine mouthwash

The ventilator care bundle was not designed specifically to reduce ventilator associated pneumonia rates. Rather it was designed to prevent several events that may cause harm to patients receiving mechanical ventilation including venous thromboembolism and gastrointestinal bleeding from stress ulcers.

The care bundle is not exclusive of other interventions that have been proven to improve outcomes for patients on ventilators such as selective decontamination of the digestive tract or lung protective ventilation but should form a basic level of reliable care.

Central line care bundle

Catheter related blood stream infections (CRBSIs) are an important preventable cause of morbidity, mortality and increased costs in intensive care units around the world.

The IHI developed a central line bundle to reduce the rate of CRBSIs and it includes the following elements.

- Hand hygiene
- Maximal barrier precautions
- Chlorhexidine skin antisepsis
- Optimal catheter site selection, with avoidance of using the femoral vein for central venous access in adult patients
- Daily review of line necessity, with prompt removal of unnecessary lines

Implementation of the central line bundle has reduced CRBSIs in a number of multi-centre studies.

Sepsis care bundle

The 'Surviving Sepsis Campaign' is an international collaboration which regularly publishes evidence based guidelines in critical care journals with the aim of reducing mortality from sepsis. The sepsis care bundle

has developed from this campaign and is one of the most widely used bundles. The most recent surviving sepsis campaign sepsis bundle has seven elements to be implemented over two time periods. It is designed to be used in conjunction with the 2013 guidelines;

To be completed within 3 h:
- Measure lactate level
- Obtain blood cultures prior to administration of antibiotics
- Administer broad spectrum antibiotics
- Administer 30 mL/kg crystalloid for hypotension or lactate $\geq$4 mmol/L

To be completed within 6 h:
- Apply vasopressors (for hypotension that does not respond to initial fluid resuscitation) to maintain a mean arterial pressure (MAP) $\geq$65 mmHg
- In the event of persistent arterial hypotension despite volume resuscitation (septic shock) or initial lactate $\geq$4 mmol/L (mg/dL):
  - Measure central venous pressure (CVP)
  - Measure central venous oxygen saturation ($ScvO_2$)
- Remeasure lactate if initial lactate was elevated

Targets for quantitative resuscitation included in the guidelines are CVP of $\geq$8 mmHg, $ScvO_2$ of $\geq$70%, and normalisation of lactate.

Several studies have reported sustained improvements in quality of sepsis care and mortality after the implementation of the sepsis care bundle.

Further reading

Resar R, Griffin FA, Haraden C, et al. Using Care Bundles to Improve Health Care Quality. IHI Innovation Series white paper. Cambridge, Massachusetts: Institute for Healthcare Improvement; 2012. (Available on www.IHI.org)

Surviving sepsis campaign sepsis bundle (www. survivingsepsis.org/Bundles/Pages/default.aspx)
Hasibeder WR. Does standardization of critical care work? Curr Opin Crit Care 2010; 16:493–498.

Related topics of interest

Central venous cannulation

Key points

- Central venous cannulation allows access to the central circulation for fluid resuscitation, drug infusion and measurement of central pressures and saturations
- Ultrasound guided placement improves safety
- Use of care bundles during and after insertion reduces infection rates and complications

Central venous cannulation

Central venous cannulation (CVC) is performed to gain access to the central venous circulation. The particular catheter inserted (single lumen, multiple lumen, wide bore and peripherally inserted central catheter) varies according to the indication. These include:

- Measurement of central venous pressure
- Infusion of multiple different drugs: Catheters with several lumens (3–5) are used frequently in critical care to allow this
- Infusion of irritant or long term treatments: e.g. total parenteral nutrition, inotropes, and vasopressors and antibiotics
- Fluid resuscitation with wide bore central venous access
- Haemofiltration/dialysis
- Insertion of pacing wires or pulmonary artery catheters
- Measurement of mixed venous or jugular bulb oxygen saturations
- Difficult peripheral access

Complications of CVCs

The insertion and use of CVCs are associated with several complications:

- Cardiac tamponade
- Vessel rupture
- Nerve damage
- Haematoma at insertion site/arterial puncture
- Thrombosis: within the same vessel or at a distant site having travelled from initial vessel
- Infection: at insertion site or blood stream, including endocarditis
- Pneumothorax/haemothorax/chylothorax

- Intravascular loss of guidewire
- Cardiac arrhythmias
- Disconnection: bleeding and infection
- Accidental drug bolus
- Malposition
- Catheter dysfunction: occlusion or leakage
- Air embolism: secondary to entrainment

Insertion sites

Internal jugular vein

Advantages: Large vessel. Easy to locate/access. Short straight path to the superior vena cava (SVC). Low rate of complications.
Disadvantages: Uncomfortable for the patient. Difficult to dress/nurse. Close to carotid artery. Risk of pneumothorax.

Subclavian vein

Advantages: Large vessel. High flow rates possible. Lowest infection rate and incidence of catheter-related thrombosis of all the sites. Easy to dress. Less restrictive for patient.
Disadvantages: Risk of pneumothorax. Close to subclavian artery. Difficult to control bleeding (non-compressible vessel). Ultrasound guided placement problematic.

Basilic vein

Advantages: Accessible during resuscitation.
Disadvantages: Increased risk of phlebitis. Catheter movement with arm movement. Greater distance to superior vena cava. High rate of misplacement.

Femoral vein

Advantages: Easy access. Large vessel. High flow rates possible. Accessible during resuscitation.
Disadvantages: Decreased patient mobility. Increased risk of thrombosis and infection. Risk of femoral artery puncture. Dressing problematic.

Insertion guidelines

CVCs are predominantly inserted percutaneously with a catheter over wire technique as described by Seldinger in 1953.

All central venous insertion sites risk air entrainment and consequent embolism.

Thus, the patient should be positioned with head down tilt (Trendelenburg). The resultant venous engorgement reduces the risk of air entrainment and increases the vessel diameter assisting insertion. Femoral venous cannulation is the exception: which does not benefit from the trendelenburg position.

Knowledge of the coagulation status of the patient determines the site of insertion. The subclavian vein which is non-compressible should be avoided in a coagulopathic or thrombocytopenic patient.

CVC insertion should always be performed as a sterile procedure to reduce the risk of central venous catheter bloodstream infection (CVC-BSI). Consideration should be given to the use of antimicrobial-impregnated catheters. Central venous catheters should be removed as soon as they are no longer needed or if there is evidence of new onset sepsis without alternative clinical cause.

The use of care bundles and quality improvement projects such as Matching Michigan can reduce the morbidity and mortality and incidence of CVC-BSIs. Elements of the CVC care bundle includes appropriate hand hygiene, 2% chlorhexidine in 70% alcohol for skin preparation, use of full barrier precautions during insertion, avoidance of femoral site, daily review of requirement and infection state with removal of unnecessary CVCs.

Use continuous ECG monitoring throughout the procedure. Insertion of wires or catheters into the right ventricle may trigger cardiac arrhythmias.

A CXR after insertion of a central venous catheter is required to exclude complications and check for catheter position.

2D ultrasound imaging guidance in central venous cannulation is advocated for placing internal jugular lines. Ultrasound guidance also has a role in catheter insertion in the femoral and basilic sites. The landmark techniques however remain important in circumstances, such as emergencies, when ultrasound equipment and/or expertise might not be immediately available.

Central venous pressure measurement

Central venous pressure (CVP) measurement is one of the most commonly used monitors in critically ill patients. The CVP is not a measure of blood volume but enables assessment of the ability of the right heart to accept and deliver blood – thus is a *reflection* of the intravascular volume and myocardial preload.

CVP is influenced by several factors:
- Venous return: Venous blood returning to the right atrium is delivered via the superior vena cava, the inferior vena cava and the coronary veins. A decrease in venous return results in a decrease in CVP
- Right heart compliance: Right ventricular compliance is the change in end-diastolic pressure with change in ventricular volume. In a healthy heart, volume administration does not cause a dramatic rise in end-diastolic pressure; the ventricle is compliant. Certain disease states cause the ventricle to be less compliant or stiff, e.g. pericardial effusion, cardiomyopathies or cardiac failure. Poor compliance leads to large CVP increases with only minimal increase in volume
- Intrathoracic pressure: If the intrathoracic pressure is elevated, e.g. positive pressure ventilation, this will be reflected in an elevation of the CVP. This does not necessarily correlate to increase in preload. As the PEEP is reduced so will the CVP but the preload (as measured by intrathoracic blood volume from cardiac output studies) will increase. ARDS and chronic lung disease may result in an increase in pulmonary pressures and thus the correlation with CVP and preload is diminished
- Patient position: An erect individual will have a lower CVP comparable to a supine one
- Obstructive shock: CVP is elevated, with no correspondence to cardiac output

The correct catheter position for valid CVP monitoring is with the tip in the superior vena cava. Radiologically, this is commonly quoted as the tip being visualised level with the right trachea-bronchial angle and carina.

It is noted however that some will place the tip within the lower SVC or upper atria to reduce the incidence of vessel erosion, but arguable increasing the risk of thrombosis.

The patient should be supine and the zero point level at the mid-axillary line in the fourth intercostal space (Right Atrium equivalence) when measuring the CVP value. A normal CVP is said to be 0–8 cmH$_2$O in spontaneous respiration and is a good indication of left atrial pressure – assuming normal myocardium and lung function. Critically ill patients frequently require a higher CVP than this to achieve an optimal cardiac output due to mechanical ventilation and reduced right heart compliance. The absolute CVP value is not as important as the response to therapy. Serial measurements are essential to enable assessment of intravascular volume. Central venous pressure is an unreliable reflection of left atrial pressure in the seriously ill.

Normal CVP waveform (**Figure 5**):
- The **'a' wave**: Occurs during atrial contraction. Some blood regurgitates into the vena cava during atrial systole; venous inflow stops and the rise in venous pressure contribute to the 'a' wave. A large 'a' wave occurs in tricuspid stenosis, pulmonary stenosis, complete heart block (cannon wave) and in severe pulmonary hypertension. There is no 'a' wave with atrial fibrillation
- The **'c' wave**: This is the transmitted pressure rise in the atria as the tricuspid valve bulges into the right atrium during isovolumetric ventricular contraction
- The **'v' wave**: Mirrors the rise in atrial pressure during atrial filling before the tricuspid valve opens. A large 'v' wave occurs in tricuspid incompetence – a giant 'v' wave
- The **'x' descent** due to atrial relaxation
- The **'y' descent** is the atria emptying into the ventricle

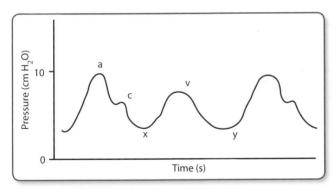

Figure 5 Venous pressure waveform. Typical waveform has an 'a' wave, 'c' wave, 'v' wave, 'x' descent and 'y' descent.

Further reading

Patient Safety First. www.patientsafetyfirst.nhs.uk.
Bersten AD, Soni N. Oh's Intensive Care Manual, 6th edn. Philadelphia: Elsevier, 2009.
National Institute for Health and Clinical Excellence (NICE). Guidance on the use of ultrasound locating devices for placing central venous catheters. Technology Appraisal Guidance - No. 49. London: NICE, 2002.
Pikwer A, Akeson J, Lindgren S. Complications associated with peripheral or central routes for central venous cannulation. Anaesthesia 2012; 67:65–71.
Smith RN, Nolan JP. Central venous catheters. Brit Med J 2013; 347:28-32.

Related topics of interest

- Arterial cannulation (p 44)
- Cardiac output measurement (p 83)
- Care bundles (p 104)

Chest tube thoracostomy

Key points

- Insertion of chest tubes into the pleural cavity involves a high risk of adverse outcomes including death
- Use ultrasound guidance whenever inserting chest tubes outside the 'safe triangle'

Indications

Chest drains are used to drain established or threatened (post thoracotomy) collections of air, blood, fluid or pus from the pleural cavity. According to British Thoracic Society guidelines, a simple, spontaneous pneumothorax can be aspirated without the need for a chest drain; however, insert a chest drain in any patient developing a pneumothorax while receiving positive pressure ventilation. Without chest drainage, 50% of these will develop into a tension pneumothorax. A tension pneumothorax requires immediate decompression. For patients *in extremis* a cannula in the second intercostal space in the mid-clavicular line of the affected side will reverse the life-threatening mediastinal compression while preparations are made for chest drainage. A patient with fractured ribs who requires intubation and positive pressure ventilation may need to have a chest tube inserted prophylactically. This is indicated particularly before interhospital transfer or prolonged anaesthesia for associated injuries; under these circumstances a developing tension pneumothorax is likely to be discovered late. If the patient has a few, undisplaced rib fractures, it is reasonable to undertake short procedures requiring positive pressure ventilation without placement of a chest tube; however, ensure easy immediate access to the chest for needle decompression and chest tube placement at the first signs of a pneumothorax developing. Computed tomography scanning of patients with serious injuries frequently reveals small anterior pneumothoraces, which are not visible plain CXR. These is no consensus on whether these 'occult pneumothoraces' should be drained routinely.

Equipment

Drainage of blood from an adult requires a large tube (e.g. at least 32 F); smaller drains will tend to become blocked. Never use sharp trocars for chest drain insertion – they may lacerate the lung or pulmonary vessels. Simple pleural effusions and simple pneumothoraces may be drained by a narrow bore (e.g. <20 F) tube using a Seldinger technique. The chest drain is usually attached to an underwater seal bottle. Some chest drainage systems will enable the re-infusion of blood collected from a massive haemothorax. A purpose-designed bag with a built-in flutter valve can be used instead of an underwater seal. This is particularly useful in the pre-hospital environment or if the patient requires interhospital transfer.

Technique

Give the patient additional oxygen to breathe and position them supine or semi-supine with the hand on the side of insertion behind the patient's head or on the hip to expose the lateral chest wall. Wherever available, use real-time bedside thoracic ultrasound for insertion of a pleural drain. Infiltrate local anaesthesia into the skin and along the proposed incision line. Under aseptic conditions, insert the drain in the fourth or fifth intercostal space just anterior to the mid-axillary line. These spaces lie within the 'triangle of safety' bordered by the anterior border of latissimus dorsi, the lateral border of the pectoralis major, a line level with the nipple below, and the apex of the axilla above; **Figure 6**. For non-Seldinger technique drains, define the track down to parietal pleura using blunt dissection, staying close to the upper border of the rib. Puncture the pleura with the blunt tip of a clamp. Remove the clamp and

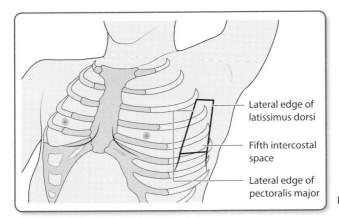

Lateral edge of
latissimus dorsi

Fifth intercostal
space

Lateral edge of
pectoralis major

Figure 6 The 'triangle of safety'.

use a finger to 'sweep' the pleural cavity and exclude adhesions or abdominal viscera prior to insertion of the drain.

Connect the drain to an underwater seal or flutter valve. Insert sutures across the skin incision. These can be tightened after drain removal. Traditional 'purse string' sutures produce very poor cosmetic results and are not used. Apply a clean dressing and obtain a CXR to confirm an acceptable position of the drain.

A Seldinger technique is used for smaller (non-surgical) drains. A needle is used to identify the pleural space; a guidewire is inserted and a chest drain is placed over the wire. The advantages of this technique are that it requires a very small or no incision, is less painful and, once the drain is placed, there is minimal leakage of blood or fluid from the insertion site. However, if the collection of fluid or air is small, or if there is adherent pleura, it is possible to inadvertently place the wire and drain into the lung.

Bronchopleural fistulae

Bronchopleural fistulae cause large air leaks. A bronchoscopy will exclude the presence of a ruptured bronchus. If the lung is non-compliant or the air leak is large, and a major airway injury has been excluded, continuous, high-flow suction (20–30 cmH$_2$O) may be applied to the drainage system. This may help to bring the visceral and parietal pleural surfaces together.

Complications

Intercostal vessels or nerves may be damaged during chest tube insertion. It is possible to lacerate the lung or pulmonary vessels, particularly if a sharp introducer is used. A common error is to place the tube outside the pleural cavity (extrapleural or intra-abdominal). Inadequately tied drains will fall out. A persistent air leak will occur if the proximal side-hole of the chest tube is outside the pleural cavity. Empyema occurs in about 2% of patients having chest tubes inserted. It is particularly likely after blunt trauma.

Removal of chest drains

Chest tubes inserted to drain a pneumothorax are removed on resolution of the pneumothorax. Assuming there is no air leak or excessive drainage of fluid (>100 mL day^{-1}), chest tubes inserted prophylactically into patients with rib fractures can probably be removed after the patient has been stabilised and any early, prolonged surgery has been completed.

Further reading

Laws D, Neveille E, Duffy J. BTS guidelines for the insertion of a chest drain. Thorax 2003; 58: ii53–59.

Related topics of interest

- Trauma – primary survey (p 380)
- Trauma – secondary survey (p 386)
- Trauma – anaesthesia and critical care (p 391)
- Pleural disease (p 260)

Chronic obstructive pulmonary disease

Key points

- Frequent exacerbations of chronic obstructive pulmonary disease are associated with poorer health and more rapid decline in lung function. Co-morbidities are common, and should be actively managed as they have a strong impact on prognosis
- Multimodal strategies can reduce exacerbation frequency
- Non-invasive or invasive ventilation can benefit patients who have reversible factors

Epidemiology

Chronic obstructive pulmonary disease (COPD) is one of the top five causes of morbidity and mortality worldwide and results in substantial social and economic burden. About 5–10 % of the population are affected, usually smokers, and 20% of cigarette smokers develop clinically significant COPD. Less common causes include occupational exposure to inhaled toxins and hereditary α_1-antitrypsin deficiency. It is more common in men than women and increases with age.

Pathophysiology

COPD is characterised by progressive lung impairment associated with chronic inflammation in the airways and lung parenchyma resulting in emphysema, chronic bronchitis and small airway fibrosis. These changes lead to progressive air flow limitation that is not fully reversible, air trapping resulting in hypoxaemia with or without hypercapnia and eventual pulmonary hypertension and cor pulmonale.

Clinical features and diagnosis of COPD

Diagnosis and assessment of severity are based on functional assessment, spirometry and complications.

Symptoms are chronic progressive breathlessness and cough, with or without sputum production, with a history of exposure to risk factors (smoking, occupational dust and inhaled chemical) or a family history α_1-antitrypsin deficiency. Airway obstruction is confirmed by spirometry showing a post-bronchodilator FEV_1/FVC of < 0.7 (the degree of reversibility is no longer recommended for diagnosis). Severe COPD is characterized by dyspnoea on minimal exertion that severely restricts daily activities, spirometry < 40% predicted, the presence of severe hypoxaemia [Pao_2 < 8 kPa (60 mmHg)], hypercapnia [$Paco_2$ > 6 kPa (45 mmHg)], pulmonary hypertension, heart failure and polycythaemia.

Investigations

- CXR. Hyperinflation with flat diaphragms and lung hyperlucency. Prominent proximal pulmonary artery shadows with peripheral tapering suggests pulmonary hypertension. The CXR does not establish the diagnosis of COPD, but is important to identify alternative diagnoses such as fibrosis, bronchiectasis, cardiac failure, pneumonia, malignancy and kyphoscoliosis
- Lung function tests demonstrate an obstructive pattern with FEV1/FVC < 70%, high residual volume and total lung capacity, and low diffusion capacity of the lung for carbon monoxide
- Oximetry/arterial blood gas analysis to objectively evaluate patient disease severity and the need for supplemental oxygen therapy. Patients with an exacerbation of COPD are often severely hypoxaemic with or without hypercapnia. A high bicarbonate and high base excess suggests chronic hypercapnia
- Blood count for polycythaemia and neutrophilia
- ECG. It is often normal but may show peaked p wave (p-pulmonale) and right ventricular hypertrophy with strain pattern

suggesting the development of pulmonary hypertension

Treatment of COPD

The management goals for COPD are to remove risk factors, prevent and treat exacerbations and complications, relieve symptoms, slow disease progression and improve exercise tolerance.

Non-pharmacological therapy

Remove risk factors: Stopping smoking improves lung function and survival. Nicotine replacement enhances smoking abstinence. Pulmonary rehabilitation: Education, nutritional counselling, exercise training and behaviour modification, helps to improve quality of life, exercise tolerance, dyspnea and fatigue.

Oxygen therapy: Home oxygen, especially with respiratory failure (arterial Po_2 <55 mmHg or oxygen saturation <88% with or without hypercapnia, or arterial Po_2 56–59 mmHg with one of the following: pulmonary hypertension, cor pulmonale or evidence of right heart failure). Survival, exercise tolerance and quality of life are improved by administration for at least 15 h per day.

Non-invasive ventilation (NIV): Especially in patients with co-existing obstructive sleep apnoea. This improves survival and reduces hospital admission.

Surgery: Lung volume reduction surgery is not widely available and only beneficial to carefully selected patients with predominantly severe upper lobe emphysema. The role of bronchoscopic lung reduction is yet to be established.

Lung transplantation: Has shown to improve quality of life and functional status of appropriately selected patients but organ availability limits numbers.

Pharmacological therapy

Bronchodilators: β_2 agonists, anticholinergics and methylxanthines are the three commonly used bronchodilators. Long or short-acting β_2-agonists stimulate β_2-adrenergic receptors of the airway. Short-acting β_2 agonists (inhaled or nebulised, e.g. salbutamol and terbutaline) act quickly and relieve symptoms for up to 6 h. Long-acting drugs (inhaled or nebulised, e.g. formoterol and salmeterol) have a duration of action of more than 12 h and are first-line maintenance therapy for symptom control. Common side effects include tachycardia, tremor and hypokalaemia. Anticholinergic drugs (inhaled or nebulized) block the effect of acetylcholine on muscarinic receptors. Short-acting drugs such as ipratropium bromide last for 4–6 h while the long-acting agents such as tiotropium last up to 24 h. Dry mouth and urinary retention are the common side effects. Methylxanthines (IV aminophylline or oral theophylline) have a narrow therapeutic range and potential toxicity includes nausea, vomiting and cardiac arrhythmia.

Corticosteroids: reduce inflammation and can be administered orally, via inhalation, or intravenously. Corticosteroids in combination with bronchodilators are mainly used in exacerbations and their role in stable COPD is limited. The long-term safety of corticosteroids is unclear. Common side effects especially in long-term use include oral candidiasis, hyperglycaemia, myopathy, osteopaenia, weight gain, fluid retention, cataract and immunosuppression.

Phosphodiesterase-4 inhibitors (Roflumilast): The National Institute for Health and Clinical Excellence (NICE) recommends this new drug is used only in the context of research trials for adults with severe COPD.

Antibiotics: Apart from treating infectious exacerbations, the use of antibiotics is not recommended. A recent trial of daily prophylactic azithromycin for 1 year reduced the frequency of exacerbations, however, the treatment is associated with hearing decrement and increased colonization of macrolide resistant bacteria.

Cough suppressant: The regular use of these drugs is not recommended as cough has a significant protective role in COPD.

Mucolytics: They provide minor benefit to patients with viscous sputum. The regular use of a mucolytic in COPD remains controversial.

Vaccination: Influenza and pneumococcal vaccines are recommended for patients with COPD.

Antitrypsin: α_1-antitrypsin may be helpful in patients with the hereditary deficiency but is not widely available and is expensive.

Treatment of exacerbation of COPD

Exacerbation of COPD is the most common reason patients with COPD are admitted to critical care units. Exacerbations are characterized by worsening symptoms and are usually caused by viral or bacterial respiratory infections.

Exclude other causes of deterioration such as pneumonia, pneumothorax, heart failure, pulmonary embolism, lung collapse or atelectasis, pleural effusion, foreign bodies causing obstruction and lung cancer. Treatment includes:

- Oxygen therapy to relieve hypoxia: titrated to target saturation and with arterial blood gases to monitor the degree of ventilator failure
- Bronchodilators to relieve dyspnea
- Corticosteroids to reduce inflammation
- Treating underlying infections with appropriate antibiotics and/or antivirals

Non-invasive ventilation is indicated in moderate to severe dyspnea with hypoxaemia, and/or respiratory acidosis. Exclusion factors include respiratory arrest, cardiovascular instability, decreased mental status, risk of aspiration, recent facial maxillary/gastro-oesophageal surgery and craniofacial trauma or burn. Decreased mental status is a relative exclusion (application of NIV may reduce $PaCO_2$ sufficiently to make the patient more alert) and many clinicians will use NIV cautiously after oesophageal surgery. Early administration of appropriate NIV reduces hospital length of stay, intubation rate and mortality.

Invasive mechanical ventilation is indicated for patients who fail or are unable to tolerate NIV, e.g. hypoxaemia, respiratory distress, acidosis (e.g. pH < 7.25), impaired consciousness, or cardiovascular failure. Many patients with severe or end-stage COPD

do not benefit from invasive ventilation and major complications include ventilator-acquired pneumonia, baro/volume trauma and failure to wean. Criteria supporting the use of intubation and mechanical ventilation include:

- A reversible reason for the current decline (e.g. pneumonia)
- A quality of life/level of activity and independence prior to this exacerbation that is acceptable to the patient

Criteria against intubation and mechanical ventilation include:

- No reversible factors
- Severe COPD unresponsive to optimal therapy
- Severe co-morbidity (e.g. heart failure, cor pulmonale and cancer)
- Poor quality of life, high dependence (e.g. continuous home oxygen) with an expected outcome that would be unacceptable to the patient

Most exacerbations in hospital are treated as infections, although commonly no causative organism is identified. Studies support the use of 5–10 days of antibiotics in moderately or severely ill patients with purulent sputum. The most common bacteria responsible for infective exacerbations are *Haemophilus influenzae, Streptococcus pneumoniae* and *Moraxella catarrhalis*. In patients with very severe COPD (FEV_1 < 30% predicted), Gram-negative organisms, particularly *Pseudomonas* and Enterobacteriaceae, are also important. Antibiotic prescribing follows local protocols that are governed by organism sensitivities. β-lactam and/or macrolides or tetracycline are common first-line treatments for exacerbations. Hospital acquired and life-threatening infections are managed more aggressively with intravenous broad spectrum antibiotics with or without MRSA or other resistant bacterial cover.

β$_2$ agonists (salbutamol or terbutaline) are best given by spacer or nebuliser (salbutamol may be given intravenously). Ipratropium is used in conjunction with β-agonists for its alternative bronchodilating action. Aminophylline may be used as an adjunct to β$_2$ agonists but is of unproven efficacy. Avoid loading doses in patients already taking theophylline preparations, and monitor levels.

Systemic corticosteroids shorten recovery time, improve lung function (FEV_1) and hypoxaemia, reduce early relapse rate and hospital length of stay. Hydrocortisone 100–200 mg 6 h is commenced, converted to oral prednisolone 30–50 mg after improvement, and withdrawn over 7–14 days.

Sputum retention is common in COPD but mucolytics are of unproven benefit. Physiotherapy and tracheal suction are important especially in intubated patients with sputum production but may be harmful in the absence of sputum production. Bronchoscopy and tracheal suction may be beneficial if mucous plugging causes lung collapse. Tracheostomy aids weaning and pulmonary toilet for those with ineffective coughs. Oxygen, diuretics and vasodilators may improve heart function. Prevent or correct electrolyte abnormalities (hypokalemia, hypomagnesaemia and hypophosphataemia) caused by diuresis and β_2 agonists. Avoid excessive carbohydrate loads in patients with hypercarbia.

Outcome

The outcome from an acute exacerbation of COPD is related to age, prehospital performance status and co-morbidities. Hospital mortality ranges from 17–50%, but long-term survival may be poor in patients with pre-existing poor respiratory reserve (FEV_1 <30%) and co-morbidity.

Further reading

Decramer M, Janssens W, Miravitlles M. Chronic obstructive pulmonary disease. Lancet 2012; 379:1341–1351.

Global initiative for Chronic Obstructive Lung Disease (GOLD). Global Strategy for the Diagnosis, Management and Prevention of COPD www.goldcopd.org.

National Institute for Health and Clinical Excellence (NICE). Management of chronic obstructive pulmonary disease in adults in primary and secondary care, Clinical guidelines CG101. London; NICE, 2010.

Patel I. Exacerbations of chronic obstructive pulmonary disease: definition, aetiology and management. Clin Med 2009; 9:170–173.

Related topics of interest

- Asthma (p 47)
- Respiratory support – invasive (p 306)
- Respiratory support – non-invasive techniques (p 311)
- Weaning from ventilation (p 413)

Coma

Key points

- Assessment and treatment of coma must be rapid because delayed correction of many causes of coma will worsen brain injury
- Many metabolic or toxic causes of coma resolve without long-term damage
- CT scanning is required to exclude intracranial pathology requiring emergency surgery

Epidemiology

Coma is the manifestation of a depressed level of consciousness. Coma is usually defined as a Glasgow Coma Scale (GCS) score of 8 or less. Coma reflects pathology in the reticular activating system of the brain stem or the cerebral cortex. The principles of critical care management of coma include:

- Protecting the patient from further injury
- Diagnosing the underlying cause
- Managing the patient to ensure an optimal outcome

Pathophysiology

There are many causes of coma:

- Primary cerebral lesion: head injury, intracranial haemorrhage, meningitis/encephalitis, abscess, tumour, hydrocephalus, cerebral oedema and epilepsy
- Secondary to systemic illness: any cause of hypoxaemia and hypotension (e.g. cardiac arrest and shock), liver failure, renal failure, CO_2 narcosis, hypoglycaemia, ketoacidosis, electrolyte abnormalities, hyper and hypo-osmolar states, myxoedema, hypothermia and sepsis (including tropical diseases)
- Drug induced: therapeutic drugs, drugs in overdose or non-therapeutic drugs and poisons, anaesthetics, benzodiazepines, opioids, antidepressants and alcohol

Clinical features

The history will often provide the likely diagnosis. Assess respiration (absent in brain stem death and following overdose of certain drugs). External signs of head injury suggest intracranial pathology (if suspicious, immobilise cervical spine). Blood in external auditory meatus or from the nose or over the mastoid is a sign of base of skull fracture. Localising neurological signs also suggest intracranial pathology.

- Examine the pupils for asymmetry, size and reactions. Bilateral unreactive pupils suggest brain stem pathology. A unilateral dilated and unreactive pupil suggests ipsilateral III nerve palsy. Meiosis suggests opioids or brain stem disease. Dysconjugate gaze suggests cranial nerve lesion (III, IV or VI) or internuclear ophthalmoplegia. Conjugate gaze deviation suggests an ipsilateral frontal lesion. Perform fundoscopy to look for retinopathy (hypertensive, diabetic) and papilledema
- Meningism suggests meningitis or subarachnoid haemorrhage
- Pyrexia suggests sepsis, meningitis or heat stroke. Hypothermia may be the sole cause of coma and a feature of myxoedema coma
- Venepuncture marks suggest drug overdose especially opioids, other illicit drugs, septicaemia and the possibility of intracerebral abscess
- Signs of liver and renal disease suggest these as underlying causes

Investigations

- Blood sugar and ketone values using a finger-prick test
- Laboratory blood sugar, urea, creatinine, electrolytes, liver function tests (ammonia concentration if hepatic encephalopathy suspected), full blood count and thyroid function
- Arterial blood gas

- Specimens for culture
- Drug screen for suspected agents and hold urine for toxicology
- Blood alcohol values
- CT/MRI scan
- Lumbar puncture is rarely required as an urgent procedure and should never be performed in the presence of signs of raised intracranial pressure (ICP)
- Electroencephalography (EEG) is useful to demonstrate abnormal activity

Treatment

- Rapidly assess and resuscitate simultaneously following the ABC format
- Direct specific therapy (including surgery) at the underlying pathology
- Correct rapidly any hypoxaemia and hypotension
- Correct hypoglycaemia with 50 mL 50% glucose IV, with thiamine 100 mg if suspicion of alcohol abuse
- Antimicrobials if infection is suspected
- GCS < 10 may require intubation to protect the airway, prevent secondary brain injury and facilitate investigation (e.g. CT scan)
- If there is ventilatory failure, ventilate the patient's lungs to achieve a normal Pao$_2$ and Paco$_2$
- Correct hypo and hyperthermia
- Correct electrolyte abnormalities and ensure adequate hydration
- Commence early enteral nutrition
- Commence DVT prophylaxis
- Consider the use of anticonvulsants
- Consider insertion of an ICP monitor and initiate therapy to reduce raised ICP if present
- Consider cerebral protective therapy (hypothermia, reduce CMRO$_2$)
- Specific antagonists: Naloxone for opioids and flumazenil for benzodiazepine overdose are of limited use because of the high risks of precipitating withdrawal and seizures that result in morbidity and difficulty managing patients

Neurosurgical emergencies

Extradural haemorrhage

Extradural haemorrhage is caused usually by a head injury. There may be an initial lucid period followed by a rapid deterioration in GCS, progressing to coma often with focal signs (lateralising weakness or pupillary signs). This is consistent with a minor brain injury with a rapid accumulation of blood from a middle meningeal artery rupture. Surgical drainage following CT scan localisation has a relatively good prognosis provided the interval to surgery was short and the initial GCS immediately after injury was high.

Subdural haemorrhage

Acute presentations of subdural haemorrhage following trauma are associated with severe underlying brain injury, initial low GCS post injury and a poor prognosis. In acute head injury, subdural haemorrhage is more common than extradural haemorrhage and the onset of coma is immediate.

Chronic subdural haematoma presents days to weeks after head trauma that is often described as trivial. Presentation may be vague with a fluctuating level of consciousness, agitation, confusion, seizures, localising signs or a slowly evolving stroke. Diagnosis is made by CT or MRI scan. Treatment is by surgical drainage.

Intracerebral haemorrhage

Intracerebral haemorrhage is associated with hypertension, haemorrhage into a neoplasm, haemorrhage into an infarct, AV malformations, vasculitis, coagulopathy (including post-thrombolysis) and mycotic aneurysms associated with bacterial endocarditis. Extensive haemorrhage presents as sudden onset of coma, drowsiness and/ or neurological deficit. The rate of evolution depends on the site and size of the bleed. Some are amenable to surgical drainage.

Intracerebral infarction

Cerebral infarction follows thrombosis or embolism. Some of these patients benefit from early intervention (within a few hours) including interventional radiology embolectomy/thrombectomy or thrombolysis and intensive care management. Selected patients may also benefit from decompressive craniectomy.

Brain death

See Brain death and organ donation.

Vegetative state

In this uncommon state, there is severe cortical damage but with preservation of some brain stem activity. Vegetative states usually follow severe hypoxic brain injury or severe head injury. Consciousness is impaired, although there may be eye opening, and there is no voluntary movement. It is a diagnosis that can be made only after a prolonged period of observation (months), at which stage it is usually permanent.

Locked-in syndrome

Locked-in syndrome is a state of normal consciousness but with impaired movement due to lower cranial nerve damage and brain stem/spinal cord damage that results in paralysis. Careful assessment of responsiveness is required and the EEG will demonstrate awake rhythms.

Pseudo-coma/psychogenic coma

This is a diagnosis of exclusion. Signs are usually not consistent with accepted neurological damage. Cranial nerve reflexes will remain intact and the EEG will show awake rhythms.

Global ischaemia

Global cerebral ischaemia is the usual result of a prolonged period of circulatory arrest but will also result from prolonged periods of severe hypoxaemia and/or hypotension from any cause. Prognosis is related to the duration of the ischaemic/hypoxic period and the presence of co-morbidity. Recovery can be delayed and prolonged, which leads to a guarded prognosis. After 6 months, the potential for major improvement in patients with severe brain injury is small: patients with potential for significant recovery will usually have demonstrated improvements within the first 72 h. If there is improvement in cranial nerve activity and motor activity during this period, continued aggressive intensive care may be indicated. EEG and evoked potentials may provide some aid to judging prognosis.

Further reading

Monti MM, Laureys S, Owen AM. The vegetative state. Br Med J 2010; 341:3765.
Angel MJ, Young GB. Metabolic encephalopathies. Neurol Clin 2011; 29:837–882.

Ferro JM, Crassard I, Coutinho JM, et al. Decompressive surgery in cerebrovenous thrombosis: a multicenter registry and a systematic review of individual patient data. Stroke 2011; 42:2825–2831.

Related topics of interest

- Brain death and organ donation (p 61)
- Post-resuscitation care (p 269)
- Seizures – status epilepticus (p 323)

Consent

Key points

- Consent serves to protect the interests of both the patient and the treating clinicians
- A well informed patient will have greater confidence in the clinicians treating them
- All adult patients should be presumed to have capacity to consent unless reasons can be shown for capacity to be lacking
- Incapacitated patients often require decisions to be taken by those treating them, in their best interests, or in exceptional circumstances by the Courts

Consent

Definition of consent

Consent is permission for something to happen or agreement to do something.

In a medical context it usually refers to permission granted by a patient to undergo an examination or procedure.

Role of consent

Consent is a necessary legal process, providing a defence in law to a potential claim for battery (refers to the application of any force upon the patient that occurs without their permission), as well as limiting exposure of the clinician to a civil claim for negligence (failure to exercise the care that a reasonable person would have done in the same circumstances).

From an ethical standpoint consent supports the principles of justice and autonomy (the patient's right to self-determination).

Consent also has a wider and arguably more important function clinically, which is to ensure that the patient is aware of what is planned, what is likely to happen, and what could possibly go wrong. By having a clear understanding of what to expect, patients are likely to have greater confidence in the treating clinicians.

Principles of consent

Informed consent is only valid if:
1. It is entirely voluntary.

2. All relevant information is provided to the patient to facilitate their decision making process.
3. The patient has capacity.

The information provided to the patient should explain both the nature and purpose of the treatment. This includes how it will benefit the patient, what is involved and why it is recommended.

The risks should include serious risks, and those which are frequently occurring (even if minor). When considering serious risks, a degree of judgement may be exercised in determining what a 'reasonable patient' would wish to know. If however, a patient should ask for every risk to be detailed, then the clinician must be forthcoming with this information.

All treatment options (including the 'no treatment' option) and their consequences should be explained. It is good practice to discuss and document the information given. The invitation of further questions and the response should also be recorded.

Consent and age

All adult patients (over 18 years of age) are presumed to have capacity to consent or refuse consent, unless it is established that they lack capacity.

Patients aged 16 or 17 years are presumed in many legal systems to have capacity to consent to treatment without parental agreement. This capacity may also exist in some patients aged under 16 years of age, as per the Gillick case, if the child can demonstrate an appropriate degree of maturity of mind.

Refusal of consent is not however binding in patients under 18 years of age and can be challenged and overruled if deemed in their best interest.

The law regarding 'young adults' aged 16–17 years remains a controversial area in most jurisdictions and there is limited case law. Discussion with a medical defence organisation and trust lawyers are advised in any case of disputes between patient, family and medical professionals.

Capacity

Capacity is an important legal principle which has been formalised since the introduction of the Mental Capacity Act 2005 for England and Wales, which provides a legal definition for mental capacity, and also provides a framework to empower and protect those who lack capacity for whatever reason. Sections 1(2) to 1(6) of the Mental Capacity Act list the five key principles of the Act:

- A person must be assumed to have capacity unless it is established that he lacks capacity
- A person is not to be treated as unable to make a decision unless all practicable steps to help him to do so have been taken without success
- A person is not to be treated as unable to make a decision merely because he makes an unwise decision
- An act done, or decision made, under this Act for or on behalf of a person who lacks capacity must be done, or made, in his best interests
- Before the act is done, or the decision is made, regard must be had to whether the purpose for which it is needed can be as effectively achieved in a way that is less restrictive of the person's rights and freedom of action

To show capacity, a patient must be able to:

- Understand information relevant to the decision
- Retain information for long enough to make a decision
- Use or weigh that information as part of the process of making a decision
- Communicate his/her decision – this can be verbal or non-verbal. The ability to express capacity should be facilitated by all reasonably practicable means (e.g. an interpreter, or devices to aid communication which may be necessary in critical care)

The patient should have the capacity, at that time, to correspond to the gravity of the decision that he/she is to make. The more serious the decision required the greater the capacity required.

No one else can consent or refuse consent on behalf of a competent adult.

Mental Health Legislation only applies to treatment of mental disorder. A person detained for treatment under the Mental Health Act (MHA) may not be treated for a physical illness without their consent. Clearly however, the mental disorder which has resulted in compulsory treatment under the MHA, may also be evidence of disordered thinking and lack of capacity – facilitating urgent treatment without consent, in their best interests, under the Mental Capacity Act.

Treatment in those who lack capacity

In England and Wales, patients aged over 16 years who lack competence, in the opinion of doctors, are treated according to the Mental Capacity Act 2005. The Mental Capacity Act creates a statutory framework in England and Wales based in large part on Common Law. Scotland uses the Adults with Incapacity Act 2001, which makes similar provisions.

Lack of capacity can be a permanent but during an intensive care admission it may be a temporary state due to their medical condition or often due to the necessary use of sedative medication.

Proxy decision-making

If a patient is unable to consent or refuse treatment, no one can grant or withhold consent on behalf of the incapacitated patient, unless proxy decision-making powers have been granted:

- Lasting Power of Attorney (England and Wales) or Welfare Attorney (Scotland)
  - Appointed by an adult patient (must be over 18 years of age) prior to losing capacity and registered with the Office of the Public Guardian
  - It must specifically state that it includes power of attorney for healthcare decisions
  - The designated person can consent or refuse to all healthcare treatments including life-sustaining treatment
- Court of Protection Appointed Deputies
  - Appointed to permanently incompetent patients or where no Power of Attorney has been granted
  - They can make judgments regarding treatment decisions but not end of life decisions

Best interests

The patient's best interests are more than just medical best interests, and any and all reasonable steps must be taken to ascertain:

- The patient's past and present wishes and feelings – including advanced decisions/directives
- The beliefs and values the patient has that are likely to influence his decisions should he have capacity
- Any other facts that would be likely to influence his decision

In addition to the Lasting Power of Attorney or the Court, the doctor must also consider, if consultation is practical and appropriate, the views of:

- Any person named by the patient as someone to be consulted on the matter in question, or of a similar kind
- Anyone engaged in the care of the person or interested in their welfare

However, the next of kin does not have a right to consent or refuse treatment.

Advance decisions

These must be made voluntarily, by an appropriately informed, adult patient and must specify which treatments are to be refused and under which circumstances. The patient must have capacity at the time of agreeing to the advance decision.

Patients cannot demand treatment that, were they to become incompetent in future, a doctor would not agree was in their best interest.

Independent mental capacity advocates

If family or friends are not available to participate in discussions, NHS institutions are required to provide an independent mental capacity advocate (IMCA). The IMCA is mandated to participate in the decision-making process by doctors, proxies or the Courts. However, the doctor is not obliged to adhere to the opinions of the IMCA, although clear documentation of this rationale would be advised.

Research

The Medicine for Human Use Regulations were introduced in 2004 to govern clinical trials of investigational medical products (CTIMP).

Non-CTIMP clinical trials are regulated either by common law (with capacity), or the Mental Capacity Act (without capacity).

All trials involving patients must be approved by the Research Ethics Committee, which includes an assessment of the consent process. In studies involving incapacitated patients the Research Ethics Committee must ensure that the research's aim is to alleviate the patient's condition, not be possible on competent patients and be beneficial for the patient or patients with the condition in future. Participation must stop if the patient objects, the patient's welfare must be of primary importance and a third person must be identified for welfare consultation.

Further reading

General Medical Council. Consent patients and doctors making decisions together. London: GMC, 2008.

Menon DK, Chatfield DA. Mental Capacity Act 2005 – Guidance for Critical Care. London: Intensive Care Society, 2011.

Department for Constitutional Affairs. Mental Capacity Act 2005 – Code of Practice. London: The Stationary Office, 2007.

Critical illness polyneuromyopathy

Key points

- Prolonged muscle weakness is common among critically ill patients
- Severe sepsis, prolonged ventilation and multiple organ failure (MOF) are major risk factors
- The underlying pathophysiology may be neuropathy, myopathy, or both; clinical features and management are not influenced by such distinction

Epidemiology

Critically ill patients may develop profound acute muscle weakness that cannot be explained by physical inactivity alone. Established risk factors are:

- Prolonged mechanical ventilation (up to 60% of patients ventilated for >7 days develop critical illness polyneuromyopathy)
- Severe sepsis and MOF
- Excessive sedation
- Muscle immobilisation – muscle mass decreases by 1–2% per day during critical illness
- Exogenous steroids
- Hyperglycaemia – the incidence is lower among postoperative patients subjected to strict blood sugar control
- Neuromuscular blocking drugs

Other possible risk factors include: parenteral nutrition, neurological disease, female gender and the elderly.

Pathophysiology

Critical illness polyneuromyopathy, also referred to as intensive care unit (ICU)-acquired weakness, describes a spectrum of disorders leading to muscle weakness. The underlying pathology may be neuropathy, myopathy or a combination; clinical presentations are indistinguishable. Proposed pathophysiological mechanisms include nerve axon ischaemia due to hypotension and microcirculatory dysfunction, decreased muscle membrane excitability and muscle atrophy.

Clinical features

Typically, there is a symmetrical, flaccid tetraparesis sparing the facial muscles, which develops after the onset of critical illness. There may be reduced or absent tendon reflexes with or without muscle wasting. Distal sensory loss of pain, temperature and vibration sensation may occur. Respiratory neuromuscular involvement can manifest as failure to wean from mechanical ventilation. Motor weakness can be assessed using the Medical Research Council (MRC) sum-score (**Table 15**). Each limb is scored from 0 to 15. The total score ranges from 0 (tetraplegia) to 60, with a sum-score of less than 48 suggesting polyneuromyopathy. However, patient cooperation is required for this assessment.

Table 15 MRC sum-score	
Movement tested on each side	**Score for each movement**
Arm abduction	0 = no movement
Flexion at the elbow	1 = flicker of movement
Wrist extension	2 = movement with gravity eliminated
Hip flexion	3 = movement against gravity
Extension at the knee	4 = movement against resistance
Foot dorsiflexion	5 = normal power

Investigations

Electromyography and nerve conduction studies may reveal a reduction in compound muscle action potentials or sensory nerve action potentials with preserved conduction velocity. Muscle biopsy is required to distinguish between neuropathy and myopathy, which frequently overlap. As clinical presentations and treatment are the same regardless of the pathophysiology, invasive investigations tend to be used only when the diagnosis is uncertain.

Differential diagnosis

- Spinal cord injury
- Guillain–Barré syndrome
- Myasthenia gravis
- Motor neurone disease
- Rhabdomyolysis
- Botulism
- Organophosphate poisoning
- Acid maltase myopathy

Treatment

Management is aimed at the treatment or avoidance of risk factors. This includes the effective prevention and treatment of sepsis and MOF, minimising the duration of assisted ventilation, and avoidance of neuromuscular blocking drugs (especially continuous infusion) and steroids wherever possible.

Strict blood sugar control using insulin is the only strategy that has been shown, in a randomised controlled trial, to reduce the incidence of acute critical illness polyneuromyopathy. However, subsequent studies have demonstrated a higher mortality in patients treated with intensive insulin therapy so this strategy is not recommended.

Early mobility therapy, e.g. bedside cycling ergometry, may reduce the incidence or severity of muscle weakness. Daily sedation interruptions and minimising the use of sedative agents are likely to be of benefit by reducing the duration of ventilation and immobility.

Physical rehabilitation and psychological support are both important in the effective management of such patients.

Complications

Duration of mechanical ventilation, ICU admission and hospital stay may all be prolonged, and hospital mortality rates are increased. Muscle weakness can persist for months and up to one third of patients have permanent severe disability.

Further reading

de Jonghe B, Lacherade JC, Sharshar T, Outin H. Intensive care unit-acquired weakness: risk factors and prevention. Crit Care Med 2009; 37:S309–315.

Hermans G, De Jonghe B, Bruyninckx F, Van den Berghe G. Clinical review: Critical illness polyneuropathy and myopathy. Crit Care 2008; 12:238.

Related topics of interest

Delirium

Key points

- Delirium is common and is under-recognised in ICU patients
- It increases both in-patient mortality and long-term morbidity
- Management is focused around a multi-component strategy

Epidemiology

Delirium is common in critically ill patients. In general, the prevalence is higher in more severely ill patients with up to 80% of mechanically ventilated patients and 50% of lower severity ICU patients affected. Delirium usually starts around day 2 and has an average duration of 4 days (± 2 days).

Male gender, increasing age, disease severity, pre-existing dementia or structural brain damage and medication-related cholinergic burden are some of the predictors for delirium.

Pathophysiology

As with many organ system failures on intensive care, the condition is likely to be a common end-result of a multitude of factors. Imbalances in the synthesis, release and degradation of multiple neurotransmitters are thought to be the common mechanism. Disruptions in neural connectivity that persist for a sufficient duration may lead to neuronal atrophy causing long-term cognitive impairment (LTCI).

Postulated causative factors include metabolic derangement, genetic susceptibility, pro-inflammatory states and micro-emboli leading to reduced cerebral perfusion. Medications (including sedatives and analgesics) are a major contributor and many of the most commonly prescribed medications have a measurable anti-cholinergic activity. The cumulative effect of this is termed the 'cholinergic burden' and is positively associated with poor cognitive function and delirium.

Clinical features

Delirium is defined as an acutely disturbed state of mind that occurs in fever, intoxication and other disorders and is characterised by restlessness, illusions, and incoherence of thought and speech.

There are three main subgroups of delirium:

Hyperactive delirium

The stereotypical image of delirium is an acutely confused patient who may be a danger to themselves and staff. However, they form the smallest proportion (approximately 1%) of the delirium spectrum. These patients are the easiest to diagnose and often receive the most attention as they cause a constant drain to nursing resources and distress to their relatives.

Hypoactive delirium

Accounting for approximately 35% of all delirium cases, these patients are passive, immobile and often ignored. They have negative symptoms such as inattention and a flat affect and as such, their clinical signs may be mistaken for depression. As they display no obvious outward signs of agitation or delirium they are harder to diagnose.

Mixed delirium

The most common form (approximately 64%), are often described as 'not themselves' and are confused and 'picky'. They will often pull out lines and drains.

Investigations

There are no laboratory or imaging investigations that are specific for delirium.

Biochemical tests

A surrogate marker for the cholinergic hypothesis has been developed; termed serum anti-cholinergic activity (SAA), it has been linked to severity of delirium but remains a research tool at present. Markers of direct neuronal injury such as neurone specific enolase (NSE) and S-100 β are elevated in delirium, but are not specific for it.

Electrophysiology studies

EEG studies of delirious patients can show non-specific slowing not dissimilar to that found with sedation or non-specific encephalopathies.

Radiology

Standard radiological imaging of the brain is unlikely to be helpful. Functional studies demonstrate a reduction in global cerebral blood flow, which improves with resolution of symptoms.

Diagnosis

In the absence of specific investigations, delirium remains a clinical diagnosis. The DSM–IV requires four diagnostic criteria for delirium:

1. Inattention and disturbance of consciousness.
2. Change in cognition.
3. Acute onset and fluctuating course.
4. Pathophysiological cause.

Several bedside scoring systems have been developed to assess delirium in intensive care patients. Those that have gained the widest acceptance in ICU patients are the ICDSC and the CAM-ICU.

Intensive care delirium screening checklist

The intensive care delirium screening checklist (ICDSC) is an eight-item scoring system, based on observations during routine patient care over a 24 h period. No patient co-operation is required. It can be performed at the bedside by ICU staff.

Confusion assessment method – ICU (CAM-ICU)

An abbreviated version of the CAM designed for use in sedated and mechanically ventilated patients, it is a simple, rapid bedside assessment tool that gives a binary answer. The CAM-ICU has a higher sensitivity than other tools, such as the ICDSC as it enables the assessment of sedated patients,

but is less specific with a higher false positive rate. It does not enable assessment of severity or sub-type of delirium. It is the most common screening tool used in UK intensive care units.

Treatment

There is no single treatment that prevents or immediately resolves delirium; instead a package of care should be instituted similar to other care bundles.

Emergency admissions already have a well-established inflammatory process and treatment is modelled around reduction of pre-disposing factors and supportive care. Regular re-orientation, use of clocks, natural daylight and sleeping patterns, cohort nursing, provision of usual visual and hearing aids, avoiding constipation and early removal of invasive catheters, along with early mobilisation are all considered best practice.

Address and correct pain and significant metabolic derangements, review prescriptions to reduce the cholinergic burden and perform daily sedation holds. There is emerging evidence that the α_2 agonist dexmedetomidine may reduce the burden of delirium compared to traditional sedatives.

When delirium is diagnosed, common practice is to use antipsychotic drugs such as haloperidol or atypical antipsychotics such as quetiapine, olanzapine or risperidone to help with symptoms. These may reduce severity and duration, but staff and relatives should be prepared that patients are likely to be delirious for several days despite treatment. It is best to avoid re-sedation or physical restraints to manage patients if possible, as this can exacerbate delirium; but is sometimes required to keep the patient safe.

Complications

In the short term, acute delirium is associated with complications such as accidental loss of invasive devices. In the medium term, there is an increased duration of mechanical ventilation, intensive care and hospital length of stay and a significant increase in healthcare costs. It is an independent risk factor for death with a threefold increase in 6-month mortality. Long-term effects are associated with increased prevalence of post-traumatic stress, increased risk of LTCI and a reduction in return to work that may be permanent with significant repercussions for both the individual and society.

Further reading

Girard TD, Pandharipande PP, Ely EW. Delirium in the intensive care unit. Crit Care 2008;12:S3.

Gusmao-Flores D, Salluh JI, Chalhub RA, Quarantini LC. The Confusion Assessment Method for the Intensive Care Unit (CAM-ICU) and Intensive Care Delirium Screening Checklist (ICDSC) for the diagnosis of delirium: a systematic review and meta-analysis of clinical studies. Crit Care 2012; 16:R115.

van den Boogaard M, Schoonhoven L, Evers AW, et al. Delirium in critically ill patients: impact on long-term health-related quality of life and cognitive functioning. Crit Care Med 2012; 40:112–118.

Related topics of interest

Diabetes mellitus

Key points

- The initial management of diabetic emergencies is aimed at airway, breathing and circulation, and not at insulin therapy
- The Joint British Diabetes Societies Inpatient Care Group has published guidelines on the management of diabetic ketoacidosis, hyperosmolar hyperglycaemic state, and hypoglycaemia in adults with diabetes mellitus
- Plasma electrolytes require frequent monitoring and careful replacement when indicated

Epidemiology

200 million people worldwide have diabetes mellitus and it affects nearly 4 million people in the UK. Insulin dependent diabetes mellitus (IDDM) accounts for around 10% and non-insulin dependent diabetes mellitus (NIDDM) accounts for 90% of diabetics. Patients with diabetes may require critical care due to end organ damage secondary to chronic disease or as an acute diabetic emergency.

Pathophysiology

IDDM is associated with autoimmune destruction of pancreatic cells leading to insulin deficiency, but it may also follow pancreatitis or pancreatectomy. In NIDDM, there is insulin resistance; insulin values are initially high but later in the disease process they are reduced and overt hyperglycaemia develops. In the critical care setting, hyperglycaemia in IDDM is managed by infusions of a short-acting insulin and frequent blood glucose measurement. The same is often true for NIDDM patients who can usually return to non-insulin control after resolution of their acute illness. Hyperglycaemia also occurs in normal individuals secondary to administration of glucose-containing solutions, corticosteroids, catecholamines and the stress response. In this non-diabetic group, the hyperglycaemia

resolves with the clinical illness and long-term anti-diabetes treatment is rarely required.

Long-standing diabetes causes end organ damage, producing severe morbidity and increased mortality.

- Vascular disease (15–60%), coronary artery disease and cerebrovascular disease
- Hypertension (30–60%)
- Cardiomyopathy
- Nephropathy
- Retinopathy
- Autonomic neuropathy (risk of arrhythmias, cardiac arrest, respiratory arrest and hypoglycaemia)
- Infection
- Increased respiratory disease
- Neuropathy

Treatment is directed at both maintaining normoglycaemia (blood glucose 6–10 mmol L^{-1}) and at associated disorders.

Specific diabetic emergencies

Diabetic ketoacidosis (DKA)

Pathophysiology
Diabetic ketoacidosis (DKA) accounts for the majority of diabetic emergencies admitted to critical care units. It is usually seen in patients with IDDM and evolves over several days. Lack of insulin combined with increases in glucagon, catecholamines and cortisol stimulates lipolysis, free fatty acid production and ketogenesis. Accumulation of ketoacids (3-β-hydroxybutyrate, acetone and acetoacetate) causes metabolic acidosis. Increased gluconeogenesis and glycolysis cause hyperglycaemia; glucose is not taken up peripherally because of the lack of insulin. The renal retention threshold for glucose is exceeded and glycosuria and ketonuria cause considerable loss of water and electrolytes. Hypovolaemia ensues and impaired tissue perfusion invokes anaerobic metabolism, which adds to the metabolic acidosis. The degree of hyperglycaemia is variable in DKA:

up to 15% may have normal or only slightly elevated blood glucose. Severe DKA has a mortality rate of 5%.

Clinical features

The clinical features of DKA include thirst, polyuria, nausea, abdominal pain, vomiting, weight loss, confusion progressing to coma, hyperventilation (Kussmaul respiration) due to acidosis, ketone breath, dehydration and hypovolaemia. DKA is commonly precipitated by infection, surgery, myocardial infarction and non-compliance with drug therapy. Ketonaemia, hyperglycaemia and acidaemia are the three biochemical markers that define a diagnosis of DKA (see **Table 16**).

Investigations

Investigations focus on assessing the severity of the underlying metabolic chaos, determining the precipitating cause and monitoring the response to treatment.

Investigations include blood ketone values, glucose, venous blood gas and urea and electrolytes. A full blood count (FBC), blood cultures, C-reactive protein (CRP), ECG, chest X-ray, urinalysis, sputum, urine, stools and wound swabs for culture are obtained as clinically indicated. A full clinical examination and regular observations are essential.

Assess blood ketone and glucose values hourly. Monitor potassium, venous bicarbonate and pH every 1–2 h during the initial phase of DKA management, decreasing the frequency of checks as the patient improves.

Table 16 Diagnostic criteria for DKA: DKA is diagnosed when all three markers are present

Marker	Value
Ketonaemia or Ketonuria	≥ 3 mmol L^{-1} >2+ on urine sticks
Blood glucose or Known diabetes mellitus	> 11 mmol L^{-1}
Venous bicarbonate +/or Venous pH	< 15 mmol L^{-1} < 7.3

Indications for consideration of care on the High Dependency Unit include:

- Blood ketones > 6 mmol L^{-1}
- Bicarbonate < 5 mmol L^{-1}
- pH < 7.1
- K$^+$ < 3.5 mmol L^{-1}
- GCS <12/15
- Arterial blood oxygen saturation <92% on air
- Systolic BP <90 mmHg
- Heart rate <60 or >100 min^{-1}
- Anion Gap >16

Treatment

Most hospitals have clear guidelines for the management of DKA (for adults and for children and young adults). The emphasis is on managing DKA at the bedside, guided by the use of point of care testing to monitor ketone, glucose, electrolyte, bicarbonate and venous pH. Inform and involve diabetic specialist teams from the outset.

The initial management of DKA focuses on fluid replacement followed by insulin therapy to restore circulating volume, to clear ketones, to suppress ketone formation and to correct electrolyte imbalance.

Targets for treatment are to:

- Decrease blood ketone level by 0.5 mmol L^{-1} h^{-1}
- Increase venous bicarbonate by 3 mmol L^{-1} h^{-1}
- Decrease capillary blood glucose by 3 mmol L^{-1} h^{-1}

Fluid resuscitation The fluid of choice for resuscitation in DKA is 0.9% sodium chloride. Hypovolaemia must be reversed rapidly to ensure adequate tissue perfusion; the overall fluid deficit can then be replaced over a longer period. Correct any hypotension (systolic blood pressure (SBP) <90 mmHg) initially with 500–1000 mL 0.9% sodium chloride given rapidly. Continue fluid replacement with 0.9% sodium chloride 1 L over 1 h, a further 1 L over 2 h followed by another 1 L over 4 h. Infuse fluid less rapidly in young adults (18–25 years) (risk of cerebral oedema), the elderly and in those with renal and cardiac failure – specialist input is advised.

Insulin infusion Treat DKA with a fixed rate insulin infusion based on the patient's weight (0.1 U Kg^{-1} h^{-1}) rather than a sliding scale. Do not give an initial insulin bolus. If the patient normally takes a long-acting insulin analogue, continue this as part of the DKA management. If the targets for correcting plasma ketone and bicarbonate values are not achieved, increase the rate of the insulin infusion. The primary role of the fixed rate insulin infusion is to clear blood ketones; however, there is a risk of inducing hypoglycaemia. Once the blood glucose is < 14 mmol L^{-1} start an infusion of 10% glucose and continue until the patient is eating and drinking. This may need to be run concurrently with the 0.9% sodium chloride. Continue the fixed rate insulin infusion until blood ketones are < 0.3 mmol L^{-1} and the venous pH is > 7.3.

Potassium and electrolytes   The potassium debt is typically 200–350 mmol. When treating DKA, maintain potassium values at 4–5 mmol L^{-1}. Hyperkalaemia may be caused by dehydration and pre-renal failure; conversely, insulin treatment may cause hypokalaemia. Supplement each bag of 0.9% sodium chloride with potassium if the plasma potassium value is ≤ 5.5 mmol/L. If the potassium values reduce to < 3.5 mmol/L despite replacement, consider inserting a central line and giving higher concentration potassium infusions.

Average losses include 5–10 L of water and 400–700 mmol of sodium. The magnesium deficit mirrors that of potassium. Phosphate deficit is also considerable at approximately 1 mmol kg^{-1}; however, phosphate is replaced only if the patient is profoundly weak.

Correction of acidosis   The metabolic acidosis will improve with restoration of tissue perfusion and reduction in ketosis. There is no role for sodium bicarbonate which is associated with numerous side effects including: adverse effects on tissue oxygenation because of increased haemoglobin oxygen affinity; increased carbon dioxide production, which will require increased minute ventilation; paradoxical intracellular and cerebrospinal acidosis; a high osmotic and sodium load, with the risk of volume overload; hypokalaemia; and hypocalcaemia.

Other supportive treatment

Initiate deep vein thrombosis prophylaxis with compression stockings or mechanical compression devices and subcutaneous heparin. Initiate stress ulcer prophylaxis. Consider a nasogastric tube and start enteral feeding early if it is indicated.

Intubation and ventilation   Tracheal intubation is required if consciousness is obtunded significantly. There is risk of aspiration because of the depressed conscious level and gastric dilation. When assisted ventilation is used, the minute ventilation must take into account the extensive respiratory compensation of the spontaneously ventilating patient; an inadequate minute volume at this stage may precipitate profound acidosis and cardiovascular decompensation.

Complications

Cerebral oedema is a common cause of death in DKA, more so in children and young adults than in older adults. Other complications include hypoglycaemia, hypokalaemia, hyperkalaemia and acute respiratory distress syndrome.

Hyperglycaemic hyperosmolar state

Pathophysiology

Hyperglycaemic hyperosmolar state (HHS), formerly known as hyperglycaemic hyperosmolar non-ketotic coma, occurs much less frequently than DKA. The new terminology reflects that an altered sensorium may be present without coma and there may be variable degrees of ketosis. The mortality associated with HHS is 15–30%. Severe hyperglycaemia and fluid depletion develops over a period of days or weeks with no or mild ketosis.

Clinical features

The classical features of HHS includes a blood glucose ≥ 30 mmol L^{-1}, raised plasma osmolality (> 320 mosmol kg^{-1}) and marked hypovolaemia, but without significant ketonaemia (< 3 mmol L^{-1}) or acidosis (pH > 7.3 , bicarbonate > 15 mmol L^{-1}).

It is seen usually in elderly patients with uncontrolled NIDDM, but may also be the first presentation of late-onset diabetes. Precipitants include infection, steroid and diuretic use, an excessive glucose intake and inter-current surgery or illness. The characteristic presentation is of non-specific anorexia, malaise and weakness, which progresses to coma, severe dehydration and renal impairment. Coma will necessitate tracheal intubation, and the patient may be obtunded for several days. Water losses are typically 6–13 L with sodium losses of 300–780 mmol.

Investigation

As for DKA above. The hyperglycaemia is often profound and infection needs to be excluded. Plasma glucose and sodium values must be monitored regularly.

Indications potential admission to a high dependency unit include:

- Osmolality > 350 mosmol kg^{-1}
- Sodium > 160 mmol L^{-1}
- pH < 7.1
- K$^+$ < 3.5 or > 6 mmol L^{-1}
- GCS < 12/15
- Oxygen saturation < 92% when breathing air
- Systolic BP < 90 mmHg
- Heart rate < 60 or > 100 bpm
- Urine output < 0.5 mL kg^{-1} h^{-1}
- Creatinine > 200 micromol L^{-1}
- Temperature < 36 °C
- Myocardial infarction, stroke or other serious co-morbidity

Treatment

Follow local guidelines and involve the diabetic team promptly. The dehydration is often more severe than occurs in DKA and replacement should be more gradual because the risk of cerebral oedema is higher. Correct the fluid deficits over a period of approximately 24 h – the electrolyte abnormalities may take many days to correct. Despite the levels of hyperglycaemia often exceeding those seen in DKA, the insulin requirements are lower than for DKA. Management recommendations include:

- Treat the causative precipitant
- Fluid replacement with 0.9% sodium chloride – aim to replace estimated fluid losses over 24 h
- Potassium replacement if K$^+$ < 5.5 mmol L^{-1}
- Sodium not to decrease by more than 10 mmol L^{-1} in 24 h
- Glucose not to decrease by more than 5 mmol L^{-1} h^{-1}
- Start a low dose insulin infusion (0.05 U kg^{-1} h^{-1}) only once glucose values are no longer decreasing with fluid resuscitation, unless ketonaemia is identified on admission when an insulin infusion is started immediately
- Monitor response to intervention with regular assessment of plasma osmolality
- Assess for potential complications including fluid overload, cerebral oedema and central pontine myelinolysis

Thrombotic events, including cardiac and cerebral events, as well as venous thrombosis, are more common in HHS and are a major cause of morbidity and mortality, therefore, prescribe prophylactic anticoagulation. Provide careful protection to prevent foot ulceration.

0.45% sodium chloride is used only if plasma osmolality fails to decrease despite adequate fluid resuscitation and optimal decrease in glucose values.

Hypoglycaemia

Life-threatening hypoglycaemia may occur in diabetics and non-diabetics. Coma in diabetics is most commonly caused by hypoglycaemia. Hypoglycaemia (blood glucose < 4.0 mmol L^{-1}) may be precipitated by:

- Inadequate carbohydrate diet, missed meals, breastfeeding, early pregnancy, malabsorption syndromes, prolonged periods without food, e.g. NBM for surgery, vomiting
- Excess glucose uptake (exercise and insulin overdose)
- Change in therapy/commencement of insulin therapy/insulin prescription or administration error
- Acute illness and sudden cessation of steroids
- Liver failure, renal failure and dialysis treatment

- Alcohol (inhibition of gluconeogenesis)
- Hypoadrenalism (including Addison's disease) and hypopituitarism

The threshold for symptoms and clinical features of hypoglycaemia varies widely:

- Nausea
- Sweating, tachycardia and palpitations, tremor (may be absent with autonomic neuropathy)
- Altered behaviour, speech abnormalities, incoordination, confusion, agitation and depressed level of consciousness
- Seizures, coma and focal neurological signs; permanent neurological damage occurs rapidly because of the brain's dependence on glucose for metabolism and the lack of any significant brain stores of glycogen

Management

Give quick-acting glucose to reverse hypoglycaemia rapidly, followed by a long-acting carbohydrate to maintain normoglycaemia. Stop any variable rate insulin infusion. In conscious patients give quick acting carbohydrate such as fruit juice or a glucose-based tablet/sweet. In conscious but uncooperative patients give a glucose-based gel to the mouth or 1 mg glucagon IM. In patients who are unconscious, having seizures, or are very uncooperative, give either 1 mg glucagon IM, 80 mL 20% glucose or 160 mL 10% glucose. Repeat the process if the blood sugar value does not increase above 4 mmol L^{-1}. Once this has been achieved, follow treatment with a longer acting carbohydrate such as milk, a meal or a glucose infusion. Patients on enteral feed should have it restarted. Measure blood glucose values frequently and, if necessary, infuse glucose continuously to maintain normoglycaemia. Cautiously restart a variable rate insulin infusion.

Intensive insulin treatment in critically ill patients

Hyperglycaemia and insulin resistance are common in critically ill patients. Hyperglycaemia is associated with increased morbidity (including infection) and mortality in critically ill patients, particularly those with myocardial infarction and stroke. The role of intensive insulin treatment to maintain tight control of blood glucose in these patients has been evaluated. A randomised controlled trial in surgical patients to target tight glycaemic control of blood glucose to 4.4–6.1 mmol L^{-1} showed reduced mortality and critical illness neuropathy, but enthusiasm for tight glucose control has been tempered by subsequent studies. In particular, the large multi-centre NICE-SUGAR study demonstrated that tight glucose control using intensive insulin therapy was associated with increased mortality among a heterogeneous population of adults in the ICU. Current practice is to maintain normoglycaemia and introduce IV insulin if the blood glucose is >10 mmol L^{-1}. There is increasing evidence that glucose variability may be almost as important as the absolute value. Continuous glucose monitoring in critically ill patients is being evaluated.

Further reading

Joint British Diabetes Societies Inpatient Care Group The management of diabetic ketoacidosis in Adults. Second Edition. Update: September 2013. http://www.diabetes.org.uk/About_us/What-we-say/Improving-diabetes-healthcare/The-Management-of-Diabetic-Ketoacidosis-in-Adults/. Accessed November 2013.

Joint British Diabetes Societies Inpatient Care Group. The management og the hypersomolar hyperglycaemic state (HHS) in adults with diabetes. August 2012. http://www.diabetes.org.uk/About_us/What-we-say/Improving-diabetes-healthcare/Management-of-the-hyperosmolar-hyperglycaemic-state-HHS-in-adults-with-diabetes/.s Accessed February 2013.

The hospital management of hypoglycaemia in adults with diabetes mellitus. March 2010. http://www.diabetes.org.uk/About_us/What-we-say/Improving-diabetes-healthcare/The-hospital-management-of-Hypoglycaemia-in-adults-with-Diabetes-Mellitus/. Accessed February 2013.

Van den Berghe G, Wouters P, Weekers F, et al. Intensive insulin therapy in critically ill patients. N Eng J Med 2001; 345:1359–1367.

Finfer S, Chittock DR, Su SY, et al. Intensive versus conventional glucose control in critically ill patients. N Engl J Med 2009; 360:1283–1297.

Savage MW. Management of diabetic ketoacidosis. Clin Med 2011; 11:154–156.

Kavanagh BP, McCowen KC. Clinical practice. Glycemic control in the ICU. N Engl J Med 2010; 363:2540–2546.

Jacobi J, Bircher N, Krinsley J, et al. Guidelines for the use of an insulin infusion for the management of hyperglycaemia in critically ill patients. Crit Care Med 2012; 40:3251–3276.

Related topics of interest

Diarrhoea

Key points

- Diarrhoea is common in the intensive care unit (ICU)
- Infectious diarrhoea needs early diagnosis and treatment
- Stopping enteral feed does not improve diarrhoea

Epidemiology

The diagnosis of diarrhoea is made difficult by the lack of a standardised definition. Definitions vary from more than 2–3 stools per day to the presence of watery stool. The incidence of diarrhoea in the ICU ranges from 25–50%. It is important to have an accurate measure of a patient's stool consistency and the use of a stool chart aids both diagnosis and management. The Bristol stool scale is frequently used.

Pathophysiology

The mechanisms by which diarrhoea is caused are as follows:

- Secretory: this is common in infectious diarrhoea, where a particle is secreted into the GI lumen that carries water with it. A good example is cholera, where sodium is secreted into the bowel
- Osmotic: a substance within the bowel lumen that cannot be absorbed draws water into the lumen. This occurs with lactose-intolerance. It is also the mechanism involved with feed-associated diarrhoea

- Hypermotility: when the transit time thorough the GI tract is too rapid for absorption
- Inflammatory: the bowel mucosa is inflamed due to infection or inflammation, with compromise of the gut integrity and impaired absorption of bowel content and exudative fluid loss leading to diarrhoea

The most important distinction is between infective and non-infective diarrhoea. The commonest cause of non-infective diarrhoea on the ICU is the use of artificial enteral feed. *Campylobacter* and *Salmonella* are causes of infective diarrhoea. The most common cause of infective intensive care induced diarrhoea is *C. difficile*. Other causes include winter GI viruses including norovirus.

See **Table 17** for causes of diarrhoea.

Clostridium difficile and antibiotic-associated diarrhoea

C. difficile is a Gram-positive anaerobic organism. It produces spores that survive for a prolonged period. It is a common and serious hospital acquired infection. It frequently arises after antibiotic use as a result of eradication of a person's normal GI tract flora. This allows clostridium to predominate and colitis develops. The colitis is known as pseudomembranous colitis and causes a discoloured offensive stool with a characteristic odour. Risk factors for progression to fulminant infective colitis include age >60, use of broad spectrum antibiotics, albumin <25 g L^{-1}, malignancy, renal disease and pulmonary disease. Certain

Table 17 Causes of diarrhoea	
Infective	*C. difficile*, campylobacter, shigella, salmonella, *E. Coli*, giardia, norovirus, rotavirus
Osmotic	Certain laxatives, enteral magnesium, bacterial overgrowth, short gut syndrome, Intestinal ischaemia
Diseases	Crohn's disease, ulcerative colitis, cystic fibrosis, chronic pancreatitis, bowel cancer
Dysmotility	Post-ileus recovery, overflow in pseudo-obstruction or faecal impaction
Drugs	Antibiotics, laxatives, NSAIDs, chemotherapy, statins, antacid medications, alcohol, enteral feed
Food Intolerance	Coeliac disease, lactose intolerance
Other	Anxiety, irritable bowel syndrome

antibiotics are more likely to precipitate *C. difficile* infection and these include cephalosporins and quinolones. The most causative antimicrobials change frequently.

Prevention is better than treatment in *C. difficile* infection.

Investigations

The mainstay of diagnosis is the exclusion of *C. difficile*.

A stool culture for microscopy, culture and sensitivity will diagnose most causes of diarrhoea. Stool ELISA diagnoses *C. difficile* toxin with high sensitivity. Send viral stool serology to exclude norovirus.

Send blood for full blood count, urea and electrolytes, clotting and C-reactive protein to monitor any associated systemic toxicity and organ failure. Erect CXR is needed if there is suspicion of perforation. Sigmoidoscopy is indicated if no cause for the diarrhoea is identified.

Examine the patient regularly. Early and frequent surgical review is indicated in patients with abdominal pain and significant tenderness, an ileus, high white cell count, those who are immunosuppressed and patients with associated organ dysfunction such as renal impairment, cardiovascular compromise and confusion. Close observation is needed to see whether there is response to conservative management or whether urgent surgery is required.

Prevention

Prevention of diarrhoea on the ICU is important. Non-infective diarrhoea is best prevented by sensible use of laxatives and early eating and drinking.

The prevention of infectious diarrhoea is a major issue in UK hospitals. The UK Department of Health has produced extensive guidance on this topic.

Prevention involves careful use of antibiotics. All hospitals should have antibiotic policies aimed at reducing *C. difficile* and policies for early testing and isolation. Rigorous infection control procedures must be applied. Alcohol hand gels do not eliminate *C. difficile* spores but handwashing with soap and water is required.

The management of patients with suspected infective diarrhoea is best summarised by using the UK Department of Health's pneumonic, SIGHT:

S Suspect that a case may be infective where there is no clear alternative cause for diarrhoea.

I Isolate the patient and consult with the infection control team while determining the cause of the diarrhoea.

G Gloves and aprons must be used for all contacts with the patient and their environment.

H Hand washing with soap and water should be carried out before and after each contact with the patient and the patient's environment.

T Test the stool for toxin, by sending a specimen immediately.

Treatment

In patients who present with diarrhoea, treatment is supportive, aimed at making a diagnosis, avoiding further contamination, maintaining hydration and avoiding systemic complications. Treat infective causes of diarrhoea with the relevant antibiotics.

C. difficile is most commonly treated with metronidazole and vancomycin. Give these drugs enterally in order to maximise effect.

Surgery may be indicated in a small proportion that has developed severe colitis.

Non-infective diarrhoea

The commonest cause of non-infective diarrhoea on the ICU is related to enteral feeding. Consider this once infection has been excluded.

The composition of enteral feeds can be adjusted to minimise diarrhoea. The most effective change is produced by increasing the fibre content of the enteral feed. Alteration from nasogastric to nasojejunal route makes no difference to diarrhoea. Bolus administration is associated with more diarrhoea than continuous administration.

The use of anti-diarrhoeal medication is controversial. The use of opioids is widespread, especially the GI specific loperamide. This is effective in slowing diarrhoea by creating a paralytic ileus but can cause toxic megacolon. It is almost completely contraindicated in cases of infective diarrhoea.

There has been recent interest in the use of probiotics and symbiotics. These are enterally delivered bacteria such as *Lactobacillus*. They are given to support GI tract colonisation with bacteria that are beneficial. They have shown some promise in preventing antibiotic-associated diarrhoea and ventilator-associated pneumonia. However, the benefit has to date not been proven and in fact has been associated with cases of systemic infection.

Complications

Diarrhoea creates a significant workload for nursing staff and puts the patient at risk of skin damage and pressure sores from frequent cleaning. The use of a bowel management system can minimise this.

Specific complications of certain types of diarrhoea occur. *C. difficile* can cause a severe infection with associated shock and organ dysfunction. The colitis can cause bowel dilatation, toxic megacolon and perforation. In fulminant *C. difficile* infection, a colectomy is sometimes indicated. Mortality is approximately 20% in fulminant pseudomembranous colitis.

Further reading

Morrow LE, Gogineni V, Malesker MA. Probiotic, prebiotic, and synbiotic use in critically ill patients. Curr Opin Crit Care 2012; 18:186–191.

Van Gossum A, Preiser JC. Diarrhoea in the critically ill. Curr Opin Crit Care 2006; 12:149–154.

Riddle DJ, Dubberke ER. *Clostridium difficile* infection in the intensive care unit. Infect Dis Clin North Am 2009; 23:727–743.

Related topics of interest

- Nutrition (p 230)
- Infection acquired in hospital (p 192)

- Infection prevention and control (p 197)

Drug overdose and poisons

Key points

- Basic and advanced life supportive measures are the mainstay of treatment
- The majority of patients will recover without specific measures
- Specific therapies are available for some drugs and involving toxicologists improves outcomes

Epidemiology

Drug overdose accounts for around 5% of admissions to general intensive care units. Overdose may be accidental or intentional as seen in suicidal or parasuicidal patients. The number of drugs available is enormous and clinical presentations vary greatly. However, basic and advanced life supportive measures remain the mainstay of treatment and the majority of patients will recover fully. A systematic approach to assessment and management comprises resuscitation, substance identification, drug elimination and specific treatment.

Resuscitation

Resuscitation should follow the well-established 'ABC' principles. However, there are specific problems:

- Hypothermia is common especially at the extremes of age. Core temperature should be measured
- Hyperthermia is relatively uncommon but is seen with salicylates, amphetamines, cocaine and anticholinergic drugs. Neuroleptic malignant syndrome and malignant hyperthermia are rare causes. Sepsis may be the cause, particularly in obtunded patients
- Rhabdomyolysis should be excluded in hypothermic, comatose or traumatised patients. It may also occur in narcotic and cocaine abuse without coma, or it may complicate prolonged seizures

Substance identification

The history is often unreliable but important information includes:

- Drug: name(s), dosage, when taken and route taken
- Circumstance: intention, witnesses, empty bottles, packets, syringes and associated trauma
- Background: previous attempt(s), past medical history and allergy
- Symptoms and signs: description and first aid prior to presentation. A full physical examination is essential

Investigations

Identify the drug (blood, urine or gastric aspirate) and decide on the need for a specific treatment. It is routine practice to check for paracetamol, aspirin and alcohol. Other helpful investigations might include:

- Blood count and coagulation. Urea, creatinine and electrolytes, liver function tests and CPK
- Serum osmolality (ethanol, methanol and ethylene glycol)
- Arterial blood gas analysis
- CXR in obtunded or intubated patients
- 12-lead ECG (assessing QRS duration and QT interval)

Treatment

Drug elimination

There are a number of strategies for drug elimination:

External decontamination is indicated for toxins that can be absorbed transdermally, e.g. organophosphates and hydrocarbons.

Induced emesis with syrup of ipecacuanha is not indicated when time of ingestion is more than 1 h. Less than 40% of ingested substance is usually recovered. It is contraindicated in children less than 6 months old, when there is coma or a depressed level of consciousness, following ingestion of caustic agents, alkalis and hydrocarbons. Potential complications include aspiration, Mallory–Weiss tears, protracted vomiting and gastric rupture. Its routine administration in the emergency department should be abandoned.

Gastric lavage is generally only useful within 1 h of ingestion but worthwhile recovery of some drugs (e.g. salicylate and theophylline) may occur later. It is not effective against alcohol ingestion and is potentially harmful following petroleum product and caustic ingestion. It should be performed only when the airway is protected. Complications include aspiration and inhalation of gastric contents, oropharyngeal trauma and oesophageal perforation. There is no certain evidence that its use improves clinical outcome and it may cause significant morbidity.

Activated charcoal (AC) is an effective adsorbent for many drugs. It is superior to emesis or lavage. Activated charcoal does not bind elemental metal (e.g. iron and lithium), alcohol (e.g. ethanol and methanol), cyanide or some pesticides (Malathion and DDT). Commercially available AC is an aqueous slurry with added cathartic and flavouring. AC should be considered only in life-threatening overdose of carbamazepine, dapsone, phenobarbital, quinine and theophylline. Its use in salicylate poisoning is controversial. No controlled study has yet demonstrated that AC reduces morbidity and mortality.

Cathartics cause diarrhoea and are used in combination with AC. Fluid and electrolyte losses may be excessive. Its sole use has no role in routine practice.

Endoscopy may be used for iron, alkali or acid ingestion, where gastric lavage and AC may cause further harm.

Surgical removal is rarely indicated (e.g. iron overdose and body packers).

Diuresis relies on bulk flow to decrease drug concentrations in blood. Intravenous fluid with or without a diuretic is used to produce a urine output of 2–5 mL kg^{-1} h^{-1}. Electrolyte and volume status must be closely monitored. There is a major risk of fluid overload. Alkalinisation with sodium bicarbonate may enhance barbiturate and salicylate elimination but is generally no longer recommended.

Haemodialysis is effective for low molecular weight compounds with small volume of distribution, low protein binding, low lipid solubility and low spontaneous clearance. Examples include methanol, ethanol, ethylene glycol, salicylates, lithium and chloral hydrate.

Haemoperfusion using either charcoal or resin columns may be useful for lipidsoluble drugs such as theophylline and barbiturates.

Specific treatments
Tricyclic antidepressants

Toxicity from tricyclic antidepressants (TCAs) remains one of the most common causes of serious drug poisoning as well as poisoning death. TCAs produce severe neurological (altered level of consciousness and seizures) and cardiovascular toxicity (atrial and ventricular arrhythmias and myocardial depression). A quinidine-like action resulting in myocardial sodium channel blockade is thought to be the underlying mechanism.

Drug levels are probably not helpful in predicting toxicity; however, ECG changes offer a more useful assessment. QRS width of 0.10–0.15 s correlates with an increased risk for seizures, whereas QRS >0.16 heralds tendency for both seizures and arrhythmias. A QRS width <0.10 does not rule out the possibility of significant toxicity. Also R_{avr} of ≥3 mm is the only ECG variable that significantly predicts adverse outcomes.

There is no specific antidote, and rapid metabolism results in recovery within 24 h. Gastric elimination and AC are effective up to 24 h after ingestion. Bicarbonate therapy is an effective treatment in reducing toxicity, particularly when arrhythmias occur. It alkalinises the blood to pH of 7.5–7.55, thus increasing protein binding of the drugs, resulting in less free drug and lower toxicity. Ventricular arrhythmias usually respond to correction of acidosis and hypoxia. When arrhythmias are resistant to bicarbonate therapy, lidocaine (lignocaine) and phenytoin may help. Magnesium is useful in the presence of torsades de pointes. Beta-blockers should be used with caution. Procainamide is contraindicated as it can worsen the cardiovascular toxicity via its shared class IA-antiarrhythmic properties.

Selective serotonin reuptake inhibitors

These drugs represent a new group of 'cleaner' antidepressants. They are safer in overdose than TCAs or monoamine oxidase inhibitors (MAOIs). Neurological and cardiovascular toxicities rarely occur. Symptoms of overdose include tachycardia, drowsiness, tremor and nausea. Serious toxicity is unlikely, and if present should alert to the possibility of co-ingestants. When selective serotonin reuptake inhibitor (SSRI) overdose patients present to the emergency department, if a careful history and examination and ECGs fail to detect co-ingestion, they should be monitored for a few hours. If no symptoms or signs appear after 1–3 h, they may be discharged from medical observation.

Serotonin syndrome is a potentially serious adverse reaction caused by excessive serotonin availability in the CNS. Drug interactions between SSRIs and other antidepressants [TCAs and monoamine oxidase inhibitors (MAOIs)] are implicated, as well as between one of the antidepressants and other drug classes such as opioid (pethidine and tramadol), pantazocine, lithium, bromocriptine, sympathomimetics (pseudoephedrine and cocaine). Signs and symptoms of serotonin syndrome include neurobehavioural (altered mental state, agitation, confusion and seizures), autonomic (hypothermia, diaphoresis, diarrhoea, salivation, tachycardia and hypertension) and neuromuscular (myoclonus, hyper-reflexia, tremor, muscle rigidity, ataxia and nystagmus). It is important to recognise the syndrome first. Once identified, the treatment becomes simpler, with discontinuation of serotonergic drugs, support care, assisted ventilation if required, temperature control, sedation and muscle relaxation. The use of serotonin receptor antagonists, cyproheptadine or propranolol offers some benefits.

Quetiapine

The second-generation atypical antipsychotic quetiapine is now the most common reason for ICU admission due to coma from drug overdose in Australia. It results in delirium progressing to coma and tachycardia with a prolonged QT interval, progression to Torsades de Pointes does not seem to occur and deaths are likely to be due to respiratory failure and obstruction, emphasizing the need for airway and ventilation management.

Paracetamol

Ingestion of >150 mg kg^{-1} by a child or >7.5 g by an adult is considered toxic. A single dose of 15 g carries great risk of liver damage, but it is possible to get liver toxicity from ingesting recommended doses, especially in the setting of fasting and malnutrition. Paracetamol is metabolised by the liver via glucuronidation and sulphation. Approximately 55% and 30% of paracetamol is normally excreted in urine in the form of glucuronide and sulphate metabolites, respectively. A small fraction is metabolised via the microsomal cytochrome P 450 mixed-function oxidase system to reactive intermediates. N-acetyl-p-benzo-quinone (NAPQI) is the reactive metabolite responsible for the observed hepatotoxicity. At recommended doses, only trace amounts of NAPQI are formed. These are readily inactivated by the endogenous store of glutathione. When a large quantity of paracetamol is ingested, or when the hepatic glutathione store is depleted, excess NAPQI binds covalently to hepatocyte proteins, causing cell death.

In the early phase (<20 h), there are relatively few symptoms apart from some abdominal pain, and nausea and vomiting. In the second phase (>20 h), clinical (pain and tenderness) and biochemical signs of hepatocellular necrosis are present. In the third phase (days 3–4) liver damage is maximal. The recovery phase lasts for 7–8 days. Treatment goals include inhibition of absorption of ingested drugs, removal of absorbed drugs, prevention of conversion of paracetamol into reactive metabolites (NAPQI) and, finally, treatment of hepatic failure and other complications once they occur.

Although gastric lavage, activated charcoal and ipecacuanha are all able to reduce the paracetamol absorption if used within the first 2 h after ingestion, gastric lavage plus activated charcoal does not seem to be superior to activated charcoal alone which has the best risk: benefit ratio, *N*-acetylcysteine (NAC) is an antidote which has demonstrated virtually total protection against hepatotoxicity if given within 8–10 h of paracetamol ingestion. It serves as a sulphur donor to replenish glutathione, and hence prevents accumulation of the toxic metabolite. Initiating NAC later than 8 h after ingestion affords less anti-dotal protection. Also, chronic ethanol abuse or concurrent use of enzyme-inducing medications may increase risk of hepatotoxicity. Delayed NAC therapy (more than 24 h after ingestion) and continuing past 72 h is considered beneficial in patients with hepatotoxicity. Methionine is an oral alternative. Activated charcoal binds acetylcysteine, and hence reduces its effectiveness. NAC is indicated if more than 10 g has been ingested, or if there is doubt about the amount taken or if the paracetamol level (taken at least 4 h after ingestion) is above the hepatotoxic line of the Rumack–Matthew nomogram. NAC may cause urticaria, bronchospasm and anaphylaxis, especially with rapid administration. Liver transplantation has the potential to be life-saving in fulminant hepatic failure.

Aspirin

Absorption may be delayed (enteric formulations) and blood concentrations within 6 h may be misleadingly low. Aspirin toxicity causes hyperventilation, tinnitus, vasodilatation and an initial respiratory alkalosis that progress to metabolic acidosis. Metabolic acidosis, non-cardiac pulmonary oedema and altered level of consciousness are typical of chronic overdose. There is no specific antidote. Gastric emptying may be useful up to 4 h after ingestion. If the plasma salicylate concentration is >350 mg L^{-1} in children or > 500 mg L^{-1} in adults, sodium bicarbonate may enhance urine excretion. Severe overdose (plasma level >700 mg L^{-1}) is an indication for haemodialysis.

Anticholinergic drugs

Atropine and other belladonna alkaloids, antihistamines, phenothiazines and tricyclic antidepressants have anticholinergic activity. This results in hyperthermia, dilated pupils, loss of sweating, delirium, visual hallucination, ataxia, dystonic reactions, seizures, coma, respiratory depression, labile blood pressure, arrhythmias, urinary retention and ileus.

Management comprises resuscitation, GI elimination and supportive care. Physostigmine, an anti-cholinesterase, crosses the blood–brain barrier and may be useful in severe cases but is not widely available.

Amphetamines and ecstasy

These drugs cause sympathomimetic effects, including arrhythmias, hypertension, seizures, coma, hyperthermia, rhabdomyolysis, renal and hepatic failure, intracerebral haemorrhage and infarction and hyponatraemia. There are no specific antidotes but beta-blockers can be used to treat arrhythmias.

Benzodiazepines

Supportive care alone will usually result in a good recovery. The antagonist flumazenil may be used but its short half-life dictates the need for an infusion and it may precipitate seizures, particularly in chronic benzodiazepine users.

Beta-blockers

Beta-blockers will cause bradyarrhythmias, atrioventricular block and hypotension. They may cause an altered mental state, delirium, coma and seizures. Sotalol may cause VT (sometimes torsades de pointes). Bradycardia is treated with atropine. Isoprenaline and cardiac pacing may also be useful in refractory cases. Intravenous glucagon, 3.5–5 mg (or 50–150 µg/kg^{-1}), is used as a β-receptor independent inotrope and chronotrope in refractory bradycardia and hypotension. An infusion of 1–5 mg h^{-1} may be required to maintain chronotropic and inotropic effects of glucagon.

Calcium channel blockers

In overdose, calcium channel blockers will cause hyperglycaemia, nausea and vomiting, coma, seizures, bradycardia, varying degrees of AV block, hypotension and cardiac arrest.

Gastric lavage may precipitate arrhythmias. Hypotension and bradycardia may respond to 10% calcium chloride. Additional calcium (bolus or infusion) is warranted in patients who responded to the initial dose of calcium chloride. Vasopressors (catecholamines) are first-line drugs for patients experiencing circulatory shock. High-dose insulin and glucose infusions have been used successfully in case reports and should be considered in large overdoses.

Digoxin

Nausea, vomiting, drowsiness and confusion are prominent. The ECG may show many types of rhythm and conduction abnormality. Management includes gastric elimination and correction of electrolytes, particularly potassium and magnesium. Digoxin-specific antibody fragments (Fab) are indicated in arrhythmias associated with haemodynamic instability. Ventricular tachyarrhythmias may respond to phenytoin, lidocaine or amiodarone. Atropine may be effective for bradycardia but temporary pacing may be required.

Ethanol

Very high doses of ethanol will cause severe cortical and brain stem depression (coma and hypoventilation) with obvious risk of aspiration of vomit. Depressed gluconeogenesis may cause hypoglycaemia and there may be a high anion gap metabolic acidosis. Management comprises supportive care with airway protection if required, intravenous thiamine and glucose and correction of fluid, electrolyte and acid-base disturbance. Gastric lavage may be effective within 1–2 h of massive ingestion. Haemodialysis is rarely indicated but is effective.

Methanol

The metabolites of methanol (formaldehyde and formic acid) are toxic. The lethal dose is 1–2 mL kg^{-1} or 80 mg dL^{-1}. A latent period of 2–18 h may occur before the onset of a triad of GI symptoms (nausea, vomiting, pain and bleeding), eye signs (blurred, cloudy vision, central scotoma, yellow spots or blindness) and metabolic acidosis. There is an elevated serum osmolality and increased anion gap. Ethanol is a competitive inhibitor for metabolism and is used as an antidote to methanol. Aim to maintain a serum ethanol level at 1 gL^{-1} or 20 mmol L^{-1}. Haemodialysis should be considered with:
- Peak methanol levels >15 mmol L^{-1} (> 50 mg dL^{-1})
- Renal failure
- Visual impairment
- Mental disturbance
- Acidosis not corrected with bicarbonate therapy

Ethylene glycol

Ethylene glycol causes an odourless intoxication with high serum osmolality, severe metabolic acidosis and oxalate crystalluria. It is associated with hyperthermia, hypoglycaemia and hypocalcaemia. Toxicity is due to hepatic metabolites (glycoaldehyde, glycolic acid, glyoxylate and oxalate). Management is as for methanol toxicity.

Opioids

An opioid overdose will cause respiratory depression, pinpoint pupils and coma. Seizures are usually due to hypoxia but can be caused by norpethidine, the neurotoxic metabolite of pethidine. Rhabdomyolysis, endocarditis and pulmonary complications are common. Naloxone is a specific antagonist that can be given i.v. and/or i.m. Its short half-life dictates the need for repeated injections or an infusion. Titration will avoid precipitating withdrawal in habitual users.

Lithium

Polyuria, thirst, vomiting, diarrhoea and agitation are common presentations of lithium overdose. Coma, seizures and nephrogenic diabetes insipidus also occur. Serum lithium levels >1.5 mmol L^{-1} are toxic. Fluid and electrolyte disturbances should be corrected. Consider haemodialysis when concentrations reach 2 mmol L^{-1}.

Organophosphates and carbonates

Toxicity is due to cholinergic overactivity and symptoms appear within 2 h of exposure.

The symptoms can be memorised with the following mnemonics:

- **DUMBELS:** **d**iarrhoea, **u**rination, **m**iosis, **b**ronchospasm, **e**mesis, **l**acrimation and **s**alivation.
- **SLUDGE:** **s**alivation and **s**weating, **l**acrimation, **u**rination, **d**iarrhoea, **g**astrointestinal pain and **e**mesis.

Observe strict isolation and avoid contact exposure. Gastric elimination is appropriate. Atropine is used treat bradycardia and pulmonary secretions. Pralidoxime is a specific reactivator of cholinesterase but is effective only if given within 24 h of exposure. Plasma cholinesterase levels require monitoring until recovery.

Further reading

Brok J, Buckley N, Gluud C. Interventions for paracetamol (acetaminophen) overdose. Cochrane Database Sys Rev 2006:CD003328.

Position statement and practice guidelines on the use of multi-dose activated charcoal in the treatment of acute poisoning. American Academy of Clinical Toxicology; European Association of Poisons Centres and Clinical Toxicologists. J Toxicol Clin Toxicol 1999; 37: 731–751.

Related topics of interest

Echocardiography for critical care

Key points

- Transthoracic and transoesophageal echocardiography are complimentary modalities which will allow the intensive care physician not only to rule out life-threatening causes of shock but also make a full cardiac anatomical assessment
- There is a trend towards focused echocardiography but all studies requested in critical care patients need to be as comprehensive as possible, this should include assessment of all five chambers, the aorta, valves, pleura and pericardium

Assessments

Left ventricular function

This can be assessed on linear, area and volume measurements of the left ventricle (LV).

- Fractional shortening (FS): The proportion that the LV diameter changes during systole. Ejection fraction can be estimated by multiplying the FS by 2. This measurement is a snap shot and will not take into account regional wall motion abnormalities
- Fractional area change (FAC): Area measurements improve the accuracy over linear measurements as more of the left ventricle is represented (see **Table 18**)
- Ejection fraction (EF): This estimates the proportion of diastolic volume that is ejected during ventricular contraction. EF is the most common measure of LV contractility. The volumes are calculated by tracing the shape of the ventricle in both systole and diastole. The machine software assumes each layer of the cross-sectional drawing to be a disc, which therefore builds up to an estimated volume. This is called 'Simpson's biplane method'. The grading of left ventricular systolic function is based on the ejection fraction obtained (**Table 20**).

Preload

- Qualitative estimations can be made by collapsibility of left ventricle cavity
- Quantitative measurements of left ventricular preload can be made by endocardial border tracing at the end of diastole
- Right atrial pressure can be estimated from evaluation of the inferior vena cava during respiration. Increased right atrial pressure causes the inferior vena cava to dilate (>1.5 cm)
- Use of Doppler flow: Pulsed wave Doppler (PW-Doppler) allows the measurement of velocities at the level of the sample volume. Two flow velocity envelopes can be seen during diastole in sinus rhythm: the E-wave, representing the early, passive filling of the left ventricle, and the A-wave, that happens late in diastole, representing the active filling, the atrial contraction

Decreased preload is indicated by:
- Decreased early diastolic filling velocity (mitral E wave) and decreased E/A ratio
- Decreased mitral E wave velocity together with decreased pulmonary flow during systole

Indicators of increased left atrial pressure:
- Normal pulmonary flow pattern with predominant S wave (systolic pulmonary venous flow)

Table 18 Causes of hypotension			
End-diastolic volume	**FAC**	**Aetiology**	
↓	↑ > 0.8	Hypovolaemia	
↑	↓ < 0.2	LV failure	
Normal	↑ > 0.8	Decreased systemic vascular resistance (SVR) severe MR, AR or VSD	

– Dominance of the D wave (diastolic pulmonary venous flow)

Aortic valve velocity variation with respiration of >12% in mechanically ventilated patients may suggest fluid responsiveness.

Regional wall motion abnormality (see Table 19)

- Myocardial damage causes wall motion abnormalities that are present at rest
- Restricted or impaired blood supply may be adequate at rest and only produce a wall motion abnormality on exertion, due to an increase in myocardial oxygen demands
- Other causes of regional wall motion abnormality (RWMA) are myocardial stunning and myocardial hibernation (improves with inotropes whereas dead myocardium does not), tethering, disturbance of regional loading conditions, epicardial pacing and left bundle branch block (LBBB)

Right ventricular function

- The right ventricle (RV) is extremely tolerant of volume loading and extremely *in*tolerant of pressure loading, e.g. high levels of PEEP and increased pulmonary vascular resistance
- The most common causes of RV dysfunction are massive PE and ARDS. However, RV infarction, fat and amniotic emboli and pulmonary contusions will also reduce function
- Ventricular interdependence: The LV and RV interact in that they share a septum. The sum of the diastolic ventricular dimensions has to remain constant. Any acute LV or RV dilatation is associated with a proportional reduction in LV or RV diastolic dimension

- RV function is notoriously difficult to assess by echocardiography. However, the two functional ways of doing this are using Tricuspid Annular Plane Systolic Excursion (TAPSE) and looking at RV free wall movement

TAPSE: This looks at the 'wringing' function of the RV and measures how much the tricuspid valve moves towards the apex during systole. RV free wall movement: the contractile inward movement of the RV free wall.

Valvular dysfunction (see Table 20)

Assessments that need to be made when assessing the various valve abnormalities include:

Aortic stenosis

- Appearance of the valve: identifies bi or tri-leaflet, calcification or thickening and normal motion
- Any secondary effects: ventricular hypertrophy, ventricular dilatation, dilated aortic root and impaired LV function
- Valve area: either by planimetry (tracing open valve orifice) or by applying the continuity equation, LV outflow tract (LVOT)
- Pressure gradient: derived from measuring the velocity across the aortic valve and then applying Bernoulli equation, it is possible to estimate pressure gradients. However, this measure will be inaccurate and thus underestimated in patients with LEFT ventricular impairment

Aortic regurgitation

- Appearance of the valve and the aortic root: Look for mechanism – dilated aortic root, leaflet prolapse, endocarditis and leaflet perforation

Table 19 Regional wall motion abnormality		
Class of motion	**Systolic wall thickening**	**Change in radius during systole**
Normal	Marked	> 30% decrease
Mild hypokinesis	Moderate	10–30% decrease
Severe hypokinesis	Minimal	< 10% decrease
Dyskinesis	None	None
Akinesis	Thinning	Increase

Table 20 British Society of Echocardiography reference values				
	Normal	Mild	Moderate	Severe
Left ventricular size, mass and function				
LV wall thickness (hypertrophy)				
IVSd/PWd (cm)	0.6–1.2	1.3–1.5	1.6–1.9	≥ 2.0
LV dimensions (dilatation), men				
LVIDd (cm)	4.2–5.9	6.0–6.3	6.4–6.8	≥ 6.9
LVIDd/BSA (cm/m^2)	2.2–3.1	3.2–3.4	3.5–3.7	≥ 3.7
LV dimensions (dilatation), women				
LVIDd (cm)	3.9–5.3	5.4–5.7	5.8–6.1	≥ 6.2
LVIDd/BSA (cm/m^2)	2.4–3.2	3.3–3.4	3.5–3.7	≥ 3.8
LV function				
Fractional Shortening (%)	25–43	20–24	15–19	< 15
Ejection fraction (%)	≥ 55	45–54	36–44	≤ 35
Right ventricular function				
Fractional area change (%)	32–60	25–31	18–24	≤ 17
TAPSE	16–20	11–15	6–10	≤ 5
Valvular lesions				
Mitral regurgitation				
Jet area/LA (%)		< 20%		> 40%
Vena contracta (cm)		< 0.3		≥ 0.7
PISA radius (Nyquist 40 cm/s)		< 0.4		> 1.0
Mitral stenosis				
Pressure half time (ms)	40–70	71–139	140–219	> 219
Mean pressure drop (mmHg)		< 5.0	5–10	> 10
Aortic regurgitation				
Jet width/LVOT diameter (%)		< 25		≥ 65
Regurgitant fraction (%)		< 30	31–49	≥ 50
Regurgitant orifice area (cm^2)		< 0.1	0.11–0.29	≥ 0.3
Aortic stenosis				
Peak velocity (m/s)		< 2.9	3.0–3.9	> 4.0
Mean pressure drop (mmHg)		< 25	25–40	> 40
Valve area (cm^2)	> 2.0	1.5–2.0	1.0–1.4	< 1.0

Reproduced with permission from The British Society of Echocardiography.

- Size of the regurgitant jet: Severe aortic regurgitation (AR) jet reaches the mitral inflow
- Diastolic flow reversal in the descending aorta implies severe AR
- Secondary effects: LV dysfunction – the LV should be hyperdynamic and dilated with secondary mitral regurgitation (MR) and pulmonary hypertension. A dilated LV is a sign of chronicity and decompensation
- Acute AR is rare but requires rapid stabilisation and often surgical repair

Mitral stenosis

- Anatomy of the valve: calcification, leaflet restriction (anterior and posterior leaflets

may not be affected equally). Classic 'hockey stick' deformity of rheumatic valves
- Pressure gradient between the left atrium (LA) and LV [using Continuous Wave Doppler (CWD)]
- Secondary effects: dilated LA with 'swirling' blood is associated with low flows (called 'SEC' – spontaneous echo contrast), clot in the LA appendage (only visible on transoesophageal echocardiography) and dilated and dysfunctional RV with raised pulmonary artery pressure

Mitral regurgitation
- What is the mechanism: leaflet prolapse, flail or perforated leaflet, or damaged chordae. It may be one or both leaflets affected
- The degree of regurgitation can be assessed by the size of the regurgitant jet in the LA, the vena contracta (the narrowest point of the neck of the regurgitant jet) and the proximal isovelocity surface area (PISA: the distance from the regurgitant orifice to the first aliasing velocity at a nyquist limit of 40 cm/s)
- Flow reversal during systole in the pulmonary veins implies severe regurgitation
- The severity of mitral regurgitation may be underestimated in patients who are ventilated with high levels of PEEP and ASB

Cardiac output
- Cardiac output can be measured by the continuity equation or by estimating the stroke volume (the machine software can do this by tracing round the LV border during end systole and end diastole – as for Simpson's method) and multiplying this by the heart rate

Clinical conditions

Cardiac tamponade
- Pericardial effusions vary in clinical significance depending on size, site and rate of accumulation. They are common in septic critically ill patients. So the key question is, is there evidence of haemodynamic compromise?

- When the pressure in the pericardium exceeds the pressure in the cardiac chambers, tamponade occurs due to impaired cardiac filling. Tamponade is a clinical diagnosis not an echocardiographic diagnosis, and is more likely with a rapid accumulation of fluid

Classical echocardiographic signs of tamponade include:
- Right atrial inversion or diastolic right ventricular collapse
- Reciprocal changes in right and left ventricular volumes with respiration
- Distended inferior vena cava (caution : IVC dilatation is common in mechanically ventilated patients)
- Respiratory variation in ventricular filling – increased RV filling and decreased LV filling on first beat after inspiration in spontaneously breathing patients. This can be assessed using CWD through the mitral valve with respiratory trace
- Ventricular interdependence: see above under 'right ventricular function'
- Respiratory changes in chambers size: pulsed or CWD across the valves can be used for the assessment of pulsus paradoxus. The maximum velocity of the flow must be measured at the first cardiac cycle after the beginning of expiration and inspiration. Tamponade physiology (=haemodynamic compromise) exists when the difference between the highest and the lowest velocity is more than 25%. It can be assessed from the right heart (tricuspid flow) or from the left heart (mitral or aortic flow)
- When a patient is mechanically ventilated, the pattern of changes observed in pulsus paradoxus is reversed; that is, the systolic BP is higher during inspiration than expiration. The airway pressure and respiratory impedance tracings can be used to demonstrate the inspiratory and expiratory phase of the respiratory cycle. Then BP can be determined with each respiratory phase. The difference in presentation of pulsus paradoxus in patients who are breathing spontaneously and with mandatory mechanical ventilation is an essential principle to be understood

Pulmonary embolus

Echo findings include:

- RV mid-cavity hypokinesia with preserved function at the apex. Wall motion is abnormal in all regions in RV dysfunction of other causes
- Dilated RV with raised pulmonary artery pressures may be seen in acute life threatening PE
- Clot may be visualised in the pulmonary arteries

Systemic embolus

- Embolic source of cerebral ischaemic event or peripheral infarction include cardiac thrombus (is usually attached to an akinetic or dyskinetic segment; colour flow will be disrupted by a true thrombus in a cardiac chamber), vegetations, tumours. Associated atrial septal defect (ASD), patent foramen ovale (PFO), aneurysms and atheromatous aortic disease may be identified

Infective endocarditis

Often requires transoesophageal echocardiogram to confirm or refute diagnosis. Infective endocarditis is a clinical diagnosis. Findings include:

- Oscillating intracardiac mass: on a valve, supporting structure, in path of regurgitant jet or iatrogenic device
- Intra-cardiac abscess are often seen as echolucent pulsatile areas (usually around the infected valve)
- New dehiscence of prosthetic valve: the valve is seen to 'rock' to and fro
- New valvular regurgitation
- Differential diagnoses include: papillary fibroma, ruptured chordae tendinae, valve thickening or calcification, Systemic Lupus Erythematosus (Libman–Sacks), non-bacterial thrombotic endocarditis, abnormalities of prosthetic valves (sewing ring, severed chordae tendinae, fibrin strands or peri-prosthetic material)

Ventilation problems: hypoxaemia

- Identifiable causes that lead to hypoxia include: poor ventricular function, mitral regurgitation, pulmonary embolus or pleural effusions

Aortic dissection

Usually require transoesophageal echocardiogram to confirm diagnosis.

- A 'flap' in the lumen of the aorta. Colour flow mapping may assist in identifying the true and false lumens
- Complications: extension into coronary arteries, presence of pericardial or mediastinal haematoma, aortic valve disruption causing regurgitation and the presence of thrombus. LV function should also be assessed

Further reading

Expert Round Table on Ultrasound in ICU. International expert statement on training standards for critical care ultrasonography. Intensive Care Med 2011; 37:1077–1083.

Related topics of interest

Extracorporeal membrane oxygenation

Key points

- Extracorporeal membrane oxygenation (ECMO) enables the lungs to be rested with a lung-protective ventilation strategy while the underlying disease process is treated
- ECMO is an expensive, complex resource that must be delivered in specialised tertiary referral ICUs
- Consider referral to an ECMO centre in patients who fail to improve despite conventional ventilation, proning and/or oscillation

Definition and description

In extracorporeal membrane oxygenation (ECMO) blood is pumped through an extracorporeal circuit while oxygen flows in a counter-current direction across a permeable membrane. It can be used to effect gas exchange when the lungs are unable to perform this function. The lungs can then be rested with minimal pressures and low F_{IO_2}, allowing time (typically 10–14 days) for them to recover.

Modes of ECMO

ECMO was developed from cardiopulmonary bypass technology and two modes are described: veno-arterial (VA) or veno-venous (VV). VA-ECMO is the older technology, pumping blood from a large vein (typically the femoral) through the oxygenator and returning it into an artery (typically the opposite femoral artery). VV-ECMO instead returns the oxygenated blood to a vein, either the femoral or the internal jugular vein. Modern ECMO cannulae have two lumens and sit in the vena cava, allowing a single cannula to provide flow both to and from the circuit, and directing the flow of oxygenated blood into the right atrium.

VA-ECMO is traditionally associated with cardiac surgery and carries the risks of arterial puncture and intimal damage, along with distal embolic phenomena. It preferentially oxygenates the lower limbs, and the upper body and brain may not receive significantly improved oxygenation. However, the extra flow from the ECMO circuit (typically around 100 mL/kg/min) can help support the cardiac output in the face of a failing left ventricle.

VV-ECMO circuits have the potential to recirculate oxygenated blood between the inflow and outflow limbs of the circuit, although this risk is lessened with an appropriately sized cannula well-positioned in the vena cava. The flow of oxygenated blood through the lungs can affect hypoxic pulmonary vasoconstriction and lead to the lungs excreting oxygen, causing the P_{aO_2} to be lower than the partial pressure of oxygen in the returned venous blood.

The ECMO Circuit

The ECMO circuit comprises a pump, heater, membrane oxygenator and venous reservoir. Connections into the circuit allow infusion of fluids and heparin anticoagulation. Modern ECMO systems use heparin-impregnated circuits to reduce the degree of systemic anticoagulation required.

Practicalities

Indications

Patients with a reversible cause of respiratory failure should be considered for ECMO if they have severe hypoxaemia (P_{aO_2}/F_{IO_2} ratio < 13.3 kPa), severe hypercapnic acidosis (pH <7.20), failure to improve with high-frequency oscillatory ventilation or with poor lung compliance that does not allow ventilation using lung-protective ventilation strategies (<6–8 mL/kg tidal volume, peak airway pressures <30 cmH$_2$O, F_{IO_2} <0.5). Alternatively, a Murray score (see **Table 21**) of 3 or more should prompt discussion with a specialist centre.

Table 21 Murray score					
	0	1	2	3	4
Pao$_2$:Fio$_2$ ratio (kPa)	≥40	30–39.9	23.3–29.9	13.3–23.2	<13.3
PEEP (cmH$_2$O)	≤5	6–8	9–11	11–14	≥15
Compliance (mL/cmH$_2$O)	≥80	60–79	40–59	20–39	≤19
CXR quadrants infiltrated	0	1	2	3	4

Contraindications

Contraindications to full anticoagulation (e.g. intracranial haemorrhage) preclude consideration for ECMO. ECMO does not reverse lung damage and patients who have been ventilated with high pressures (>30 cmH$_2$O) or Fio$_2$ >0.8 for more than seven days have very little chance of recovery and should not be considered.

Complications

The complications of ECMO are largely related to the requirement for anticoagulation (gastrointestinal bleeding, intracranial bleeding and heparin-induced thrombocytopenia) and large-bore cannulation (pneumothorax, embolic phenomena, vascular disruption and infection). There is also the possibility of exsanguination due to circuit disconnection. Failure of the oxygenator or of the pumping system will lead to a failure of oxygenation and rapid decline and death in a patient dependent on ECMO. For these reasons ECMO patients need very high nurse:patient ratios (usually 2:1) including a dedicated, specially trained ECMO nurse in addition to the usual ICU nursing staff.

Evidence supporting the use of ECMO

Early studies of ECMO were complicated by methodological and ethical concerns, such that in most cases patients in the conventional therapy arms were allowed to cross over into the ECMO arm for 'rescue therapy' if they failed to improve. ECMO was also not considered as a treatment option until patients had undergone long periods of conventional therapy and had high predicted mortality (>90%). ECMO gained acceptance in neonatal and paediatric intensive care settings while remaining an experimental and unproven therapy in adults.

The CESAR trial was the first modern ECMO trial and compared ECMO to conventional ventilation in adults, using death or serious neurological disability at 6 months as its primary outcome. Adults aged 18–65 years with a reversible cause of respiratory failure and a Murray score >3 or pH <7.2 were randomised to ECMO or conventional management. Those who had been ventilated at pressures >30 cmH$_2$O or Fio$_2$ >0.8 for >7 days were excluded. One hundred and eighty patients were enrolled, and of the 90 patients in the ECMO group 5 died before or during transfer to the ECMO centre and 16 improved without the need for ECMO after transfer. Analysis on an intention-to-treat basis showed a significant reduction in death or serious disability in the ECMO arm [37% vs. 53%, RR 0.69 (95% CI 0.05–0.97)], although the ECMO patients had a longer hospital stay and higher costs.

In an analysis of outcomes in patients referred to ECMO centres during the 2009–10 influenza A(H1N1) outbreak in the UK, patients who were transferred to an ECMO centre were matched with patients with similar disease severity who were not transferred. Survival to hospital discharge was significantly increased in the ECMO group [hospital mortality 24.0% vs. 46.7% for propensity matched pairs (RR 0.51, 95% CI 0.31–0.84)] although only 86% of the patients transferred to the ECMO centres actually underwent ECMO.

The use of modern ECMO circuits, lower levels of anticoagulation and the ability to set up mobile ECMO prior to transferring patients are some of the reasons why these papers have shown better results than earlier studies. Despite criticism of these studies, ECMO has become widely accepted as a beneficial intervention in selected patients, and it is unlikely that further randomised controlled trials would now be feasible due to ethical objections to withholding ECMO in the conventional treatment arm.

Extracorporeal carbon dioxide removal

Correcting respiratory acidosis permits lung-protective ventilation strategies despite severe impairment of gas exchange, thereby reducing ventilator-induced lung injury. Carbon dioxide is much more soluble than oxygen so the blood flows required to normalise the $Pa\text{co}_2$ are lower than those required for oxygenation (typically around 0.5–1.0 L/min). Arterio-venous systems use the patient's own blood pressure to perfuse the circuit without the use of a pump. However, they have been criticised for causing high rates of arterial damage and making patient mobilisation difficult, leading to the development of newer, veno-venous systems using a modified ECMO circuit including a pump. Although these systems may produce a degree of improvement in oxygenation they do not approach the flow rates required for full ECMO.

Further reading

Combes A, Bacchetta M, Brodie D et al. Extracorporeal membrane oxygenation for respiratory failure in adults. Curr Opin Crit Care 2012; 18:99–104.

Noah M, Peek G, Finney SJ, et al. Referral to an extracorporeal membrane oxygenation center and mortality among patients with severe 2009 influenza A(H1N1). JAMA 2011; 306:1659–1668.

Peek GJ, Mugford M, Tiruvoipati R, et al. Efficacy and economic assessment of conventional ventilatory support versus extracorporeal membrane oxygenation for severe adult respiratory failure (CESAR): a multicentre randomised controlled trial. Lancet 2009; 374:1351–1363.

Related topics of interest

Endocarditis

Key points

- Infective endocarditis is associated with significant morbidity and mortality, and is increasingly the result of nosocomial infections
- Prolonged antibiotic therapy, and surgery in selected patients, are the main treatments
- Prophylaxis is limited to dental treatment in high-risk patients

Epidemiology

Infective endocarditis (IE) results in the formation of infective vegetations on the endocardium. The cardiac valves are most commonly involved but other areas of endocardium may also be affected, e.g. ventricular septal defect, atrial septal defect (ASD) and coarctation.

In developing countries rheumatic heart disease remains the major risk factor for IE. In developed countries increasing age with associated degenerative heart disease, and use of cardiac and intravascular devices are major risk factors. Other risk factors include intravenous drug use, HIV, diabetes, prosthetic valves, structural heart disease and a previous history of IE.

Causative organisms

Staphylococcus aureus is the most common organism overall; other organisms are shown in **Table 22**.

Endocarditis occurs in one of two groups of patients: native valve endocarditis and prosthetic valve endocarditis.

Native valve endocarditis

The frequency of causative organisms by age group is given in **Table 22**.

- *Streptococcus bovis* is frequently associated with malignancy.
- HACEK organisms (*Haemophilus parainfluenzae, Haemophilus aphrophilus, Actinobacillus actinomycetemcomitans, Cardiobacterium hominis, Eikenella corrodens* and *Kingella kingae*) account for 2% of all native valve endocarditis patients.
- Rare: *Rickettsia* (Q fever), *Brucella, Mycoplasma, Legionella* and *Histoplasma*.

In intravenous drug users fungi infections account for 5% of IE.

1% of patients will have more than one organism.

8% of patients remain culture negative.

Prosthetic valve endocarditis

Early (within 60 days):
- *Staphylococcus aureus* (35%)
- Coagulase-negative staphylococci (17%)
- Enterocci (5–10%)
- Gram-negative organisms (10–15%)
- Fungi (5–10%)

Late onset (after 60 days):
- *Staphylococcus aureus* (18%)
- Coagulase-negative staphylococci (20%)
- Streptococci (7–10%)
- Enterococci (10–15%)
- Gram-negative organisms (2–4%)

There is an increased incidence of resistant organisms causing IE.

Table 22 Organisms causing native valve endocarditis: frequency within different age groups				
Organism	Neonate	2 months to 15 years	16–60 years	>60 years
Streptococcus spp.	20%	45%	50%	35%
Staphylococcus aureus	45%	22%	35%	25%
Coagulase-negative *Staphylococcus*	10%	5%	6%	4%
Enterococcus	<1%	5%	6%	15%
Gram-negative bacilli	10%	2%	2%	2%

Pathophysiology

Infective endocarditis most commonly involves the left side of the heart, with the mitral valve most commonly affected. Drug addicts often have right-sided involvement, most commonly of the tricuspid valve. Vegetations consisting of fibrin, platelets and infecting organisms form in areas with endothelial disruption and high velocity and abnormal blood flow. Prosthetic valve endocarditis accounts for 7–25% of all cases. There is no difference in incidence between mechanical and bio prosthetic valves, although mechanical valves have a greater risk of early infection.

Nosocomial IE accounts for 7–29% of all cases of endocarditis in tertiary hospitals. At least 50% are a result of infected intravascular devices.

Clinical features

Low-virulence organisms such as *Streptococcus viridans* tend to have insidious clinical courses. Virulent organisms such as *Staphylococcus aureus* and fungi cause more dramatic presentations. Fever is present in up to 90% of patients, and new murmurs or changing murmurs are detected in 48% and 20% of cases, respectively. Myalgia, arthralgia, fatigue, anorexia and anaemia are common presenting features. In patients with a prosthetic valve, an unexplained fever should lead to a search for endocarditis. Embolic phenomena are common, especially if vegetations are larger than 10 mm. Splenomegaly (40%) and clubbing are both late signs. Neurological signs occur in 20–40% due to embolism and haemorrhage from mycotic aneurysms. Heart failure due to fulminant valvular regurgitation and cardiac conduction abnormalities also occurs.

Immune complex deposition causes vasculitis, splinter haemorrhages, Osler's nodes in the finger pulp, Roth spots in the retina and microscopic hematuria (due to either proliferative glomerulonephritis or focal embolic glomerulonephritis) may be present. In severe cases, shock and multi-organ failure are features.

Nosocomial endocarditis has an acute onset and classic signs are often absent. A persistent bacteraemia before treatment, or for >72 h after removal of an infected intevenous cannula, device, should raise suspicion of endocarditis.

Investigations

- Blood count may show neutrophilia and anaemia.
- Urinalysis for haematuria and casts.
- Blood cultures – at least three from different sites 1 h apart and before antibiotics are given. Cultures are positive in up to 90% of patients. Culture may be negative because of prior antibiotic exposure, fastidious organisms, e.g. *Coxiella burnetii* (Q fever), fungi, anaerobes, right-sided endocarditis or non-IE, e.g. Libman-Sacks disease in SLE or marantic endocarditis (non-thrombotic endocarditis usually seen in patients with terminal malignant disease). In patients with confirmed endocarditis or a high probability of endocarditis with negative cultures, consider further tests such as lysis centrifugation and special enriched growth mediums looking for fastidious organisms.
- Transthoracic echocardiography detects vegetations larger than 2–3 mm (**Figure 7**) and in appropriate patients is the first-line technique. Transoesophageal echocardiography (TOE) is more sensitive. Most experts would use a TOE in patients with prosthetic heart valves, if transthoracic echocardiography is technically difficult, or if the probability of endocarditis is high. Patients should all have Doppler studies.

Diagnosis

1. **Definite infective endocarditis**
   a. Pathological criteria
   - Micro-organisms on culture or histology in a vegetation (local or embolic) or in an intracardiac abscess.
   - Pathological lesions on histology confirming endocarditis.

b. Clinical diagnosis based on major and minor criteria
- 2 major criteria, or
- major and 3 minor criteria, or
- 5 minor criteria.
2. **Possible infective endocarditis.** Clinical findings fall short of a definite diagnosis, but endocarditis is not rejected.
3. **Rejected.** Firm alternative diagnosis, or resolution of clinical manifestations with 4 days or less of antibiotics, or no evidence of endocarditis at autopsy or surgery.
4. **Definitions**
   a. Major criteria
   Positive blood culture with typical micro-organism for IE from:
   - Blood cultures more than 12 h apart, or
   - All three or a majority of four or more blood cultures with first and last at least 1 h apart, or
   - Micro-organisms consistent with endocarditis isolated from persistently positive blood cultures, or
   - Single positive blood culture for *Coxiella burnetii.*
   Evidence of endocardial involvement – positive echocardiogram for endocarditis (a TOE is recommended for patients with a prosthetic valve):
   - Oscillating intracardiac mass on a valve or supporting structures, in the path of regurgitant jets or on implanted material in the absence of an alternative explanation.
   - Abscess.
   - New partial dehiscence of prosthetic valve or new valvular regurgitation.
   b. Minor criteria
   - Predisposing heart lesion or i.v. drug use.
   - Fever > 38.0 °C.
   - Vascular phenomena.
   - Immunological phenomena: e.g. glomerulonephritis, Osler's nodes, rheumatoid factor, Roth spots
   - Microbiological evidence: positive blood cultures not meeting major criteria or serological evidence of active infection with organisms consistent with IE.
   - Echocardiogram consistent with endocarditis but not meeting major criteria.

Treatment

General resuscitative management following the ABC priorities.

Aggressive antimicrobial therapy particularly covering resistant organisms if they are suspected.

Repeated assessment for worsening valvular function, heart failure, abscess formation and embolicphenomena (especially cerebral).

Cardiac surgery is indicated for acute valvular regurgitation or stenosis leading to heart failure, acute aortic or mitral regurgitation with early closure of the mitral valve, myocardial abscess or fistula, fungal endocarditis, valve dysfunction and persistent infection despite 7–10 days of appropriate therapy, high risk of emboli (vegetations >10 mm) and persistent positive blood cultures despite treatment.

Surgery for prosthetic valve endocarditis may be needed for early infection, heart failure with prosthetic valve dysfunction, fungal infection, staphylococcal infection not responding to antibiotics, perivalvular leak or abscess formation, infection with Gram negative organisms and persistent bacteraemia after 7–10 days of appropriate antibiotics.

There is no role for routine anticoagulation.

Principles of antimicrobial therapy:
Antimicrobial therapy is started only after blood cultures are performed.
- Empirical therapy is commenced and then modified depending on organisms isolated from blood cultures. Rifampicin is added if prosthetic valve endocarditis is suspected.
- Prolonged treatment is required (4–6 weeks) because the high density of micro-organisms protected in vegetations is associated with a high relapse rate.
- A persistent fever may reflect ineffective treatment, abscess formation, septic emboli or antibiotic fever.

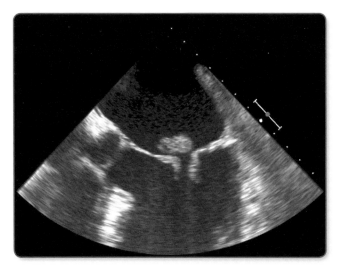

Figure 7 Echocardiogram from the same patient demonstrating a large mitral valve vegetation, managed by mitral valve replacement and antibiotics.

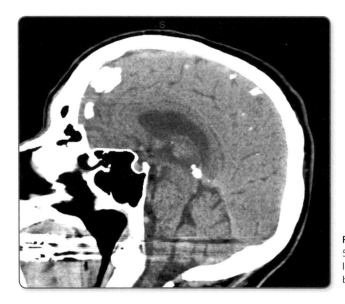

Figure 8 Sagittal CT scan of 56 years male showing multiple leptomeningeal lesions, open biopsy grew *Streptococcus mitis*

Complications

Complications include septic emboli (**Figure 8**), secondary haemorrhage, multi-organ failure, valve rupture or regurgitation resulting in cardiogenic shock, valve obstruction and abscess formation. Streptococcal and tricuspid endocarditis carries a 10% mortality. The prognosis is poor (>20% mortality) in non-streptococcal disease, severe heart failure, aortic and prosthetic valve involvement, age > 65, diabetic patients, valve ring or myocardial abscess and large vegetations. Death is usually due to heart failure and embolic events, in particular cerebral mycotic aneurysmal bleeds. Prognosis is worst (60% mortality) in early prosthetic valve endocarditis. Recurrent or second episodes are seen in 6% of patients.

Prophylaxis

Prophylaxis is reserved for patients undergoing dental procedures who are at high risk of IE, e.g. prosthetic valve, congenital heart disease or in patients who have had previous IE.

Further reading

Hoen B, Duval X. Clinical practice. Infective endocarditis. N Engl J Med 2013; 368:1425–1433.

Thuny F, Grisoli D, Collart F, Habib G, Raoult D. Management of infective endocarditis: challenges and perspectives. Lancet 2012; 379:965–975.

Murdoch DR, Corey GR, Hoen B, et al. Clinical presentation, etiology, and outcome of infective endocarditis in the 21st century: the International Collaboration on Endocarditis-Prospective Cohort Study. Arch Intern Med 2009; 169:463–473.

Habib G, Hoen B, Tornos P, et al. Guidelines on the prevention, diagnosis, and treatment of infective endocarditis (new version 2009): the Task Force on the Prevention, Diagnosis, and Treatment of Infective Endocarditis of the European Society of Cardiology (ESC). Endorsed by the European Society of Clinical Microbiology and Infectious Diseases (ESCMID) and the International Society of Chemotherapy (ISC) for Infection and Cancer. Eur Heart J 2009; 30:2369–2413.

Related topics of interest

- Cardiac failure – acute (p 80)
- Cardiac valve disease (p 97)
- Sepsis – management (p 329)

End-of-life care

Key points

- Studies on end-of-life care in the ICU have identified shortcomings; including poor pain control, frequent aggressive treatments, late discussion and documentation of 'Do Not Attempt Resuscitation' orders, patient and proxy dissatisfaction with communication and lack of acknowledgement of patient treatment preferences
- Wide variations in the practice and patterns of end-of-life care have been noted within different cultures
- Deficiencies can be improved by establishing a standard of care for the dying patient in the ICU that addresses issues relating to decision making, communication, family support, symptom control and terminal care

Decision making

The decision to make the transition from curative to palliative care is not always an easy one and is influenced by several factors:

Patient autonomy versus paternalism

Informed patients with decision making capacity can choose to accept or refuse therapies; however, problems may arise when they are unable to make decisions due to illness or sedation, of which less than 5% of patients in ICU maintain capacity. In these cases, patients may have designated a specific individual to act for them. When no individual has been designated, it may sometimes be appropriate to appoint a legal guardian. (See Consent Topic). A consensus of Critical Care Societies encourages a 'shared decision-making' approach with patient, family and physicians contributing to decisions.

Conflict arises when doctors and patients (or their surrogates) have opposing views on what constitutes futile treatment. In these instances, patients (or their surrogates) should determine what the wishes of the patient are/would be and physicians should provide information about the patient's prognosis and what can or cannot be achieved by specific therapies. Where agreement is not possible, physicians are not obliged to provide or continue therapies that they believe to be futile. However, every effort should be made to resolve any conflict and disagreement, which may require the involvement of a mediator or legal services.

Communication

Patients and their caregivers must be adequately informed of their options to help them choose their treatments, set their priorities and prepare for death. Clinicians must impart information in a way that best assists them to do so and in a manner sensitive to their cultural and spiritual needs. Time must be made to discuss and identify the patient's wishes and values and sufficient time must also be given for important decisions to be reached. There is increasing evidence regarding the importance of communication skills for caregiver outcomes, including reduced psychological morbidity. In light of this, guidelines for communicating prognosis and end-of-life issues are now being systematically reviewed and developed.

Family support

In their definition of palliative care, the World Health Organization stresses the holistic nature of treatment and the importance of achieving the best quality of life for families as well as patients. The needs of the family have been assessed by a number of studies and include:

- Information to clarify the dying patient's condition, treatment and prognosis
- Discussions on expectations and preferences for treatment and decision making
- Assurance that the patient is comfortable
- Psychosocial support
- Physical support such as nutrition and sleep
- Lenient visitation rights and privacy
- Opportunity to say goodbye
- Bereavement support

Cultural and spiritual differences

The cultural and spiritual values of patients and families may have an impact on treatment choices.

In some countries, laws on advanced care directives or DNAR orders do not exist and withdrawal of therapies is not readily discussed. It has also been observed that a physician's age and gender, experience with dying, religion, country of work and speciality may influence end-of-life decision making.

Spirituality, which is not synonymous with religion, plays a role in how patients and their caregivers make choices and cope with death. Each patient's understanding of spirituality should therefore be explored. Intensive care staff should also be aware of cultural differences in grieving and bereavement and consider involvement of relevant counsellors or clergy and accommodate for end-of-life customs and rituals as best as possible.

Withdrawing life support

Withdrawing ventilator support varies from terminal extubation to leaving the tracheal tube in place while weaning from ventilation. There is no evidence to recommend the use of one method over the other and clinicians should work with the team and caregivers in making this decision for individual cases. Non-invasive ventilation may be used as a palliative measure for dyspnoea. It should be stopped when it is no longer effective in symptom control and the dyspnoea has been relieved by other methods.

Withdrawal should always proceed with comfort measures in place and plans in place to address distress, pain, anxiety and delirium if they occur.

Symptom control

Pain

Pain can be assessed with good history taking and pain scales. In the case of the incapacitated patient, motor activity (grimacing and agitation) and haemodynamic signs (tachycardia and hypertension) in association with autonomic signs (diaphoresis and lacrimation) could be indicators of pain. Examples of pain scales include the Behavioural Pain Scale and the Pain Assessment Behaviour Scale.

Pain in the ICU is often related to procedures and interventions and minimising these sources should be part of the management plan.

Morphine is the standard drug of choice due to its familiarity, efficacy and cost. It can be given by oral, intravenous, subcutaneous, epidural, intrathecal and intracerebroventricular routes. The half life of 2–3 h after intravenous administration will be prolonged in renal failure. In terminal care, it is most commonly given by continuous infusion. Alternatively fentanyl is a potent synthetic opioid which can be given by intravenous, intramuscular, subcutaneous, epidural, intrathecal, sublingual and transdermal routes. It has a half life of 30–60 min after an intravenous dose and should be administered by continuous infusion in this setting. It is metabolised by the liver and is therefore potentially useful for patients with renal failure. It causes less histamine release and has a lower incidence of hypotension than morphine. Hydromorphone is a semi synthetic opioid structurally similar to morphine. Its higher solubility enables large doses to be administered in low volumes of solution.

Dyspnoea

Signs of respiratory distress in mechanically ventilated patients include tachypnoea, tachycardia, fearful facial expression, accessory muscle use, diaphragmatic breathing and nasal flaring.

There is little data to support specific treatment approaches for dyspnoea in the terminal setting. Treatment should be individualised and aimed at removing the cause of dyspnoea. If this is not possible, the perception of dyspnoea should be altered.

Oxygen may relieve dyspnoea by relieving hypoxaemia. Its efficacy in dyspnoeic non-hypoxaemic patients is currently being evaluated.

Opioids are the drugs of choice to relieve dyspnoea. Their effects are postulated to be secondary to effects on ventilatory response to CO_2, decreased O_2 consumption, hypoxia and inspiratory flow loading.

Delirium

Delirium is common among ICU patients who are dying. In up to 50% of cases, no cause will be found and when one is found it is often irreversible.

Pain or dyspnoea may contribute to delirium and treatments for these should be optimised before using antipsychotics and sedatives. Non-pharmacological management includes removing restraints, promoting sleep, dimming lights, reducing noise and encouraging family or caregiver involvement.

Haloperidol is the neuroleptic agent of choice and has proven efficacy in managing agitated delirium. It can be given orally, subcutaneously, intramuscularly and intravenously.

Midazolam can be used in conjunction with haloperidol in agitated delirium and can be given as a continuous intravenous, subcutaneous infusion or as PRN boluses. It is highly lipophilic and has a rapid onset of effect, with response within 5–10 min of intravenous administration. It has no specific effects on delirium but its benefit derives from its sedative, hypnotic and amnesic effects.

Propofol, which is widely used in the ICU for sedation may be used but may cause pain on administration.

For the rare patient who does not settle with the above medications, other treatment options include barbiturates, chlorpromazine and levomepromazine.

Death rattles

Swallowing difficulties, infection and general debility cause secretions to accumulate in the oropharynx and airways. In the terminal setting, noisy breathing can be very distressing for the family and staff. Cessation of parenteral fluids and treatment with anticholinergic agents, such as hyoscine hydrobromide or glycopyrrolate, may be effective. Families should also be reassured that noisy and agonal breathing is part of the normal dying process rather than signs of discomfort.

Terminal care

During the terminal phase, interventions which do not add to comfort should be stopped. These interventions include monitoring, alarms, unnecessary medications, antibiotics, blood products, hydration and cardiovascular support. The environment should also be altered to ensure peace and privacy.

Other considerations at the time of death include notification of death to caregivers and other relevant medical teams, potential organ donation and bereavement support for families. Equally important is self care for clinicians by way of debriefing sessions and access to spiritual and psychosocial resources.

Further reading

Prendergast TJ, Luce JM. Increasing incidence of withholding and withdrawal of life support from the critically ill. Am J Respir Crit Care Med 1997; 155:15–20.

Carlet J, Thijs LG, Antonelli M, et al. Challenges in end-of-life care in the ICU Statement of the 5th International Consensus Conference in Critical Care: Brussels, Belgium, April 2003. Intensive Care Med 2004; 30:770–784.

Miccinesi G, Fischer S, Paci E, et al. Physicians' attitudes towards end-of-life decisions: a comparison between seven countries. Soc Sci Med 2005; 60:1961–1974.

A controlled trial to improve care for seriously ill hospitalized patients. The study to understand prognoses and preferences for outcomes and risks of treatments (SUPPORT). The SUPPORT Principal Investigators. JAMA 1995; 274:1591–1598.

Truog RD, Campbell ML, Curtis JR, et al. Recommendations for end-of-life care in the intensive care unit: A consensus statement by the American College of Critical Care Medicine. Crit Care Med 2008; 36:953–963.

Lanken PN, Terry PB, DeLisser HM, et al. An Official American Thoracic Society Clinical Policy Statement: Palliative Care for Patients with Respiratory Diseases and Critical Illnesses. Am J Respir Crit Care Med 2008; 177:912–927.

Clayton JM, Hancock KM, Butow PN, et al. Clinical practice guidelines for communicating prognosis and end-of-life issues with adults in the advanced stages of a life-limiting illness, and their caregivers. Med J Aust 2007; 186:S77–108.

New South Wales Ministry of Health. End-of-life care and decision-making – guidelines. Sydney; Ministry of Health, 2005.

Related topics of interest

• Analgesia in critical care – advanced (p 28)

• Sedation (p 319)

Ethics

Key points

Biomedical ethics is based on four key principles:
- Respect for autonomy and the right to self-determination
- Non-maleficence
- Beneficence
- Justice

Basic principles

The area of ethics concerned with medical practice is termed biomedical ethics. In 1978, Beauchamp and Childress described its four key principles (**Table 23**).

Particular challenges arise in critical care. Most patients are sedated, unconscious or lack capacity, resources are limited and end of life decision making is common.

Withholding and withdrawing treatment

The difference between withholding and withdrawing treatment is based on the distinction between omission and commission. Ethically, the distinction is unclear and both can be considered justifiable depending on the circumstances. To withhold or withdraw care in those who are benefiting from it would be unethical. Equally the initiation and prolongation of improper treatment where there is no benefit would also be unethical. The limiting of life sustaining treatment in European critical care units is common. In the 2003, Ethicus study 72.6% of patients who died had limitations of treatment (10% of all ITU admissions). Perhaps more importantly Rocker et al. (2004) described that in Canada most patients were perceived by family members to die in comfort during withdrawal of life support. When life support was withdrawn it was most commonly via the withdrawal of mechanical ventilation.

It is sensible that medical resources, especially scarce resources, should be distributed only to those who have a reasonable chance of benefit. To distribute resources to those with a negligible chance of success would be wasteful and may deny others more likely to succeed the opportunity of that benefit. In view of this, care should not be initiated or continued where the prospect of success is futile.

In cases where doubt exists regarding suitability for critical care or in emergency situations where important information is lacking, a pragmatic approach is required. In these cases, a tendency towards initiating critical care treatment is preferable. In using this approach, the balance between the risk of under-treating those who may benefit from critical care can be avoided. In those who continuation of care is felt to be futile care can be withdrawn in a caring and companionate way.

Rationing

Per patient, critical care costs on average six times more per day than a non-critically ill patient on the ward (Edbrooke et al). Costs are increased due to high staff to patient ratios, intensive monitoring and expensive drugs and equipment. Rationing of beds varies between countries. When faced with an overcapacity unit, it may be necessary to undertake transfers for non-clinical reasons, in order to create bed capacity. This requires a balance between an individual's right for

---

Table 23 Key principles of biomedical ethics
• **Respect for autonomy** – The respect and support of autonomous decisions.
• **Nonmalaficence** – Avoiding the causation of harm.
• **Beneficence** – Relieving, lessening or preventing harm.
• **Justice** – The fair distribution of benefits, risks and costs.

autonomy against the broader need for justice and the fair allocation of limited resources.

Chance and queuing: A 'first come, first served' system requires that those already receiving treatment take priority over those who present later. It may be that a sick unstable patient presents to the emergency department requiring critical care, when no beds are available. In such circumstances, this patient could be transferred to another intensive care unit by weighing the greater risk of this transfer against the fact that there is no capacity available to treat them. Conversely, an existing but stable critical care patient could be transferred to another unit to create a bed space. In this case, the stable patient would be taking on the risk of transfer (albeit probably a risk of lower magnitude) but on behalf of another patient. This argument weighs the loss of autonomy of the stable patient against the justice and fair allocation towards the sicker patient who has a more urgent need.

Triage: The delivery of care during disasters and major incidents may necessitate an extreme form of rationing. Resources may be inadequate to care for all injured and in these cases rationing may occur based on prospect of success. As a result of the 2009, H1N1 influenza pandemic the United Kingdom Department of Health produced guidelines on the ethical principles for pandemic preparedness. This recognised that governments, organisations and individuals might face difficult decisions and choices that may impact on the freedom, health and in some cases prospects of survival of individuals. Clinicians were not expected to make decisions alone but to be guided by the Department of Health, local approaches to triage and the use of shared decision-making. Use of the sequential organ failure assessment scoring system as a possible strategy to identify those who were most benefiting from treatment was considered as a triage system. This was never required as local and regional surge capacity plans coped with the demands on critical care at that time.

Organ donation

Currently three people die every day in the UK whilst waiting for an organ donation. This puts considerable pressure on health organizations and clinicians to maximise organ donation. Whilst donation after cardiac death has been on-going since the 1960s donation after brainstem death was only made possible following the consensus definition of brainstem death testing in 1976. There are two guiding principles behind the work of the UK Donation Ethics Committee.

1. The offer of organ donation should be a routine part of the planning of end of life care.
2. That once it has been agreed that organ donation is in the patient's best interests, the ethical imperative is to enable the most successful outcome of that donation.

Controversies exist around the form of consent for donation (opt in or opt out systems) and the ethics of admitting patients to intensive care purely to facilitate organ donation.

Many countries such as England use an organ donor register, to identify a patient's individual wishes and also then require assent from relatives. Others such as Wales are moving to introduce a system of presumed consent. This is akin to an opt-out system whereby patients are assumed to want to donate their organs unless they previously registered an objection or family members decline on their behalf. Proponents argue that presumed consent would increase organ donation numbers while objectors feel it has the potential to undermine the concept of donation as a gift.

Delaying withdrawal of care for the purpose of facilitating organ donation is considered to be in the best interest of someone who wanted to be a donor, if it facilitates donation and does not cause them harm or distress. Equally delaying the withdrawal of treatment and changing a patient's location may be considered in the best interests of a person who wanted to be a donor if this facilitates donation. Guidance is provided by the UK Donation Ethics Committee 2011.

Informed consent for research

Most critical care patients are sedated, unconscious or lack capacity. This prevents the ability to obtain informed consent to enter research studies. In most Western countries when a patient is declared, incompetent 'assent' is obtained from a surrogate. Here, the surrogate assumes the patients choice from previous knowledge of the patient to choose what they would have chosen themselves. The surrogate may not be the closest relative or even a relative at all. When the patient regains capacity they can then give or decline consent.

In emergency situations where time constrains prevent informed consent from being obtained research may be conducted without consent from patients or a surrogate. In these cases, research must be planned in advanced, be approved by an ethics committee and involve minimal risk to the patient. Consent from the patient or surrogate at the earliest possible opportunity is needed to continue in the study.

Dealing with difficult decisions

When ethical dilemmas occur, decisions regarding care should be shared amongst clinicians. This can alleviate the stress on individuals of making difficult decisions. Regular multidisciplinary team meetings provide a forum to discuss issues and share viewpoints.

Where guidance from governing bodies or legal frameworks exists these should be followed. Failure to do so without very good reason would undoubtedly be looked upon unfavourably by the courts. In the rare situation that guidance is unclear or when clinicians, families or patients are in dispute, ethical and legal advice can be sought. This can be obtained from hospital lawyers, medical defence unions, governing bodies or in extreme cases from the courts.

Further reading

Beauchamp T, Childress J. Principles of Biomedical Ethics, 6th edn. Oxford University Press, 2009.

Luce JM, White DB. A History of ethics and Law in the intensive care Unit. Critical Care Clinician 2009; 25: 221–237.

Academy of Medical Royal Colleges, UK Donation Ethics Committee (UKDEC). An ethical framework for controlled donation after circulatory death. London; Academy of Medical Royal Colleges, UKDEC, 2011.

General Medical Council (GMC). Good practice in research and consent to research. London; GMC, 2014.

Related topics of interest

Fibreoptic bronchoscopy

Key points

- Fibreoptic bronchoscopy is used for diagnosis and treatment
- Bronchoalveolar lavage enables samples to be obtained from the distal airways
- Bronchoscopic aspiration of mucous plugs may enable re-inflation of a collapsed lobe
- Use of bronchoscope during percutaneous dilatational tracheostomy reduces the risk of misplacing the tracheostomy tube

Diagnostic uses

Fibreoptic bronchoscopy enables the direct inspection and instrumentation of the upper and lower airway. Its versatility and portability enable the technique to be performed at the bedside within the critical care unit and it is increasingly used in the management of critically ill patients.

Diagnostic indications

1. Diagnosis of pneumonia. Successful treatment of pneumonia depends on correct antimicrobial coverage against the causative organism. Bronchoscopy enables samples to be obtained directly from the lower respiratory tract, minimising contamination from the colonised upper airway. Microbiological analysis of these samples enables the identification of the infectious agent and the prescription of the appropriate treatment. It is particularly useful in immunocompromised patients with pulmonary infiltrates as it has a high diagnostic yield, especially in the identification of *Pneumocystis jirovecci*, mycobacteria and fungi. Two main techniques are used:
   i. Bronchoalveolar lavage: the fibreoptic bronchoscope (FOB) is wedged into an airway, isolating that airway from the rest of the lung. Saline is injected in aliquots of 20 mL (total 150–200 mL) through the FOB and suction is then used to retrieve this fluid, which is then sent for analysis
   ii. Protected specimen brush: a catheter, housing a retracted brush system, is passed down the channel of the FOB. The retracted brush is protected from contamination during its passage through the FOB, and then advanced beyond the tip of the catheter, into the distal respiratory tract to sample the secretions. The brush is then retracted to protect it from further contamination as the catheter is withdrawn up the FOB

   Oxygenation frequently worsens after lavage because of epithelial surface changes and the release of pro-inflammatory cytokines. This effect is generally transient lasting from 15 min in normal lung to several hours in severe parenchymal disease
2. Evaluation of haemoptysis. Bronchoscopic evaluation in the first 12–18 h usually enables identification of the site of bleeding. If the source of bleeding is not initially visible, segmental lavage can be performed looking for blood within the recovered fluid
3. Evaluation of radiological abnormalities. Lesions can be biopsied but the incidence of complications, particularly pneumothorax, is as high as 20% among those receiving mechanical ventilation
4. Localisation of the tracheal tube tip
5. Evaluation of major airway trauma and thermal injury

Therapeutic indications

1. Aspiration of mucous plugs. Chest physiotherapy and suctioning are normally successful in treating mucous plugs and resultant atelectasis. If these techniques fail, bronchoscopy with bronchoalveolar lavage can be used to remove the plugs and re-expand the atelectic lung. However, the relatively narrow suction channel in the FOB can limit its efficacy

in the presence of very thick mucous and studies have failed to consistently demonstrate an advantage over aggressive physiotherapy. Although the technique is controversial, it is indicated in lobar collapse unresponsive to chest physiotherapy and in total lung collapse

2. Local treatment of haemoptysis. A bronchial blocker, passed down the channel of the FOB, can be used to isolate and tamponade a bleeding sub-segment. Alternatively endobronchial intubation of the non-bleeding lung can be life saving. However in massive haemoptysis it is often preferable to use a rigid bronchoscope to broaden the therapeutic options available

3. Removal of aspirated foreign bodies. Although the rigid bronchoscope traditionally is the preferred instrument for the removal of foreign bodies, the FOB used with a variety of forceps and baskets, has been shown to be safe and effective

4. Treatment of bronchopulmonary fistula. Proximally located fistulas may be directly visualised, whereas more distal fistulas may be localised by systematically passing an occluding balloon into each bronchial segment. When the correct segment is located inflation of the balloon will result in reduction of the air leak

5. Bronchoscopic placement of stents (cancer) and valves (COPD lung reduction surgery)

Airway management

Indications for bronchoscopic airway management include:

1. Tracheal intubation
   Especially useful in the setting of difficult intubation, anatomical deformity, head and neck immobility and upper airway obstruction. The need for a skilled bronchoscopist is a major drawback of this technique since in unskilled hands, bronchoscopy may simply extend the period of hypoxia and cause trauma to the upper airway

2. Percutaneous dilational tracheostomy
   The tip of the FOB is placed distally in the tracheal tube enabling the needle puncture and dilation of the trachea to be visualised in real time. This reduces the risk of needle damage to the posterior wall of the trachea and paratracheal insertion of the tracheostomy tube

3. Bronchial intubation (double lumen tube)

4. Placement of a nasogastric tube

Complications

Fibreoptic bronchoscopy is generally a safe procedure when performed in the ICU on critically ill patients. The outer diameter of a standard FOB occupies about 10% of the cross-sectional area of the trachea; hence, in a spontaneously breathing non-intubated patient, the increased airway resistance is small and bronchoscopy is well tolerated. However, the same scope will occupy about 50% of the diameter of an 8.0-mm tracheal tube. This degree of obstruction leads to a significant increase in airway resistance, which can lead to the development of high auto-PEEP and alveolar hypoventilation. Additionally, continuous and excessive application of suction during FOB will exacerbate small airway collapse and cause derecruitment.

Other common complications are oxygen desaturation, hypotension, frequent premature ventricular beats, and pulmonary haemorrhage. These are generally transient and rarely life-threatening. Relative contraindications include difficult ventilation or oxygenation, severe coagulopathy, acute myocardial infarction or ischaemia and status asthmaticus.

Recently, there has been interest in the use of non-invasive ventilation during FOB in non-intubated patients, in which bronchoscopy would traditionally been contraindicated due to the significant risk of oxygen desaturation.

Further reading

Ovassapian A, Randel GI. The role of the fiberscope in the critically ill patient. Crit Care Clin 1995; 11:29–51.

Snell A, Mackay J. Bronchoscopic anatomy. Anaesth Intensive Care Med 2008; 9:542–544.

Guerreiro da Cunha Fragoso E, Gonçalves JM. Role of fiberoptic bronchoscopy in intensive care unit: current practice. J Bronchology Interv Pulmonol 2011; 18:69–83.

Related topics of interests

- Tracheostomy (p 368)

Fluid therapy

Key points

- Intravenous fluid therapy is not innocuous – the right fluid must be used for the right situation in the right volume
- There are few high quality randomised trials with significant patient centred outcomes (e.g. mortality and morbidity) to provide evidence-based recommendations for fluid therapies in the critically ill
- Hydroxyethyl starch solutions increase the incidence of acute kidney injury and mortality in critically ill patients

Physiology

Total body water represents about 60% of the body weight of a young adult male. The distribution of this fluid across the primary fluid spaces is depicted in **Figure 9**.

Intracellular fluid (ICF) is separated from extracellular fluid (ECF) by a cell membrane that is highly permeable to water but not to most electrolytes. Intracellular volume is maintained by the membrane sodium-potassium pump, which moves sodium out of the cell (carrying water with it) in exchange for potassium. Thus, there are significant differences in the electrolytic composition of intracellular and ECF.

The intravascular space and the interstitial fluid (ISF) are separated by the endothelial cells of the capillary wall (the capillary membrane). This wall is permeable to water and small molecules, including ions. It is impermeable to larger molecules such as proteins.

The higher hydrostatic pressure inside capillaries (compared with that in the ISF) tends to force fluid out of the vessel into the ISF.

The osmotic pressure of a solution is related directly to the number of osmotically active particles it contains. The total osmolarity of each of the fluid compartments is approximately 280 mOsml^{-1}. Oncotic pressure is that component of osmotic pressure provided by large molecules. The higher osmotic pressure inside capillaries tends to pull fluid back in to the vessels.

Electrolyte concentrations differ markedly between fluid compartments. Notably, sodium and chloride are chiefly extracellular while the majority of total body potassium is within the intracellular compartment. There is also a relatively low content of protein

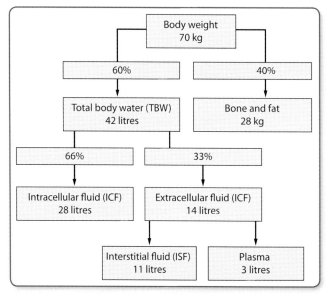

Figure 9 Distribution of fluid in the body.

anions in ISF compared with ICF and plasma.

Crystalloids

The composition of some of the commonly prescribed crystalloids is given in **Table 24**.

A crystalloid is a solution of small non-ionic or ionic particles (e.g. sodium chloride). After intravenous administration, the distribution of a crystalloid is determined chiefly by its sodium concentration. Since sodium is confined mainly to the ECF, fluids with high sodium concentrations (e.g. 0.9% sodium chloride) will be distributed mainly through the ECF. Solutions with lower sodium concentrations (e.g. 5% glucose) will be distributed throughout both ECF and the intracellular compartment. In comparison with Hartmann's solution, the higher sodium content of 0.9% sodium chloride will result in slightly better intravascular volume expansion. However, large quantities of 0.9% sodium chloride will cause hyperchloraemic acidosis, and probably leads to adverse outcomes. After head injury, 0.9% sodium chloride is the preferred resuscitation fluid because Hartmann's solution is slightly hypotonic relative to plasma and may worsen cerebral oedema.

Colloids

Colloid solutions are fluids containing large molecules that exert an oncotic pressure at the capillary membrane. Natural colloids include blood and albumin. Artificial colloids contain large molecules such as gelatin, dextran, starch and haemoglobin. It has been thought that since colloids are larger molecules that they remain within the intravascular compartment longer than equivalent volumes of crystalloid solutions. However, many studies have shown this effect to be minimal, and there appear to be significant unwanted effects, particularly concerning mortality, allergic reactions, renal function, coagulation and long-term pruritis.

Blood

Blood is now commonly used in hospitals as the primary resuscitation fluid in massive haemorrhage. Experience from military studies has shown that rapid replacement of red blood cells (RBCs) and other blood components decreases overall transfusion requirements and saves lives by preventing other complications. The ideal blood product is probably fresh whole blood, but is currently used only in military settings. Many institutions have implemented massive haemorrhage protocols, where 'shock packs', typically consisting of O Rhesus negative (for females) or O Rhesus positive (for males) RBCs, fresh frozen plasma with or without platelets, are provided by blood bank as soon as the massive haemorrhage protocol is activated. Depending on continued blood loss and subsequent blood and coagulation

Table 24 Composition of commonly prescribed crystalloids							
Crystalloid (mosmol kg^{-1})	Osmolality	pH	Na$^+$ (mmol L^{-1})	K$^+$ (mmol L^{-1})	HCO$_3^-$ (mmol L^{-1})	Cl$^-$ (mmol L^{-1})	Ca^{2+}
0.9% sodium chloride solution	308	5.0	154	0	0	154	0
Hartmann's solution	280	6.5	131	5.0	29[a]	111	2
PlasmaLyte 148	299	5.5	140	5	50[b]	98	0
5% glucose	278	4.0	0	0	0	0	0
4% glucose in 0.18% sodium chloride solution	286	4.5	31	0	0	31	0

[a]HCO$_3^-$ is provided as lactate.
[b]27 mmol L^{-1} as acetate and 23 mmol L^{-1} as gluconate.

results further shock packs are released with additional RBCs, FFP, and platelets and cryoprecipitate, or additional specific coagulation products are then given aiming to prevent further coagulopathy and impaired tissue perfusion.

There is emerging evidence that using RBCs following longer storage times may lead to worse outcomes. This may have implications on blood transfusion services in the future.

Albumin

Human albumin is a single polypeptide with a molecular weight of around 68 kDa. It is a negatively charged substance and is repelled by the negatively charged endothelial glycocalyx, thus extending its intravascular duration. Albumin has transport functions, is able to scavenge free radicals and has anticoagulant properties. In health, it contributes about 80% of oncotic pressure but, in the critically ill, serum albumin correlates poorly with colloid oncotic pressure. In the United Kingdom (UK), albumin is prepared in two concentrations (4.5% and 20%) from many thousands of pooled donors. Although albumin supplied in the UK is sourced from the United States, there remains a theoretical risk of transmission of the prion causing variant Creutzfeldt–Jakob disease. The half-life of exogenous albumin in the circulating compartment is 5–10 days assuming an intact capillary wall membrane. It is expensive to prepare but has a long shelf life. The role of albumin as a resuscitation fluid remains controversial. A meta-analysis of the use of albumin-containing solutions for the resuscitation of patients with sepsis has documented lower mortality compared with other fluid resuscitation regimens but conversely subset analysis of a randomised controlled trial showed that mortality may be increased in patients with traumatic brain injury.

Gelatins

Gelatins are modified bovine collagens suspended in ionic solutions. The collagen is sourced from outside the UK. Gelatin solutions have long shelf lives and, based on current knowledge, do not transmit infection. Gelatin solutions contain molecules of widely varying molecular weight. Despite a quoted average molecular weight of approximately 35 kDa, most of the molecules are considerably smaller than this and are excreted rapidly by the kidney. Thus, gelatin solutions remain in the circulating compartment for a short period. They maintain their maximal volume effect for only 1.5 h, and only 15% remains in the intravascular space 24 h after administration. Although anaphylaxis to colloids is rare, recent data indicate that gelatins are the most common to be implicated. There is no evidence for improved outcomes with the use of gelatin.

Hydroxyethyl starch

Hydroxyethyl starch (HES) is manufactured from either corn or potato starch. Several HES solutions are available, each with a different average molecular weight. Most HES solutions have a longer intravascular half-life than other synthetic colloids, with a significant volume effect for at least 6h. The higher molecular weight starch solutions (450 kDa), particularly when combined with high substitution ratios (e.g. 0.7 or 7 hydroxyethyl groups for every 10 glucose rings), prolong clotting time by impairing factor VIII and von Willebrand factor and have not been used in the UK for many years. Lower molecular weight solutions (130 kDa) with a lower substitution ratio (typically 0.4 – known as tetrastarches) are associated with fewer adverse effects than the high molecular weight solutions. Recent studies of different HES solutions [Scandinavian Starch for Severe Sepsis/Septic Shock Trial (6S trial) and Crystalloid Versus Hydroxyethyl Starch Trials (CHEST)] have shown increased incidence of renal failure and mortality (6S trial) in critically ill patients. Other adverse effects include prolonged coagulation and long-term itching. The Medicines and Healthcare Products Regulatory Agency (UK) suspended the licences for all HES products in June 2013, other licensing authorities are reviewing HES licences.

Artificial oxygen carriers

Haemoglobin-based oxygen carriers (HBOCs)

Blood is the only fluid in routine use that has significant oxygen-carrying capability. While this property makes it indispensable during resuscitation of haemorrhagic shock, it is expensive, in short supply, antigenic, requires cross-matching, has a limited shelf life, requires a storage facility and carries a risk of disease transmission. Free haemoglobin causes severe renal injury. Polymerisation of the haemoglobin overcomes this problem and improves intravascular persistence. Haemoglobin solutions under development are derived from one of three sources: bovine blood, out-of-date human blood (5–13% of blood donated in the United States is discarded) and recombinant haemoglobin. The products currently under investigation do not require crossmatching, have similar oxygen dissociation curves to blood and are apparently free from risk of transmitting viral or bacterial infections. They have an intravascular half-life of up to 24 h. Some haemoglobin solutions have a significant vasopressor effect which is thought to result from scavenging endothelial nitric oxide. Polymerised bovine haemoglobin [haemoglobin-based oxygen carrier (HBOC)-201] is licensed for clinical use in South Africa. MP4OX, a pegylated human haemoglobin-based colloid has recently completed a phase IIb study in adult trauma patients.

Perfluorocarbon emulsions

Perfluorocarbons (PFCs) are inert chemicals consisting mainly of carbon and fluorine atoms. PFCs are excreted unchanged via the lungs following plasma clearance by the reticuloendothelial system. Oxygen can dissolve 20 times more effectively in PFCs than plasma. The linear oxygen dissociation curves of these compounds means that significant oxygen carriage occurs only at an F_{IO_2} approaching 1.0. The emulsions consist of micro-droplets of < 0.2 μm that can pass through very small capillaries non-traversable by red cells. This may increase oxygen carriage to critically ischaemic tissues. Modest efficacy and a high incidence of flu-like symptoms are holding up the introduction of these solutions to clinical practice.

How much is enough?

After consideration of beneficial and adverse effects of each necessary fluid compound, the universal question of volume remains. Traditionally, whilst a patient has remained responsive to a fluid challenge then further fluid has been administered, aiming to minimise requirement of vasopressors or inotropes. However normal individuals display characteristics of fluid responsiveness, and ameliorating these may result in over-administration. A number of potential markers of end-points of resuscitation, including fluid responsiveness, lactate, pulse-pressure variation or cardiac output indices have been studied, and no single one has been identified as being better than others. However, adverse effects of tissue oedema in critically ill patients include gut dysfunction, myopathy and neuropathy, infections and failure to wean from ventilation and therefore establishing the right balance between volume resuscitation and reliance on vasopressors is crucial.

Further reading

Reinhart K, Perner A, Sprung CL, et al. Consensus statement of the ESICM task force on colloid volume therapy in critically ill patients. Intensive Care Med 2012; 38:368–383.

Bunn R, Trivedi D. Colloid solutions for fluid resuscitation. Cochrane Database Syst Rev 2012; 7:CD001319.

Cecconi M, Parsons AK, Rhodes A. What is a fluid challenge? Curr Opin Crit Care 2011; 17:290–295.

Delaney AP, Dan A, McCaffrey J, Finfer S. The role of albumin as a resuscitation fluid for patients with sepsis: A systematic review and meta-analysis. Crit Care Med 2011; 39:386–391.

Related topics of interest

Guillain–Barré syndrome

Key points

- 30% of patients with Guillain–Barré syndrome (GBS) require ventilatory support
- Autonomic dysfunction occurs in 70% of cases
- 5% of all patients diagnosed with GBS die within a year despite ICU support

Epidemiology

The incidence of Guillain–Barré syndrome (GBS) is 1–2 per 100,000 per year. Males are more frequently affected than females. There is geographical variation in the incidence of subtypes of GBS.

Pathophysiology

GBS was originally described as a single clinical disorder, occurring typically after a preceding infection induced an immune-mediated response with cross-reactivity to antigens expressed on peripheral nerves causing an acute polyneuropathy. It is now recognised that a variety of neurone components can develop immune-mediated pathology, depending on the particular clinical subtype of GBS.

Clinical features

The classical key features of GBS are symmetrical progressive muscular weakness with hypo- or areflexia with associated sensory and autonomic disturbances. The syndrome is typically preceded by an acute respiratory or gastrointestinal infection which may be viral or bacterial (e.g. *Campylobacter jejuni, Mycoplasma pneumoniae,* and Cytomegalovirus [CMV]). GBS can also occur after vaccination. Symptoms progress typically for 2 weeks; by 4 weeks 90% of patients reach maximal weakness after which a recovery phase starts.

Acute inflammatory demyelinating polyneuropathy (AIDP) is the most commonly described variant (85% of cases). The clinical features of AIDP are described above.

Miller–Fisher syndrome (MFS) presents with a triad of ophthalmoplegia, ataxia and areflexia. Limb weakness may occur in up to 30% of patients. The incidence of MFS varies by geographical location (25% in the eastern Asia; 5% in the USA).

Acute motor axonal neuropathy (AMAN) is seen in eastern Asia often following *Campylobacter jejuni* infection. It has clinical features similar to AIDP although sensory neurones remain unaffected. Acute motor and sensory axonal neuropathy (AMSAN) is similar to AMAN but also involves sensory neurones.

Several rare forms of GBS have also been described including pure sensory GBS which may lead to severe sensory ataxia, and Bickerstaff encephalitis characterised by some features of MFS together with hyperreflexia and encephalopathy.

Up to 30% of patients require invasive mechanical ventilation and 50% develop oropharyngeal weakness. Autonomic instability is common and can affect the cardiovascular (tachy- or bradycardias, arrhythmias, labile blood pressure and orthostatic hypotension), genitourinary (urinary retention) and gastrointestinal (ileus) systems. Severe neuropathic pain may also occur affecting typically the lower limbs and back.

Investigations

In addition to the history and clinical examination, cerebrospinal fluid (CSF) analysis, neurophysiology studies and neuronal antibody testing are also used to support or refute a diagnosis of GBS.

Typical CSF findings following lumbar puncture (LP) one week after symptom onset are a raised protein with a normal white cell count. A normal protein may be found in some patients if a LP is undertaken less than 7 days after onset of symptoms. A CSF pleocytosis (increased white cell count) suggests either an alternative diagnosis or intercurrent HIV infection.

Neurophysiological studies assist in both diagnosis and prognosis. Sequential nerve conduction studies (NCS) may be used as axonal pathology progresses with time. A variety of abnormalities may be seen on NCS, depending on the variant of GBS.

In AIDP, initial involvement of nerve roots by inflammatory demyelination results in absent or delayed F waves and loss of H waves. Slowing of conduction velocities occurs by about 4 weeks. In contrast, with AMAN, in which sensory involvement is absent, there is no slowing of conduction because there is no peripheral nerve demyelination.

Several neuronal antibody tests are available, reflecting the different GBS subtypes. Up to 90% of patients with MFS have antibodies directed against the ganglioside GQ1b. *Campylobacter jejuni* infection can induce antibodies against several gangliosides (GM1, GD1a and GD1b) leading to AMAN and AMSAN.

Magnetic resonance imaging is usually normal in GBS although there may be post-contrast nerve root enhancement.

Microbiological and immunological investigations help to identify any precipitating infection. These include serology for *Campylobacter jejuni, Mycoplasma pneumoniae,* CMV, Epstein-Barr virus (EBV), HIV, herpes simplex virus (HSV), Hepatitis A, B and C, together with testing of the stool for *C. jejuni* and poliovirus.

Diagnosis

The diagnostic criteria for GBS are areflexia, together with progressive muscular weakness of two or more limbs, and may also include facial muscle weakness and ophthalmoplegia. Several features are supportive (but not diagnostic) of GBS and include progressive, symmetrical symptoms evolving over 4 weeks followed by a plateau phase and subsequent recovery, autonomic dysfunction, albuminocytological dissociation on CSF analysis (raised protein but normal white cell count) and GBS consistent findings on neurophysiological testing.

Differential diagnoses for the various subtypes of GBS include vasculitis, beriberi, porphyria, diphtheria, Lyme disease, toxin-induced neuropathy, botulism, brain stem stroke or encephalitis, myasthenia gravis or Wernicke's encephalopathy. A raised white blood cell count in the CSF, a sensory level, severe bowel and bladder dysfunction, or persistent asymmetrical weakness should raise the possibility of alternative spinal cord pathology including epidural abscess formation, transverse myelitis or corda equina syndrome.

Treatment

Treatment options are divided into general supportive measures and those directed specifically against modifying the disease process.

Invasive ventilatory support (together with associated care bundles) is required in 30% of patients because of respiratory failure, which may develop rapidly. Intubation is required if clinical respiratory distress is present, or if one major or two minor criteria are met. Major criteria for intubation include hypercarbia, hypoxaemia or a vital capacity of less than 15 mL kg^{-1}. Minor criteria are atelectasis, unsafe swallow or impaired cough. Tracheostomy is usually required.

Hypertension often requires treatment with labetolol or esmolol. Sinus tachycardia is common and may require treatment, particularly if malignant arrhythmias occur. Urinary catheterisation is required for bladder atony, and prokinetic drugs are often required to treat ileus. Neuropathic pain is common. Extensive rehabilitation is required during the recovery phase.

Plasma exchange and intravenous immunoglobulin (IVIG) therapy can shorten the recovery period; they are equally effective and the choice of therapy depends generally on local availability. Plasma exchange is provided typically up to six times over a period of up to 10 days. IVIG 400 mg kg^{-1} is given daily for five days. There is no role for glucocorticoids.

Complications

The key complications of GBS are respiratory failure, autonomic instability and neuropathic pain. Invasive ventilatory support, intravascular access techniques, tracheostomy insertion and prolonged ICU stay all carry additional risks. Fourteen percent of patients have long-term motor problems and 5% of patients die in the first year despite ICU treatment. Chronic inflammatory demyelinating polyneuropathy (a continuum of AIDP which lasts longer than 8 weeks) occurs in 2% of patients.

Further reading

Yuki N, Hartung HP. Guillain-Barré syndrome. New Engl J Med 2012; 366:2294–2304.

Patwa HS, Chaudhry V, Katzberg H, Rae-Grant AD, So YT. Evidence-based guideline: intravenous immunoglobulin in the treatment of neuromuscular disorders: report of the Therapeutics and Technology Assessment Subcommittee of the American Academy of Neurology. Neurology 2012; 78:1009–1015.

Cornblath DR, Hughes RA. Treatment for Guillain-Barré syndrome. Ann Neurol 2009; 66:569–570.

Kissel JT, Cornblath DR, Mendell JR. Guillain-Barré syndrome. In: Diagnosis and management of peripheral nerve disorders. New York: Oxford University Press, 2001.

Related topics of interest

- Neurological diseases (p 226)
- Respiratory support – invasive (p 306)
- Weaning from ventilation (p 413)

Haematological disorders

Key points

- Haematological malignancies are heterogenous and affect many systems
- Haematological and renal support is commonly required
- Neutropenic sepsis is a medical emergency

The haematological malignancies, leukaemia, lymphoma and myeloma, make up a small proportion of all malignancies and often respond well to treatment. However, relapse is common and treatment is associated with significant morbidity and mortality.

Leukaemias are malignancies of bone marrow resulting in abnormally high numbers of leucocytes or their progenitors in the blood. They are classified by the rate of disease progression and further sub-divided according to cell type – e.g. acute lymphoblastic leukaemia (ALL) or chronic myeloid leukaemia (CML).

Lymphomas are malignancies of lymphocytes occurring in the lymphatic system, divided into Hodgkin's disease (HD) and non-Hodgkin's lymphoma (NHL). NHL can be further sub-classified according to cell type. The 2008 WHO classification has over 80 subtypes of lymphoma.

Multiple myeloma is a disease of plasma cells in the marrow, resulting in abnormally high levels of immunoglobulins.

Other haematological malignancies include myelodysplasia, myeloproliferative disorders and monoclonal gammopathy of unknown significance.

Epidemiology

Haematological malignancies account for 9% of new cancer diagnoses in the United States and United Kingdom (UK). The UK incidence is 63 per 100,000 whereas global incidence is lower at 15 per 100,000, illustrating that most haematological malignancies are diseases of old age. Median age at diagnosis is 70, although two forms of ALL (Precursor B and T) are diseases of young people. Lymphomas account for around a third of all haematological malignancies; quarter

are leukaemias and the rest myeloma, myelodysplasia and myeloproliferative disorders.

Pathophysiology

Leukaemias and lymphomas develop when progenitor cells undergo genetic transformation leading to clonal expansion. This can occur at any stage from pluripotent stem cell to specialized progenitor cell. Multiple mutations are required for malignant proliferation, affecting the expression of oncogenes and tumour-suppressor genes. Genetic transformations range from point mutations and deletions to chromosomal translocations. Translocations are often associated with particular diseases, such as the Philadelphia chromosome t(9;22) in CML; t(8;14) in Burkitt's lymphoma.

Most mutations are random but there are risk factors. Environmental factors linked to leukaemia and lymphoma include ionizing radiation (particularly AML and CML), chemicals (e.g. benzene and polychlorinated phenyls) and infective agents (e.g. human T-lymphotropic virus type 1 (HTLV-1) and adult T-cell leukaemia; Epstein-Barr virus (EBV) and Burkitt's lymphoma). Heritable risk factors include Down's syndrome (20–30 times risk of acute leukaemia), Fanconi's anaemia and Kleinfelter's syndrome. Most familial associations are weak and have no identifiable culprit gene.

Leukaemia

Acute leukaemias tend to involve earlier progenitors or stem cells than chronic leukaemias, and the first genetic mutation may occur in utero, with a second event (e.g. infection) in childhood precipitating disease. Cellular proliferation results in replacement of bone marrow by abnormal cells and pancytopenia. The abnormal cells then infiltrate other tissues such as meninges, testes and skin.

Lymphoma

Most (85%) lymphomas are B-cell disorders. The lymphoma subtype is determined by the stage of lymphocyte development at which mutation occurs. Disease usually starts in lymph nodes before spreading to lymphoid tissue in other organs.

Myeloma

Multiple myeloma is a neoplastic proliferation of mature plasma cells in bone marrow, which secrete a monoclonal immunoglobulin (paraprotein). Paraprotein causes hyperviscosity, renal failure and amyloidosis. Bone marrow infiltration leads to osteolysis, reduced haemopoiesis and hypercalcaemia.

Clinical features
Acute leukaemias

There is a short (<12 week) history of symptoms with bone marrow failure, tiredness and pallor, susceptibility to infections and abnormal bruising or bleeding. Increased catabolism leads to lethargy, sweating and fever. Organ infiltration can cause bone pain, lymphadenopathy, hepatosplenomegaly and meningism.

Chronic leukaemias

Hypermetabolism causes weight loss, night sweats and malaise. Splenomegaly (often massive) is common in CML, causing pain or digestive disturbance. Bleeding tendency or signs of anaemia are common, but often, an incidental finding of an abnormal white cell count leads to diagnosis, particularly in CLL. Lymphadenopathy is common in CLL.

Lymphomas

The commonest presentation is asymmetric, painless lymphadenopathy, with moderate splenomegaly in about half of cases. Signs of systemic disease (malaise, sweats, fever and pruritus) are more common in HD.

Myeloma

Bone pain, vertebral collapse and pathological fractures are common presentations, along with signs of anaemia and/or bone marrow failure. Renal failure and hypercalcaemia may cause oliguria or polyuria, thirst, oedema and confusion.

Investigations

Normochromic, normocytic anaemia with thrombocytopenia is common. White cell count is usually over 30–$50 \times 10^9 \, L^{-1}$ in chronic leukaemia and raised in acute leukaemias (but can be normal or low). Acute leukaemias may have blast cells visible on blood film. Lumbar puncture should be performed to assess CNS involvement.

In all cases, renal and hepatic function, calcium and phosphate levels should be checked. Blood cultures and infective markers should be taken if there is any suggestion of infection.

Imaging can identify complications of disease (e.g. pneumonia) or stage diseases (CT in lymphoma). A skeletal survey identifies lytic lesions in myeloma.

Diagnosis

The diagnosis of leukaemia relies on microscopic analysis of blood and bone marrow (aspirate or biopsy); determination of cell type, karyotype and immunological markers help determine appropriate treatment and prognosis.

Lymph node biopsy and histology with immunological markers and genetic analysis is required for a diagnosis and sub-typing of lymphoma. Reed-Sternberg cells are present in HD.

Myeloma is diagnosed with findings of monoclonal serum IgM and infiltration of marrow or lymph nodes with plasma cells.

Treatment
General supportive care

- Central venous access for sampling and access; preferably tunnelled
- Protection from infection with meticulous (reverse) barrier nursing
- Prophylactic antibiotics, anti-virals, antifungals and anti-pneumocystis
- Blood products and coagulation factors as clinically indicated
- Analgesia and anti-emesis
- Fluid and nutritional support
- Respiratory and cardiac support as needed

Disease specific

Radiotherapy and cytotoxic agents are the mainstay of treatment along with immunosuppressant agents such as corticosteroids or interferon. Granulocyte colony-stimulating factor to promote neutrophil recovery in neutropenic patients, should be considered in conjunction with the Haematologists.

Complications

ARDS

This can be related to cytokines associated with the malignancy, transfusion, radiotherapy or chemotherapy (particularly all trans-retinoic acid). Early use of corticosteroids is important in treatment.

Bone marrow failure

Anaemia, thrombocytopenia and neutropenia are common at presentation and almost universal after commencing treatment. Neutropenia requires isolation and strict barrier nursing with meticulous attention to sterility for all procedures. Prophylactic antibiotics have been shown to help. The febrile neutropenic patient is a medical emergency requiring urgent sampling, isolation and urgent (within 1 h) empirical antibiotic therapy. Neutropenic septic shock has a mortality >36%.

Renal failure

Myeloma often causes renal failure due to amyloid deposition and can require renal support. Some chemotherapeutic regimens can also induce renal failure.

Metabolic derangement

Tumour lysis syndrome is associated with hyperkalaemia, hypercalcaemia and hyperuricaemia. Myeloma is also associated with hypercalcaemia requiring treatment or renal support.

Further reading

Hoffbrand AV, Moss PAH. Essential haematology, 6th edn. Hoboke; Wiley Blackwell, 2011.

Sekeres MA, Stone RM. The acute leukemias. In Irwin RS, Rippe JM. Intensive Care Medicine. 6th edn. Philadelphia; Lippincott, Williams & Wilkins, 2008:1408–1417.

Bird GT, Farquhar-Smith P, Wigmore T, Potter M, Gruber PC. Outcomes and prognostic factors in patients with haematological malignancy admitted to a specialist cancer intensive care unit: a 5 year study. Br J Anaesth 2012; 108:452–459.

Beed M, Levitt M, Bokhari SW. Intensive care management of patients with haematological malignancy. Contin Educ Anaesth Crit Care Pain 2010; 10:167–171.

Related topics of interest

HIV and critical care

Key points

- Highly active antiretroviral therapy (HAART) has transformed the long-term prognosis of HIV infection
- Respiratory failure is the commonest indication for ICU admission
- *Pneumocystis jirovecii* pneumonia remains a major cause of morbidity
- The optimal use of HAART in critical care requires awareness of the complex management issues and involvement of an HIV specialist

Epidemiology

First reported in 1981, the HIV/AIDS pandemic has spread worldwide, affecting 34 million people including over 90,000 cases in the UK, nearly a quarter of whom are unaware of their infection. HIV is transmitted by sexual contact, blood or blood products and from mother-to-child. Heterosexual transmission now accounts for the vast majority of new infections worldwide.

The outlook for patients with HIV has dramatically improved over the last decade with the development of HAART. High death rates and the perceived futility of ICU treatment observed in the early days have declined. Despite an increase in the number of people living with HIV there has been a 24% fall in AIDS-related mortality since 2005 and the lifespan of an adult with HIV is now only slight reduced. HIV infection has been transformed into a chronic, treatable health condition.

Pathophysiology

HIV is a cytopathic retrovirus with a long latent period and chronic course. Interactions between HIV and the host response are complex. The virus preferentially infects T-helper cells (CD4-receptor positive), gradually destroying them, reducing immune surveillance, resulting in progressive susceptibility to characteristic opportunistic infections and malignancies. Activation of numerous elements of the immune system results in functional immunosuppression.

Diagnosis

The CDC staging system assesses severity of HIV disease by CD4 counts and by the presence of specific HIV-related conditions. The definition of AIDS includes all HIV-infected individuals with CD4 <200 cells/mm^3 (or CD4 percentage <14%) or with AIDS-indicator conditions.

HIV testing in critical care

A significant number of individuals are unaware of their HIV status and most deaths now occur in individuals diagnosed too late for effective treatment. There is an increasing imperative for early diagnosis and a low threshold for HIV testing. Obtaining informed consent is often impossible in ICU, testing usually undertaken on the basis of best interests when clinically indicated. CD4 counts can be misleading, as they may be low in critical illness irrespective of HIV status.

Presentation

As HAART has altered the long-term prognosis in HIV so the spectrum and outcome of critical illness has changed. Non-AIDS associated diagnoses, including incidental medical and surgical conditions, have become more common and are associated with better survival. ITU mortality has progressively improved, now variably reported between 20–30%, and comparable to outcomes in non-HIV-infected patients.

Respiratory failure remains the most common reason for ICU admission and *Pneumocystis jirovecii* pneumonia (PJP, previously referred to as *Pneumocystis carinii* pneumonia) is still frequently identified as the responsible pathogen (see below). In many centres, bacterial pneumonia and sepsis are overtaking PJP becoming the most common admitting diagnoses.

Tuberculosis (TB) is another common presentation. Co-infection with HIV increases the risk of active TB in exposed individuals. This combination also results in rapid clinical progression and unusual presentations making diagnosis difficult, encouraging resistance and culminating in a poor prognosis.

Non-HIV causes of respiratory failure, such as asthma and COPD, are increasingly common. A rising rate of cardiovascular disease is being reported, the artherogenic metabolic complications of HAART are thought to be contributory. Other presentations include end-stage liver disease secondary to co-infection with viral hepatitis and end-stage renal failure from HIV associated nephropathy, diabetes and hypertension. Dialysis and transplantation are used in appropriate patients. Neurological complications, particularly intractable seizures and reduced GCS are also common.

Treatment

The potential role of HAART in treating HIV patients in ICU remains unclear and is challenging because of difficulties with drug delivery, dosage, interactions and toxic side effects. Few oral suspensions or intravenous preparations are available. Variable absorption and frequent co-existing renal and hepatic impairment make dosing unpredictable. There are numerous interactions of HAART with other HIV-associated medications and common ICU drugs. Erratic plasma levels raise concerns of promoting toxicity and HIV resistance. There is also a risk of precipitating immune reconstitution inflammatory syndrome (IRIS) following the introduction of HAART. This can cause a paradoxical clinical worsening, in an already critical illness, as the immune system is restored. Given the complexities it is crucial that HIV experts and specialist pharmacists are involved in the care of these patients.

No consensus guidelines currently exist and decisions should be made on a case-by-case review. Patients already receiving HAART should continue therapy wherever possible due to the risk of selecting drug resistant virus. Patients admitted with non-HIV related conditions and CD4 count >200 cells/mm^3 can potentially defer treatment, short-term prognosis depending on successful resolution of the non-HIV related condition. Commencing HAART should be considered in all patients presenting with an AIDS-associated illness, those with CD4 counts <200, an anticipated prolonged ITU stay or deterioration despite optimal ICU management. Monitoring viral load (VL) may be helpful. Vigilance for HIV drug resistance, altered pharmacokinetics, interactions, toxic effects and IRIS is necessary.

Prognosis

Factors associated with poor outcome for HIV-infected patients in ICU are illness severity, organ failure (particularly the need for mechanical ventilation), an AIDS-defining diagnosis and sepsis. Other suggested indicators of poor prognosis include prolonged hospital to ITU admission interval, low serum albumin, poor functional status and history of significant weight loss. Immunovirological factors including HIV RNA VL and low CD4 count may also worsen prognosis.

Pneumocystis jiroveci pneumonia

Presentation

Typically a slow indolent course with progressive dyspnoea, fever and a dry cough. Findings on examination are often minimal.

Investigations

CXR is either normal or reveals diffuse interstitial infiltrates. Atypical patterns can occur and pneumatoceles may be visible. Blood gases indicate severity. Exercise oximerty may be useful in less severe disease. Definitive diagnosis is made by detection of the organism in samples obtained from induced sputum, bronchoalveolar lavage or lung biopsy.

Complications

The risk of pneumothorax is high, especially in those who have had previous episodes of *Pneumocystis jiroveci* pneumonia (PJP) or received prophylactic nebulised pentamidine. Prognosis of PJP complicated by pneumothorax is poor.

Treatment

First line therapy is intravenous co-trimoxazole 120 mg kg^{-1} day^{-1} in divided doses for 14–21 days. Adverse reactions are common including severe GI upset, rashes, pancreatitis, bone marrow suppression, nephrotoxicity and hepatotoxicity. FBC, U&Es and LFTs need to be closely monitored. Intravenous pentamidine 4 mg/kg/day or a combination of clindamycin and primaquine are commonly used as second-line agents.

Adjuvant glucocorticoids reduce the risk of respiratory failure, mechanical ventilation and death in patients with severe HIV-related PJP. Steroids are indicated if Pao_2 <70 mmHg or arterial/alveolar gradient >35 mmHg and should be started as early as possible. A common regime is oral prednisolone 40 mg 12 h for 5 days, with a reducing dose continued for the duration of treatment. IV methylprednisolone can also be used.

Intensive, early non-invasive ventilation (NIV) has been successfully used in patients with PJP-associated respiratory failure. Mechanical ventilation is usually reserved for those who have failed a trial of NIV. Standard lung-protective ventilatory strategies should be employed, avoiding excessive fluid administration and maintaining a high index of suspicion for pneumothorax.

Further reading

Huang L, Quartin A, Jones D, Havlir DV. Intensive care of patients with HIV infection. N Engl J Med 2006; 355:173–181.

Dickson SJ, Bateson S, Copas AJ, et al. Survival of HIV-infected patients in the intensive care unit in the era of highly active antiretroviral therapy. Thorax 2007; 62:964–968.

Crothers K, Huang L. Critical care of patients with HIV. HIV InSite Knowledge Base Chapter, May 2006. University of California, San Francisco.

Related topics of interest

- Infection prevention and control (p 197)
- Infection acquired in hospital (p 192)
- Refractory hypoxaemia (p 295)

Hypertension

Key points

- Hypertension (HTN) is a significant risk factor for stroke, myocardial infarction and kidney disease
- Approximately 90% of cases are due to essential hypertension
- Most cases of secondary hypertension are due to a renal cause

Epidemiology

In the UK, approximately 25% of adults have HTN. This increases to greater than 50% for patients over the age of 60. There is a 7% and 10% increase risk of mortality from ischaemic heart disease and stroke respectively with each 2 mmHg systolic blood pressure increase.

Where clinic BP readings are used, HTN is classified accordingly:

Grade/stage 1	HTN	140–159 and/or 90–99 mmHg
Grade/stage 2	HTN	160–179 and/or 100–109 mmHg
Severe/grade 3	HTN	>=180 and/or >=110 mmHg

Pathophysiology

There is an increase in systemic vascular resistance secondary to increased vascular tone. The arterial walls thicken and atheroma may develop in larger vessels. This increases afterload to the left ventricle which hypertrophies.

Salt and water excretion may be impaired by a reduction in glomerular filtration rate (GFR) secondary to a reduction in renal blood flow. The Renin–Angiotensin–Aldosterone System is stimulated which encourages further sodium and water retention.

Causes of hypertension

Essential hypertension

Many factors may be responsible which include genetic predisposition, environmental factors, obesity, alcohol intake and salt intake. Essential HTN accounts for approximately 90% of patients with HTN.

Secondary hypertension

There are many causes of secondary HTN:
- Coarctation of the aorta
- Drugs:
  - Carbenoxolone, cyclosporin, erythropoietin, MAOIs and tyramine, oestrogen containing contraceptives, NSAIDs and steroids
- Endocrine:
  - Acromegaly, congenital adrenal hyperplasia, Conn's, Cushing's, hyperparathyroidism, hyperthyroidism, hypothyroidism and phaeochromocytoma
- Pregnancy-induced hypertension
- Obstructive sleep apnoea
- Obesity
- Renal:
  - Renal causes account for approximately 80% of secondary HTN and include diabetic nephropathy, glomerulonephritides, polycystic kidneys, renal transplant and renovascular disease
- Hypertension in critical care:
  - Anxiety, fluid overload, hypercarbia, hypoxia, hypothermia, measurement error, pain, pyrexia and raised intracranial pressure

Clinical features

Patients may be entirely asymptomatic but may present with features of end organ disease such as acute kidney injury, heart failure, myocardial infarction or stroke.

Investigations

A full history and examination should be carried out including fundoscopy to assess for hypertensive retinopathy.

Urinanalysis – to assess for presence of blood or protein. If protein is evident an albumin:creatinine ratio should be assessed.

Blood samples for plasma glucose, urea and electrolytes, estimated GFR (eGFR), haemoglobin, uric acid, serum total cholesterol and HDL cholesterol.

CXR and ECG – to look for any end organ damage.

Investigations for causes of secondary HTN should include 24 h urinary catecholamines/metanephrines collection, thyroid function tests, aldosterone, renin, cortisol and growth hormone levels, aldosterone:renin ratio and renal imaging.

Diagnosis

If clinic blood pressure is 140/90 mmHg or greater, a diagnosis of hypertension should be confirmed through ambulatory blood pressure monitoring (ABPM) or home blood pressure monitoring (HBPM).

If ABPM is used, 2 measurements per patient's waking hour should be made. A minimum of 14 measurements should be averaged to confirm a diagnosis of hypertension.

When using HBPM, blood pressure should be taken in the morning and evening. Recordings should be taken over a minimum of 4 days and ideally over 7. The average value of the readings diagnoses the presence of hypertension.

Treatment

Treatment of HTN varies according to the patient population, the response to pre-existing treatments and with disease severity.

Lifestyle alterations include improving diet and exercise regime, weight loss, decreasing alcohol consumption, limiting caffeine intake, low salt intake and stopping smoking.

Patients < 55 years old:
Step 1 – Angiotensin-converting enzyme (ACE) inhibitor or Angiotensin receptor blocker (ARB).
Step 2 – ACE inhibitor or ARB with a calcium channel blocker (CCB).
Step 3 – As step 2 but add thiazide-like diuretic.
Step 4 – As step 3 but consider further diuretics, alpha or beta-blockers. Seek expert advice.

Patients = or >55 years old or black patients of African or Caribbean family origin:
Step 1 – CCB
Step 2 – ACE inhibitor or ARB with a CCB. An ARB is advised in black patients of African or Caribbean family origin.
Subsequent steps are as above.

Elderly patients:
Elderly patients should be treated as per 55–80 years old guidelines but adjusting for co-morbidities.

Diabetic patients:
ACE inhibitor or ARB therapy in this group of patients confers a renoprotective action. Patients with established proteinuria should have lower blood pressure levels targeted to those without.

Malignant hypertension

This is a hypertensive emergency. It is diagnosed as severe HTN with retinopathy associated with encephalopathy, microangiopathic haemolytic anaemia, nephropathy and papilloedema.

Initially the diastolic blood pressure should be reduced to 100–105 mmHg, to be achieved in 2–6 h. A reduction of 15–25% (but not exceeding 25%) should be achieved in this acute phase. Further gradual reductions may be attempted over a more prolonged timescale (12–24 h).

Sodium nitroprusside, Glyceryl trinitrate, Esmolol or Labetalol may be used for the treatment of malignant hypertension.

In the absence of therapy, 1-year survival is only 10–20%. Five-year survival rates of more than 70% are typical with appropriate treatment.

Complications

Heart failure, hypertensive encephalopathy, ischaemic heart disease, malignant hypertension and stroke.

Further reading

National Institute for Health and Clinical Excellence (NICE). Hypertension: clinical management of primary hypertension in adults. Clinical Guideline 127. London: NICE, 2011.

Mancia G, Fagard R, Narkiewicz K, et al. 2013 ESH/ESC Guidelines for the management of arterial hypertension: The Task Force for the management of arterial hypertension of the European Society of Hypertension (ESH) and of the European Society of Cardiology (ESC). Eur Heart J 2013; 34:2159–2219.

Kumar P, Clark M. Kumar and Clark's Clinical Medicine, 8th edn. London: Saunders Elsevier, 2012.

Related topics of interest

- Acute coronary syndrome (p 4)
- Cardiac failure – acute (p 80)
- Stroke (p 356)

Hyperthermia

Key points

- Normal body temperature ranges between 35.6 °C and 37.5 °C, depending on the time of day, body site measured and measurement technique used
- Pyrexia is any body temperature over 37.5 °C
- Fever, hyperpyrexia and hyperthermia are used interchangeably to represent a raised body temperature but are separate entities with different treatment strategies

Pathophysiology

- Fever represents an upward resetting of the hypothalamus, triggered by elevated prostaglandin E2 (PGE2) values, secondary to either infectious or non-infectious causes (**Table 25**). It may respond to antipyretics such as non-steroidal anti-inflammatory drugs (NSAIDs) or paracetamol, although their use for temperature control is controversial
- Hyperpyrexia represents an extremely high temperature (> 41.0 °C) with severe infections or brain injury with hypothalamic damage
- Hyperthermia represents an elevated temperature with a normal hypothalamic set point, indicating an imbalance between metabolic heat production and normal heat loss (**Table 26**). Consequently, there is no response to antipyretics

Clinical features

Hyperthermia is a core temperature > 37.5 °C (severe if greater than 40 °C or increasing at more than 2 °C per hour). It increases metabolic rate and oxygen consumption, which precipitates an increased cardiac output and minute ventilation to meet demand. The increased carbon dioxide production is initially compensated for by tachypnoea but the patient soon starts to develop a respiratory acidosis. This is compounded by the metabolic acidosis, which is caused by an increasing oxygen debt and lactic acidosis. Sweating and vasodilation cause hypovolaemia, which exacerbates the metabolic derangement if left untreated. Central nervous system dysfunction (delirium, seizures coma and permanent damage), rhabdomyolysis, acute renal failure, myocardial ischaemia and dysfunction may all follow.

Treatment

- General cooling measures: decreased ambient temperature, patient exposure, skin wetting in combination with cold air fans, commercial cooling blankets, etc. (application of ice packs to the extremities is less efficient due to vasoconstriction). More invasive measures include cold fluid given intravenously or intraperitoneally, intravascular cooling devices, or cardiac

Table 25 Causes of fever	
Infectious	**Non-infectious**
Bacterial infection	Burns
Viral infection	Pancreatitis
Fungal infection	Transfusion reactions
Device-related infection Consider: Central line-associated bacteraemia, infection associated with peripheral IV lines, drains and implanted devices	Vasculitis Gout Malignancy (haematological) Thrombo-embolic disease Intra-cranial injury: trauma, vascular, infection, tumour

Table 26 Causes of hyperthermia		
Increased heat production	Drug reaction: excessive dosage or abnormal reaction to normal dose	MDMA (ecstacy), thyroxine, MAOIs, tricyclic antidepressants, amphetamines, cocaine
	Malignant hyperthermia	Halogenated volatile anaesthetic agents, succinylcholine
	Neuroleptic malignant syndrome	Butyrophenones, phenothiazines
	Serotonin syndrome	SSRIs, excess serotonin precursors/agonists, drug interactions
	Endocrine disorders	Hyperthyroidism, phaeochromocytoma, adrenal insufficiency
Decreased heat loss	Excessive conservation	Neonates and children
	Classic (non-exertional) heat stroke – thermoregulatory failure	High environmental temperature
	Exertional heat stroke	Strenuous exercise/over-exertion
	Drug effects	Anticholinergic administration

bypass and direct cooling of blood volume
- Definitive treatment: dantrolene (for malignant hyperthermia, neuroleptic malignant syndrome, MDMA poisoning), mannitol (rhabdomyolysis) and renal replacement therapy (acute renal failure)
- General critical care: invasive monitoring to optimise fluid balance, sedation and ventilation if required

3,4-methylenedioxymetha-mphetamine (MDMA, Ecstasy) poisoning

3,4-methylenedioxymethamphetamine (MDMA) is an amphetamine derivative that was first used as an appetite suppressant but is now a recreational substance of abuse. There is a wide range of adverse effects unrelated to dose or frequency of use. Psychosis, sudden cardiac death, seizures, tachycardia, hepatitis, subarachnoid haemorrhage and acute renal failure may all occur. An acute syndrome comprising hyperthermia, disseminated intravascular coagulation (DIC), rhabdomyolysis, acute renal failure and death may present in patients with a pre-existing metabolic myopathy or genetic predisposition.

Hyperpyrexia and myoglobulinuria are triggered by a combination of sympathetic over activity, vigorous muscular activity as well as disturbance of central control. The aetiology is an augmentation of central serotonin function by stimulation of neuronal serotonin release.

The peak temperature and duration of hyperthermia are important prognostic factors and any temperature over 40 °C must be treated aggressively. Due to the similarity between this condition and malignant hyperthermia, dantrolene has been accepted as part of the treatment. Serotonin antagonists or inhibitors of serotonin synthesis have been suggested as alternative therapies.

Serotonin syndrome

A potentially severe adverse drug reaction, characterised by an altered mental state, autonomic dysfunction (including hyperthermia) and neuro-muscular abnormalities. The syndrome may follow administration of selective serotonin re-uptake inhibitors (SSRIs) such as sertraline, fluoxetine, paroxetine and fluvoxamine. It occurs either in over dosage, in interaction with excess serotonin pre-cursors or agonists (tryptophan, LSD, lithium and L-dopa), in interaction with agents enhancing serotonin (MDMA) or in drug interactions with non-SSRIs (clomipramine) or with monoamine oxidase inhibitors (MAOIs).

The cause of the syndrome appears to be excessive stimulation of serotonin receptors and as such, shows some similarity to both MDMA poisoning and neuroleptic malignant syndrome. Treatment involves withdrawal of the precipitating agents and general supportive measures, although in severe cases serotonin antagonists (chlorpromazine, cyproheptadine and methysergide) as well as dantrolene may be used.

Neuroleptic malignant syndrome

This is an idiosyncratic complication of treatment with neuroleptic drugs such as the butyrophenones and phenothiazines. Patients are usually catatonic with extrapyramidal and autonomic effects including hyperthermia. The aetiology of neuroleptic malignant syndrome (NMS) is unknown but appears to be related to antidopaminergic activity of the precipitating drug on dopamine receptors in the striatum and hypothalamus, suggesting a possible imbalance between noradrenaline (norepinephrine) and dopamine. There is no evidence of an association with malignant hyperthermia.

Clinical features include hyperthermia, muscle rigidity and sympathetic over activity. Treatment involves withdrawal of the agent and general supportive and cooling measures.

Malignant hyperthermia

This is a rare pharmacogenetic syndrome with an incidence of between 1:10,000 and 1:200,000. Most recent estimates of the population prevalence of the genetic susceptibility are between 1:5000 and 1:10,000. It shows autosomal dominant inheritance with variable penetrance. The associated gene is on the long arm of chromosome 19. Other gene sites have been proposed and there may be considerable genetic heterogeneity. MH presents either during or immediately following general anaesthesia. The cardinal signs are hyperthermia and a combined respiratory and metabolic acidosis with associated muscle rigidity. Dysfunction of the sarcoplasmic reticulum increases intracellular ionic calcium and results in depletion of high-energy muscle phosphate stores, increased metabolic rate, hypercapnia and heat production, increased oxygen consumption and a metabolic acidosis. It results from exposure to the trigger agents, namely succinylcholine and volatile anaesthetics.

On suspicion of MH, stop all trigger agents immediately. Monitor the temperature, ECG, BP and end-tidal CO_2 levels and analyse an arterial blood gas sample. Sample venous blood immediately for potassium, creatine kinase and myoglobin, as well as FBC and a clotting screen. Monitor the urine output and test for myoglobin.

Give dantrolene in bolus doses of 1 mg kg^{-1} at 10 min intervals until the patient responds, up to a maximum dose of 10 mg kg^{-1}. The average required dose is around 3 mg kg^{-1}. Dantrolene uncouples the excitation-contraction mechanism by acting at the interface between the t-tubular system and sarcoplasmic reticulum. It is a yellow/orange powder stored in a vial of 20 mg with 3 g of mannitol and sodium hydroxide. It is stored below 30 °C and protected from light. Reconstitution is with 60 mL of sterile water (it takes some time to dissolve) and forms an alkaline solution of pH 9.5.

Start general cooling measures and treat hyperkalaemia. Rehydration with intravenous fluids and promotion of a diuresis will help to prevent any myoglobin-induced renal damage. DIC may develop. After successful treatment of a suspected MH reaction, refer the patient to a specialist centre for confirmation of the diagnosis and counselling.

Further reading

Bouchama A, Knochel JP. Heat stroke. N Engl J Med 2002; 346:1978–1988.

Capacchione JF, Muldoon SM. The relationship between exertional heat illness, exertional rhabdomyolysis, and malignant hyperthermia. Anesth Analg 2009; 109:1065–1069.

Halsall PJ, Hopkins PM. Malignant Hyperthermia. Br J Anaesth CEPD Rev 2003; 3:5–9.

Related topics of interest

- Adrenal disease (p 14)
- Drug overdose and poisons (p 136)
- Hypothermia (p 186)
- Infection prevention and control (p 197)
- Thyroid gland disorders (p 365)

Hypothermia

Key points

- Accidental hypothermia occurs typically in individuals who have significant co-morbidities, who have been exposed to cold, and in whom the ability to remain euthermic is impaired
- Induced hypothermia is used to treat a variety of medical conditions
- Accidental hypothermia affects all organs

Epidemiology

In the UK, accidental hypothermia accounts for approximately 1400 hospital admissions per year. It is more common in the elderly, in those who are socially isolated, deprived or chronically debilitated, and as a result of prescribed or recreationally abused depressant drugs. There is a predictable seasonal association with more deaths in the winter. It is, however, a relatively uncommon cause of death, accounting for about 300 deaths per year in the United Kingdom. Those who die from hypothermia are more likely to be aged ≥ 70 years.

Pathophysiology

Normal morning core temperature is between 36.3 and 37.1 °C and there is a circadian fluctuation of 0.5–0.7 °C. Accidental hypothermia is defined as a core temperature of less than 35 °C and is divided into mild (35–32 °C), moderate (32–28 °C) or severe (28 °C or less). Therapeutic hypothermia has been defined as a core temperature of less than 35 °C: mild (34–34.9 °C), moderate (32–33.9 °C) and deep (< 30 °C). Normal temperature regulation is an intricate physiological process that matches heat production and dissipation, involving a variety of body systems and mechanisms. Accordingly, hypothermia may be viewed as a multi-system disorder.

Drowning

Immersion in cold water in outdoor clothing results in a slow reduction in core temperature falls slowly (one hour to decrease 2 °C in water temperature of 5 °C in laboratory conditions). When core temperature decreases to 33–35 °C, muscles are usually considerably colder; thus, neuromuscular performance is poor and there is significant risk of aspiration and hypoxia long before any temperature-related cerebral protection, which occurs only at much lower temperatures. Head immersion speeds cooling and children cool more quickly because of their large surface area to mass ratio and lack of subcutaneous fat; however, the cerebral protection sometimes seen in immersed children cannot be explained by cerebral hypothermia alone. The primitive mammalian diving reflex, where sudden cooling of the face causes intense vasoconstriction, bradycardia and decreased metabolic rate, may play a part in these rare cases.

Clinical features

These depend principally on the temperature of the patient on initial presentation, together with their responsiveness to warming interventions and the presence or absence of complications.

Cardiovascular

Cold generally induces peripheral vasoconstriction; however, hypothermia has different effects on myocardial contractility, heart rate and vascular tone such that, as body temperature falls, alterations in cardiac output may be complex, particularly because the volume loading of the heart is unlikely to remain constant. Decreasing temperature is generally accompanied by bradycardia; below 33 °C the ECG may show 'J' ('Osborn') waves at the junction of the QRS and T waves. Atrial fibrillation is relatively common. Once the temperature reaches 28–30 °C, the heart becomes prone to ventricular tachyarrhythmias including VF, less responsive to anti-arrhythmic agents, and more difficult to defibrillate.

Respiratory

Hypothermia depresses usual ventilatory responses and the protective cough reflex may be impaired. Apnoea occurs below 24 °C.

Central nervous system

Hypothermia has a depressant effect on the CNS, which may manifest as confusion, apathy, and amnesia. Consciousness is lost around 30 °C.

Metabolic

Cerebral metabolism decreases by 6–10% per 1 °C reduction in temperature. Once the core temperature is 32 °C, 'whole-body' metabolism will be between 50% and 65% lower, with consequent reduction in oxygen consumption, CO_2 production and glucose and other substrate metabolism. Fat metabolism is also affected. The overall result is a metabolic acidosis which also influences the serum potassium value. Hypothermia impairs drug metabolism: at 33 °C the clearance of many drugs is reduced by about one third.

Oxygen consumption and CO_2 production is increased by shivering but this ceases below 30 °C.

Renal

Hypothermia impairs secretion of ADH and increases resistance to its action, which results in polyuria. Peripheral vasoconstriction increases central intravascular volume, which also causes polyuria.

Haematological

Since the coagulation system comprises several temperature-sensitive enzyme systems, a hypothermia-related coagulopathy is common. Blood viscosity increases with decreasing temperature; this may be compounded by a diuresis-related increase in haematocrit. Thrombocytopenia may develop as a consequence of sequestration, bone marrow depression and platelet activation and aggregation.

Endocrine

Hypothermia causes pancreatitis and increases insulin resistance. Patients with hypoadrenalism or hypothyroidism may have

impaired thermoregulation and are more susceptible to hypothermia.

Infection and immunity

Immunity is impaired with the result that infections (wounds and respiratory tract) are more common.

Gastrointestinal

Gastric motility is impaired and reduced hepatic blood will slow drug metabolism.

Investigations

Baseline investigations for the patient presenting with hypothermia include full blood count, coagulation and routine biochemistry, together with arterial blood gas analysis, 12-lead ECG, and chest radiograph. Additional investigations may be indicated in specific patients (e.g. toxicology, thyroid and adrenal function tests).

Diagnosis

The diagnosis of accidental hypothermia is made by measuring core temperature (rectum and tympanic membrane) and by recognising cold exposure and the presence of relevant factors in the patient's history.

Treatment

Patients who present with accidental hypothermia can be returned to a normal temperature reasonably rapidly (2–3 °C per hour), while avoiding or managing complications.

- Rewarming techniques include the use of infused warmed fluids and forced-air warming; patients with severe hypothermia may require rewarming with extracorporeal membrane oxygenation or cardiopulmonary bypass
- For hypothermia-associated cardiac arrest, defibrillation is unlikely to be successful. If up to three defibrillation attempts are unsuccessful, delay further attempts until the core temperature is > 31 °C. Circulation is maintained with high-quality basic life support or other circulatory support

methods, e.g. mechanical devices or extracorporeal life support
- Patient movement and handling, intubation, and other invasive procedures are undertaken gently to avoid precipitating VF.
- Adjust mechanical ventilation to account for the decreased CO_2 production at lower body temperature and thereby avoid marked hypocapnia

Therapeutic hypothermia

Mild therapeutic hypothermia is recommended for cardiac arrest victims that remain comatose after ROSC (see Post-resuscitation care). Initially recommended for out of hospital VF cardiac arrest victims it is also often used for other cardiac arrest victims. It is also used in neonatal intensive care for hypoxic-ischaemic brain injury.

Further reading

Brown DJ, Brugger H, Boyd J, Paal P. Accidental hypothermia. N Engl J Med 2012; 367:1930–1938.
Polderman KH. Mechanisms of action, physiological effects, and complications of hypothermia. Crit Care Med 2009; 37:S186–202.
Nolan JP, Morley PT, Vanden Hoek TL. Therapeutic hypothermia after cardiac arrest. An advisory statement by the Advanced Life Support Task Force of the International Liaison Committee on Resuscitation. Resuscitation 2003; 57:231–235.
Brugger H, Durrer B, Elsensohn F, et al. Resuscitation of avalanche victims: Evidence-based guidelines of the international commission for mountain emergency medicine (ICAR MEDCOM) Intended for physicians and other advanced life support personnel. Resuscitation 2013; 84:539–546.

Related topics of interest

ICP monitoring

Key points

- ICP monitoring is recommended in many patients with severe traumatic brain injury. Other conditions where it may be useful include fulminant hepatic failure, intracranial haemorrhage, hydrocephalus and benign intracranial hypertension
- ICP monitoring allows early diagnosis and treatment of intracranial hypertension to prevent secondary neuronal injury. Relying on clinical signs alone would make early intervention impossible
- Invasive methods of monitoring ICP include parenchymal catheters and intraventricular catheters

Introduction

The rationale for monitoring ICP is that elevated ICP is a cause of secondary brain injury that is amenable to treatment. The Brain Trauma Foundation recommends monitoring of intra-cranial pressure in all salvageable patients with severe traumatic brain injury, defined as GCS 3–8 after resuscitation, who have abnormalities (haematomas, contusions, herniation or compressed basal cisterns) on CT. Some 50% of these patients will have elevated ICP. A lower level recommendation is made for ICP monitoring in severe TBI patients with a normal CT and two of the following risk factors: age>40, motor posturing, or systolic blood pressure < 90 mmHg. Only 15% of these patients will have elevated ICP. Other conditions where ICP monitoring may be useful in guiding treatment or prognostication of comatose patients include fulminant hepatic failure, intra-cerebral haemorrhage, subarachnoid haemorrhage, hypoxic brain injury, hydrocephalus and benign intracranial hypertension.

The most commonly used methods are intra-parenchymal monitor and external ventricular drain (EVD). The advantage of a ventricular catheter is that it allows drainage of CSF to treat intracranial hypertension. Although the traditional EVD with external transducer would only allow measurement of intracranial pressure when the drain was closed, newer systems with transducers within the EVD lumen allow simultaneous drainage and measurement of ICP. These catheters may underestimate ICP if the drainage holes are partially blocked. The zero point of these transducers is the foramen of Munro, which is approximated by the external auditory meatus. Intra-parenchymal monitors (e.g. Neurovent-P or Codman) are small-bore microprocessor-tipped wires inserted via a small burr hole or skull bolt, or via an even smaller specially designed 'cranial access device'. The monitor is zeroed to atmospheric pressure prior to insertion. Transducer drift is small so recalibration is not necessary. The monitor is usually placed in the non-dominant frontal lobe to reduce risk of injury to eloquent brain. Less commonly, the monitor may be placed in the pericontusional grey matter in focal injury. Monitoring on the contra-lateral side to an expanding haematoma may significantly underestimate intracranial pressure.

Sub-dural catheters have been used historically to measure ICP, but are less accurate than other invasive methods. Non-invasive methods used to estimate ICP include transcranial Doppler measurement of blood flow (pulsatility index), measurement of tympanic membrane displacement, and ultrasound measurement of the optic nerve sheath diameter. None of these are accurate enough to substitute for invasive monitoring, but they may have a future role in selecting patients for ICP monitoring where there is uncertainty, or in guiding the early institution of ICP-lowering therapy whilst awaiting placement of an invasive monitor.

ICP physiology and pathophysiology

The interpretation of the ICP value is context-sensitive. The normal resting ICP is 0–10 mmHg. Raised ICP, even over 50 mmHg commonly occurs with coughing or straining without any adverse effect. However, sustained ICP of greater than

20 mmHg is strongly associated with poor outcome following traumatic brain injury. This is because compensatory mechanisms that would normally maintain cerebral blood flow across a wide range of cerebral perfusion pressures have been exhausted in this context. In addition, pressure difference between intracranial compartments, with consequent shift of brain structures is an important cause of secondary neuronal injury. ICP monitoring allows diagnosis and treatment of these changes in a timely and targeted fashion. In the sedated patient, relying on clinical signs such as papillary dilatation or the Cushing response would only detect late rises in ICP making early treatment impossible.

The shape of the ICP waveform is similar to an arterial pressure waveform. There are three peaks: P1 is the percussion wave caused by the transmitted arterial systolic pressure, P2 is the tidal wave thought to indicate brain compliance, P3 is the dicrotic wave caused by the transmitted pressure of aortic valve closure. With an expanding intracranial space-occupying lesion with in the rigid skull box, as brain compliance reduces, the amplitude of the IPC waveforms rises, the P2 wave exceeds P1 and mean ICP begins to rise (**Figure 10**).

ICP-guided management of traumatic brain injury

The Brain Trauma Foundation guidelines recommend that ICP lowering treatments are given at a threshold of 20 mmHg, with a combination of ICP values, clinical findings and radiologic appearances used to determine the appropriate treatments. It should be noted that some interventions to lower the ICP may worsen the metabolic state of the brain, and thus continuous ICP monitoring prevents the potential harm associated with indiscriminate use of these treatments. Using ICP monitoring in combination with invasive blood pressure monitoring, cerebral perfusion pressure (CPP) can be continuously calculated allowing targeted vasopressor use. Initial CPP targets of 60 mmHg are recommended, with adjustment based on brain chemistry and cerebrovascular reactivity where these modalities are also monitored.

Measures to prevent secondary brain injury used for all patients during the early treatment of severe TBI include maintaining adequate CPP, ensuring adequate arterial oxygenation and low-normal carbon dioxide levels ($Paco_2$ 4.5–5.0 kPa), 10°–15° head up positioning and avoidance of obstruction to venous drainage, adequate sedation, normothermia and consideration of seizure prophylaxis. Where intracranial pressure rises above the threshold despite these treatments, surgical options such as CSF drainage via EVD and evacuation of space occupying lesions should be considered. Additional medical treatments that may be used as a temporising measure or where no further surgical option is available include osmotic agents (mannitol or hypertonic

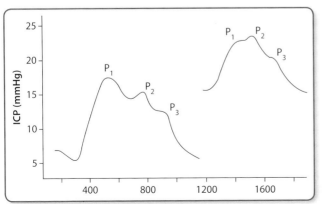

Figure 10 Intracranial Pressure Waveform. A: Normal waveform, B: reduced intracranial compliance. P1: percussion wave, P2: tidal wave, P3: dicrotic wave.

saline), hyperventilation to $Paco_2$ 4.0–4.5 kPa, induced hypothermia and barbituate coma. Decompressive craniectomy is an alternative to medical therapy for uncontrolled intracranial hypertension but its use is controversial and was associated with an increased risk of unfavourable outcome in the Early Decompressive Craniectomy in Patients With Severe Traumatic Brain Injury (DECRA) study.

Cerebrovascular pressure reactivity

Cerebrovascular pressure reactivity (PRx) is the correlation coefficient between mean ICP and mean arterial pressure averaged over a time window of 3–4 min. This can be used as a measure of cerebrovascular autoregulation. Where autoregulation is intact, a rise in MAP will lead to a fall in ICP. This is due to the reactive vasoconstriction which reduces the intra-cerebral blood volume. In a non-reactive vascular bed, increase in MAP will lead to passive vasodilation and a rise in ICP. In other words, good cerebrovascular reactivity leads to a negative PRx, whilst impaired autoregulation leads to a positive PRx. In many patients, a U shaped relationship can be demonstrated between CPP and PRx, where the CPP leading to the most negative PRx value can be termed 'optimal CPP' and used as a target in the treatment of TBI.

Further reading

Brain Trauma Foundation. Guidelines for the management of severe traumatic brain injury, 3rd edn. New York: Brain Trauma Foundation, 2010.
Forsyth RJ, Wolny S, Rodrigues B. Routine intracranial pressure monitoring in acute coma. Cochrane Database Syst Rev 2010; 2:CD002043.

Cooper DJ, Rosenfeld JV, Murray L et al. Decompressive craniectomy in diffuse traumatic brain injury. New Eng J Med. 2011; 364: 1993–1502.

Related topics of interest

Infection acquired in hospital

Key points

- Compared with community-acquired infections, infections acquired in ICU are more often caused by antibiotic resistant pathogens
- The focus of infection and prior antibiotic exposure should be sought as these inform management
- Collaboration between the critical care physicians and hospital microbiologists is required to guide appropriate empiric antibiotic choices and diagnostics

Epidemiology

Although antimicrobial resistance in the community is increasing, community-acquired infections are usually caused by relatively antibiotic sensitive organisms. In contrast, hospital-acquired infections are more likely to be caused by antibiotic resistant nosocomial bacteria or the patient's endogenous resistant flora selected by previous antibiotic therapy. Infection diagnosed 48–72 h after admission to hospital is generally considered nosocomial, rather than community acquired infection.

Results from the European Prevalence of Infection in Intensive Care (EPIC) study showed that 21% of critical care inpatients had at least one infection acquired in a critical care unit. The more recent EPIC II study showed that the predominant sites of infection were respiratory tract (63.5%), abdominal (19.6%), bacteraemia (15.1%) and urinary tract (14.3%).

Pathophysiology

Patients in critical care units are at high risk of infection because their defences are compromised by:
- Breach of the skin from intravascular cannulation, surgery or trauma
- Loss of protective commensal bacteria caused by broad-spectrum antimicrobials
- Ischaemic damage to the gut mucosa enabling translocation of bacteria and their products (e.g. endotoxins)
- Compromise of the respiratory tract through intubation and suppression of the cough reflex
- Irritation and inflammation of the uroepithelium, and pooling of urine secondary to urinary tract catheterisation
- Insertion of prosthetic material at any site causing ineffectual immune clearance of microbes and formation of biofilm
- Retrograde movement of bacteria from lower GI tract up to oropharynx due to ileus, nasogastric tube insertion and gastric acid suppression
- Depression of immune function due to immunosuppressive medication, poor nutrition and chronic disease

Diagnosis

Assessment of the systemic inflammatory response syndrome, and potential foci of infection is difficult in ICU as the classic symptoms and signs are often masked by treatment or sedation. Intensivists often rely on a low index of suspicion, blood markers of inflammation and radiological evidence of infection to institute therapy. Before antibiotics are given or changed appropriate specimens must be collected for culture to aid diagnosis and guide further treatment.

Treatment

Treatment of focus

Drainage of infected collections will result in much more rapid resolution of the infection than antibiotics alone, and may save the patient the detrimental effects of long courses of antibiotics, and long periods of inflammation.

Antibiotic choice

Most critically ill patients with nosocomial infection will need antibiotic therapy before the microbiological diagnosis is confirmed. The choice of antibiotics will be influenced by:
- The most likely site of infection and therefore the infecting organism
- Likelihood of antibiotic resistant flora as assessed by antibiotic exposure over the

last 3 months, duration of inpatient stay, normal place of residence and occupation

- Results of surveillance cultures and infection screens
- The severity of the infection. Rapidly progressing life-threatening infections warrant greater breadth of cover to include less likely pathogens while narrower spectrum antibiotics are more appropriate where the patient is stable
- The patient's vulnerability to known antimicrobial side effects, including allergies, and risk of *Clostridium difficile* infection
- Drug interactions
- Local and national resistance patterns.
- The pharmacokinetic properties of each antibiotic, especially in meningeal and urinary tract infections

Because of the importance of local population and environmental microbiology in determining likely pathogens for any given presentation, close collaboration between the critical care physicians and hospital microbiologists is required to guide appropriate empiric antibiotic choices and diagnostic opportunities.

Pathogens of particular importance

Coagulase negative staphylococci

These skin commensals cause infections of prosthetic material (commonly intravascular catheters), producing biofilm. They are generally of low virulence but often resistant to multiple antibiotics. Glycopeptides (e.g. vancomycin or teicoplanin) are usually the empiric treatment of choice.

Staphylococcus aureus

Staphylococcus aureus is a skin commensal of approximately 30% of adults. It is virulent, capable of causing destructive deep foci of infection in immunocompetent hosts, and is very difficult to eradicate from prosthetic material. A *S. aureus* bacteraemia should prompt a search for a deep focus, including a thorough clinical examination

and an echocardiogram. Blood culture is repeated 48–72 h after initiation of appropriate antibiotics to guide further investigation. In countries with a high prevalence of nosocomial methicillin resistant *Staphylococcus aureus* (MRSA), empiric antibiotic regimens must cover MRSA, but this is not required in countries or institutions where prevalence is low. The antibiotic of choice for methicillin sensitive *Staphylococcus aureus* infection is generally flucloxacillin or other anti-staphylococcal penicillin. Empiric MRSA cover can be provided by glycopeptides. Several newer Gram-positive active drugs, such as daptomycin, linezolid and tigecycline have shown non-inferiority to vancomycin for selected indications, and can be considered as alternatives. Linezolid has demonstrated improved clinical response for MRSA nosocomial pneumonia compared to vancomycin (clinical success rates 58% versus 47%, respectively). Importantly MRSA isolates are also often susceptible to other antimicrobials with Gram-positive activity and antibiotic choice should be based on sensitivity testing and patient factors.

Enterobacteriaceae

These Gram-negative organisms inhabit the gastrointestinal tract and cause intra-abdominal and urinary tract infections (UTIs), and ventilator associated pneumonia. Resistance to multiple classes of antibiotic is frequently encoded on mobile genetic elements that can be transferred between strains and between species. Enterobacteriaceae – producing extended spectrum β-lactamases, which confer resistance to almost all β-lactams except carbapenems are now commonplace in ICUs across the globe. The recent isolation of enterobacteriaceae carrying carbapenemases is of great concern. They are relatively common in hospitals in some countries, and all patients transferring from ICUs in areas of high prevalence should be isolated until screens for multi-resistant Gram-negative organisms are clear.

Reasonable empiric drugs where resistance is not expected would include, β-lactam β-lactamase inhibitor combinations or aminoglycosides, quinolones and second or third generation cephalosporins, depending on local antibiotic policy. Where there are risk factors for resistance, empiric treatment is tailored to the likely resistance pattern. Definitive treatment is guided by antibiotic sensitivities, and there is no evidence that dual therapy is more effective than monotherapy.

Pseudomonas aeruginosa

This environmental organism thrives in wet habitats. It may cause outbreaks related to colonisation of hospital water distribution systems, but more often causes sporadic colonisation of skin, gastrointestinal and respiratory tract of patients exposed to antibiotics. It can invade to cause serious infection particularly in the immunocompromised. *Pseudomonas aeruginosa* easily develops antibiotic resistance on treatment, and therefore serious infections should be treated with two anti-pseudomonal antibiotics such as an aminoglycoside plus an anti-pseudomonal β-lactam.

Acinetobacter spp. and Stenotrophomonas maltophilia

These antibiotic resistant environmental organisms are selected in settings of high broad-spectrum antimicrobial use, and can survive for long periods in dust or on hospital surfaces or equipment. They have low virulence and usually cause disease in debilitated patients previously exposed to multiple antibiotics. *Acinetobacter* spp. have variable antibiotic susceptibility, but highly resistant clones are widespread, often susceptible only to polymyxins (e.g. colistin) and variably to tigecycline and amikacin. They may colonise ICU ventilation systems necessitating ward closure. *Stenotrophomonas maltophilia* is challenging to treat, because antimicrobial susceptibility testing does not predict clinical response to treatment. First line therapy is high dose co-trimoxazole.

Clostridium difficile

Clostridium difficile causes a toxin-mediated colitis with high mortality. Approximately 2–5% of adults in the community are colonised, and risk factors for disease are age, antibiotic use and hospital admission. Once the diagnosis is suspected, scrupulous infection control is vital to avoid transfer of infectious spores to another patient. Stop broad-spectrum antibiotics or switch to a narrower spectrum drug. In the ICU setting oral vancomycin is the current treatment of choice, though fidoxamicin has similar efficacy with a lower recurrence rate and may be preferred in some cases. In patients with a non-functioning gut, vancomycin can be administered rectally or via a stoma. If a section of colon or rectum cannot be reached, IV metronidazole in addition to oral vancomycin may be given.

Enterococci

Enterococci are environmental Gram-positive bacteria and commensals of the gastrointestinal tract. They are relatively low virulence organisms, and when present as part of a mixed infection of urine or abdominal collections, specific anti-enterococcal therapy is often not required. However, they can cause significant infection, notably bacteraemia (often associated with intravascular catheters) and endocarditis. Enterococci are inherently resistant to several antibiotic classes, including cephalosporins. Resistance to glycopeptides (e.g. vancomycin or teicoplanin) can be acquired, and is more common in units with high rates of glycopeptide use. The resulting isolates are termed glycopeptide-resistant enterococci, or vancomycin-resistant enterococci, with these terms used interchangeably. Treatment can be challenging as antibiotic options are limited, and infection control procedures are important.

Candida

Candida spp. are commensals of the GI tract and colonise skin, upper respiratory tract and urinary catheters, especially in patients on antibiotics. They are frequent isolates from respiratory specimens but this usually indicates oropharyngeal colonisation because they very rarely cause pneumonia. *Candida* spp. can cause severe invasive disease, most commonly fungaemias (often secondary to vascular catheters) or deep tissue infections including endocarditis. Risk factors for invasive disease include duration of broad-spectrum antibiotics, duration of intensive care, gastrointestinal perforation or surgery, presence of intravascular catheters and isolation of *Candida* from more than one site. Fluconazole is generally the drug of choice for sensitive strains, with a 12 mg kg⁻¹ loading dose then 6 mg kg⁻¹ daily. Colonisation with fluconazole resistant strains (often non-albicans species) may occur during prolonged azole therapy. Recent Infectious Diseases Society of America guidelines (2009) recommend that, unless local surveillance demonstrates very low levels of fluconazole resistance, patients with severe infection or previous azole exposure should be treated with an echinocandin until sensitivity is known. All patients with candidaemia should have dilated fundoscopy looking for endophthalmitis, and repeat blood cultures to ensure clearance. Seek specialist advice for treatment of candida endocarditis, CNS infection or endophthalmitis.

Foci of infection

Respiratory tract infections

Epiglottitis

Nosocomial pneumonia including ventilator associated pneumonia.

In the presence of large-bore nasogastric tubes or nasotracheal tubes, consider sinusitis.

Urinary tract infection

Most patients in critical care units will have a urinary catheter *in situ*. The likelihood of the catheter becoming colonised with nosocomial bacteria increases with the duration of catheterisation. Do not treat asymptomatic bacteriuria, but if a UTI is suspected clinically send a urine specimen for culture to guide antimicrobial selection. Empirical antibiotic therapy should cover enterobacteriaceae (see pathogen section). Do not use drugs which do not reach therapeutic concentrations in urine (e.g. tigecycline).

Bloodstream infection

Bacteraemias and fungaemias are relatively common in intensive care and should prompt a search for an infected focus especially intravascular catheters, and appropriate antimicrobial therapy given.

Catheter-associated bloodstream infection

Intravascular catheters are a significant focus of infection in critically ill patients, with coagulase negative staphylococci (CONS) and *Staphylococcus aureus* the commonest isolates. Where there is sepsis in a patient with intravascular catheters, take blood cultures peripherally and through the catheters before starting empiric therapy. Empiric therapy should include a glycopeptide or alternative anti-staphylococcal drug if a catheter focus is suspected. Where catheter blood cultures are positive, confident diagnosis of catheter infection versus an alternative focus is difficult. Various microbiological criteria have been developed, but in practice the catheter is often implicated on the basis of the organism isolated, the age of the catheter and the site and conditions of catheter insertion.

Removal of the implicated intravascular catheter is preferred for most infections, but the importance of removal varies with the causative pathogen. In *S. aureus* or *Candida*, infection removal is strongly recommended as delayed removal is associated with increased mortality. Conversely with CONS infection, 7 days intravenous treatment with a glycopeptide will lead to cure in around 80% of cases, and is preferred where line replacement would be difficult. The need for ongoing antibiotic therapy after line removal also varies with pathogen. For CONS infection, no further antibiotics are usually required, but for *S. aureus* or *Candida* infection a standard course of treatment is recommended because of the risk of seeding to deep tissues.

Central nervous system infection

Consider nosocomial central nervous system infection in patients who either have CSF leak secondary to basal skull fractures, or who have CSF shunts or drains. In the latter, obtain CSF samples for culture to guide therapy, avoiding collection from a non-sterile site in CSF leak.

Abdominal sepsis including *C. difficile*

In sepsis with a presumed abdominal focus, *C. difficile* (see pathogen section) must be considered. *C. difficile* can cause an ileus instead of diarrhoea, and often presents as a new neutrophilia and abdominal pain in patients on broad-spectrum antibiotics. Where infection other than *C. difficile* is suspected, abdominal sepsis is treated with empiric antibiotics covering enterobacteriaceae (see pathogen section) and usually anaerobes. Anaerobe cover is more important where the source of infection is the distal small bowel or large bowel. Breadth of spectrum will depend on risk factors for resistant organisms (including antibiotics used for surgical prophylaxis) and risk of *Candida* infection (see pathogen section). Oesophageal rupture or leak is a specific risk factor for *Candida* infection, and cover is generally recommended. Anaerobe cover can be provided by metronidazole, or broad-spectrum drugs such as co-amoxiclav, piperacillin/tazobactam or carbapenems.

Wound infection

Post surgical wound infection is usually caused by *S. aureus* (see pathogen section) and β-haemolytic streptococci (groups A, C and G). Flucloxacillin is usually the preferred empirical antibiotic where MRSA is not suspected. Alternatives include clindamycin, cefuroxime or glycopeptides. Abdominal, groin or perineal wounds may become infected with anaerobes, and less commonly enterobacteriaceae, requiring broader spectrum antibacterials.

Further reading

Clark NM, Patterson J, Lynch JP. Antimicrobial resistance among Gram-negative organisms in the intensive care unit. Curr Opin Crit Care 2003; 9:413–423.

Pagani L, Afshari A, Harbarth H. Year in review 2010: Critical Care – Infection. Crit Care 2011, 15:238.

Raad I, Hend H, Maki D. Intravascular Catheter-related infections: advances in diagnosis, prevention and management. Lancet Infect Dis 2007; 7:645–657.

Clark NM, Patterson J, Lynch JP. Antimicrobial resistance among Gram-negative organisms in the intensive care unit. Curr Opin Crit Care 2003; 9:413–423.

Vincent JL, Rello J, Marshall J, et al. International study of the prevalence and outcomes of infection in intensive care units. JAMA 2009; 302:2323–2329.

Related topics of interest

Infection prevention and control

Key points

- Controlling nosocomial infection improves morbidity and mortality, and helps to contain healthcare costs
- Strict hygiene measures are important and are categorised as environmental, hand-washing and personal protective equipment (PPE)
- The responsible use of antibiotics has greatly increased in recent years

Introduction

Infection prevention and control is an essential and integral part of any health care service; to be effective it must be interdisciplinary and interdepartmental, with all members of staff understanding their responsibility. Controlling nosocomial infection not only improves morbidity and mortality, but also helps to contain healthcare costs. Public awareness has increased, with outbreaks of healthcare acquired infections widely reported in the media. The appearance of multi-resistant untreatable organisms is a serious concern.

Cornerstones of infection prevention and control are surveillance, hygiene, barrier nursing/isolation and antimicrobial stewardship.

Alert organisms

Infection and colonisation with certain organisms are alerts to potential hazards in the ward. Other organisms, if a particular problem in an individual unit, can be added to the list as appropriate.

- Meticillin-resistant *Staphylococcus aureus* (MRSA)
- Group A β-haemolytic streptococci (*Streptococcus pyogenes*)
- Glycopeptide resistant enterococci (e.g. vancomycin resistant *Enterococcus*)
- Multi-resistant Gram-negative organisms (e.g. extended spectrum β-lactamase or carbapenemase producers)
- *Legionella* spp.
- *Neisseria meningitidis*
- *Clostridium difficile*
- *Salmonella* spp., *Shigella* spp., *E.coli* 0157, *Campylobacter* spp.
- *Mycobacterium tuberculosis*
- Influenza, RSV
- Varicella zoster (chicken pox), measles, rubella, parvovirus, mumps
- Norovirus, rotavirus
- Creutzfeldt–Jakob disease and other prion diseases

Surveillance

Surveillance is an important part of infection control; it facilitates recognition of acute problems that demand immediate action, as well as long-term trends to guide decision making (e.g. on empirical antibiotic policies). In the UK, mandatory surveillance systems are now in place for:

- *Staphylococcus aureus* (MSSA and MRSA) bacteraemia
- Glycopeptide resistant enterococci bacteraemia
- *E. coli* bacteraemia
- *Clostridium difficile* associated disease
- Surgical site infection

Risk factors for acquiring an infection

- Critical care unit admission for more than 48 h
- Trauma
- Assisted ventilation
- Urinary catheterisation
- Vascular cannulae
- Stress ulcer prophylaxis (where gastric pH is raised)

- Poor general condition of patient, e.g. malnutrition and organ failure
- Contaminated surgical procedure

The antibiotics given to the patient will drive the selection of resistant organisms, but the likelihood of the patient becoming infected is dependent on the above risk factors and the infection prevention and control practices adhered to in the unit.

Policies and procedures

Effective infection prevention and control in the critical care unit requires adherence to the following policies and procedures:
- Antibiotic policies tailored to individual units
- Hand hygiene policies
- Asepsis and antisepsis policies tailored to individual procedures
- Isolation procedures and indications
- Decontamination policies
- Disposal of waste policies

Hygiene

Environmental

The patient and the medical staff are the most likely source of nosocomial infection but the quality of the environment also impacts on this. The air quality of a critical care unit must be of a high standard and the air in most units is filtered and diluted by a high number of air exchanges per hour. Some critical care units are equipped with high-efficiency particulate air filtration, which filters out matter down to 0.5 μm (most bacteria are larger than this). The cleanliness of the environment is as important as the quality of the air. Obvious dirt and dust is highly contaminated and linked strongly with outbreaks of MRSA and *Clostridium difficile*.

Hand washing

The choice of hand preparation (hand wash, antiseptic hand preparation or surgical scrub) is dependant on the degree of hand contamination and whether or not it is important to merely remove dirt and transient flora, or to reduce residual flora to minimum counts. This decision is dependant on the

procedure to be undertaken. All clinical staff should perform hand washing before and after contact with a patient. Hand washing is defined as the removal of soil and transient organisms from the hands. Plain soap and water is used for simple hand washing. There is no evidence that antibacterial soaps are of superior benefit in this process. Soap does not kill the resident flora but does reduce transient flora. The duration of hand washing is also important, because anti-microbial agents require sufficient time to be effective. All soap and dirt/bacteria are then rinsed off and the hands dried thoroughly with paper towels. Cloth towels harbour organisms. The tap is turned off using either elbows or a paper towel, which is then discarded.

Greater reduction of transient organisms necessitates hand antisepsis – this is achieved at the same time as hand washing by using soaps or detergents that contain antiseptics. It can also be achieved by using alcohol hand rub after removal of dirt, i.e. when hands are clean after initial hand washing. Large amounts of organic matter reduce the efficacy of alcohol. When dealing with more than one patient, hands can be cleansed between patients with alcohol alone provided all dirt is removed initially and subsequently if used up to three times. The application of 70% ethanol to hands will reduce viable organism counts by 99.7%; however, spores of *Clostridium difficile* and some viruses (e.g. norovirus) are not killed by the use of alcohol hand rub; soap and water are required in this clinical setting.

Surgical hand scrub removes or destroys transient micro-organisms and reduce resident flora for the duration of the procedure. The optimal duration of surgical scrub is about 5 min but may be agent dependant. The moist and warm atmosphere inside latex surgical gloves is ideal for the proliferation of micro-organisms; this risk is reduced by agents that have a prolonged duration of action. Alcohol-based lotions are preferred in Europe and chlorhexidine or iodophors are more popular in the United States. Poor compliance is common: health care workers do not wash their hands as thoroughly or as frequently as they should and doctors and nurses over estimate the efficacy of their hand washing. Many hospitals have adopted a 'bare below the elbow' policy to enhance thorough hand hygiene.

Personal protective equipment

Use of PPE is essential but not a substitute for careful hand hygiene. Gloves are used during invasive procedures when they provide a barrier against microbial transmission to and from the patient. Gloves must be discarded after contamination and after each patient. Transmission of organisms occurs even when gloves are used; thus, hands are washed after removal of gloves, and they are also changed between procedures on the same patient.

Isolation

The spread of infection between patients is reduced by isolating patients with transmissible infections (source or barrier isolation). This can be done in dedicated side rooms, or segregation/cohort nursing. Some infections (e.g. multi-drug-resistant tuberculosis) necessitate the use of negative pressure ventilation rooms. Patients who are colonised or infected with resistant organisms (e.g. MRSA and ESBL), or have conditions that pose a high cross-infection risk (e.g.

vomiting and diarrhoea) should be nursed in isolation. This is also considered for patients who are at an increased risk of harbouring multi-resistant organisms. Such patients are those with a history of recent hospitalisation, or a prolonged duration of hospital stay. This is a serious concern where there are high rates of resistant organisms, an outbreak at a facility, or if the patient is transferred from a geographical area with a high prevalence of multi-resistant organisms (e.g. some parts of India, South East Asia and Africa).

Antibiotic stewardship

Awareness of the need for responsible use of antibiotics has greatly increased in recent years. Key issues are:

- Association of certain classes of antibiotics with an increased risk of *Clostridium difficile* associated disease
- Selection of resistant organisms by the use of broad spectrum antibiotics
- Cost containment

Broad spectrum empirical antibiotic cover is usually initiated in critically ill patients but the spectrum is narrowed as soon as possible, following local antibiotic guidelines. ('Start smart – then focus').

Further reading

Goldmann D. System failure versus personal accountability - the case for clean hands. N Engl J Med 2006; 355:121–123.

Pratt RJ1, Pellowe CM, Wilson JA, et al. epic2: National evidence-based guidelines for preventing healthcare-associated infections in NHS hospitals in England. J Hosp Infect 2007; 65:S1–64.

Related Topics of Interest

Inotropes and vasopressors

Key points

- Inotropes primarily increase the force of contraction of the myocardium
- Vasopressors primarily increase peripheral vascular resistance
- After optimal volume loading, inotropes and vasopressors play a major role in the management of critically ill patients with circulatory failure

Introduction

Inotropes increase the force of contraction of the myocardium thereby increasing cardiac output. Vasopressors increase vascular tone. Many of the drugs used commonly in the intensive care unit (ICU) exert both inotropic and vasopressor effects, and often affect heart rate. A classification for inotropes is shown in **Table 27**; most of the drugs in clinical use are in Class 1 and act by increasing intracellular calcium.

Sympathomimetic amines

Noradrenaline (norepinephrine), adrenaline (epinephrine) and dopamine occur naturally and exert potent inotropic effects via adrenergic and/or dopaminergic receptors.

Noradrenaline (norepinephrine)

Noradrenaline is the precursor of adrenaline. It stimulates predominantly α_1-adrenergic receptors but also has significant action at β_1-adrenergic receptors. As a result, it is a powerful vasoconstrictor but also has moderate positive inotropic effects. Noradrenaline is the drug of choice to treat hypotension associated peripheral vasodilation – classically septic shock.

Adrenaline (epinephrine)

Adrenaline is used in cardiopulmonary resuscitation, where it increases the rate of return of spontaneous circulation; however, it has yet to be shown to increase long-term survival rates. It has powerful α_1- and β_1-adrenergic receptor stimulating effects. It may be used as a positive inotrope in the treatment of septic shock and cardiogenic shock (usually as a second line drug), but may increase lactic acidosis.

Dopamine

Dopamine is the immediate biosynthetic precursor of noradrenaline. It increases cardiac contractility by direct stimulation of myocardial β_1-adrenergic receptors and indirectly through sympathetic nerve terminal release of noradrenaline. It also

Table 27 Classification of inotropes	

Class 1. Drugs that increase intracellular calcium	• Calcium ion
	• Calcium channel agonists
	• Drugs that increase caradiac cyclic adenosine monophophate (cAMP)
	   – β-adrenergic agonists (adrenaline, noradrenaline, dopamine, dobutamine, dopexamine, isoprenaline, ephedrine)
	   – Phosphodiesterase inhibitors (milrinone, enoximone)
	   – Glucagon
	• Drugs that inhibit the Na^+-K^+ pump (digoxin)
	• Drugs that prolong the action potential (β-adrenergic agonists)

Class 2. Drugs that increase sensitivity of actomyosin to calcium ions	• α-adrenergic agonists, levosimendan
Class 3. Drugs that act through metabolic or endocrine pathways	Triiodothyronine

stimulates dopamine$_1$ receptors, causing coronary, renal, mesenteric and cerebral arterial vasodilation, as well as dopamine$_2$ receptors, resulting in vasodilation by inhibiting sympathetic nerve terminals. Although 'low-dose' dopamine infusion can increase renal blood flow and urine output, there is no evidence that it reduces the incidence of renal dysfunction in the critically ill and is no longer used for this purpose.

Isoprenaline

Isoprenaline is a synthetic catecholamine that increases both heart rate and contractility. It is used for the short-term emergency treatment of heart block or severe bradycardia; however, low-dose adrenaline can achieve the same goal.

Dobutamine

Dobutamine is a synthetic derivative of isoprenaline and is available in a racemic mixture. L-dobutamine is primarily an α_1-adrenergic agonist with some vasoconstrictive effects, while D-dobutamine stimulates β_1- and β_2-adrenergic receptors, thus increasing myocardial contractility while producing marked vasodilation. Use of dobutamine is popular after myocardial infarction and in cardiogenic shock because myocardial oxygen consumption is lower than other inotropes. It is often used in combination with noradrenaline – even small doses of dobutamine can restore cardiac output, which may have been reduced in response to the potent vasoconstriction produced by noradrenaline.

Dopexamine

Dopexamine is a synthetic analogue of dopamine. It acts on cardiac β_2-receptors to produce positive inotropic effect and on peripheral dopamine receptors to increase renal and gut perfusion.

Administration

All catecholamines (**Table 28**) are infused continuously through a central venous catheter because their half life is short (1–2 min) and extravasation may cause tissue necrosis. They achieve steady state plasma concentration within about 5–10 min. Infusions are titrated against clinical end points, such as cardiac output, mean arterial pressure, base deficit and lactate.

Cardiac glycosides

Digoxin

Cardiac glycosides increase the force of myocardial contraction and slow conduction through the atrioventricular node. Digoxin is the most commonly used cardiac glycoside. The effects are mediated largely by an increase in intracellular calcium concentration and by inhibition of the membrane sodium-potassium pump. Peripheral resistance is also increased by a direct mechanism and by increased sympathetic activity. Normal half-life of about 35 h to 5 days can be prolonged by renal impairment. It has a small inotropic effect. Digoxin may reduce cardiac output in cardiogenic shock because of its effect on after-load.

The potential for toxicity in the critically ill patient is increased by hypokalaemia, hypomagnesaemia, hypercalcaemia, hypoxia and acidosis. The use of digoxin in acute congestive heart failure is limited by its delayed onset of action, except in patients with atrial fibrillation and a rapid ventricular rate, in whom it may help to control the ventricular response.

Phosphodiesterase inhibitors

Amrinone, milrinone and enoximone

These drugs increase cyclic adenosine monophosphate (cAMP) by inhibiting phosphodiesterase III, the enzyme responsible for the breakdown of cAMP producing positive inotropic and lusitropic (improved diastolic relaxation) effect. They may be beneficial in patients with reduced ventricular compliance or predominant diastolic failure. They cause a dose-dependent increase in cardiac output and reduction in right- and left-sided

Table 28 Dose range, receptor of action and effect on cardiac output (CO) and systemic vascular resistance (SVR) of the mainly used cathecolamines

Inotrope and dose range	Adrenergic receptor α_1	Adrenergic receptor β_1	Adrenergic receptor β_2	Dopaminergic receptor$_{1,2}$	CO	SVR
Dopamine low dose ($0.5–2\ \mu g\ kg^{-1}\ min^{-1}$)	–	+	–	+++	↑	↓
Dopamine medium dose ($2–5\ \mu g\ kg^{-1}\ min^{-1}$)	+	++	–	+	↑	↑
Dopamine high dose ($5–10\ \mu g\ kg^{-1}\ min^{-1}$)	++	+	–	++	↔	↑↑
Noradrenaline ($0.03–0.2\ \mu g\ kg^{-1}\ min^{-1}$)	+++	++		–	↔	↑↑
Adrenaline ($0.01–0.15\ \mu g\ kg^{-1}\ min^{-1}$)	+++	+++	++	–	↔	↔/↑
Dobutamine ($2.5–10\ \mu g\ kg^{-1}\ min^{-1}$)	+/–	+++	++	–	↑	↓

– = no stimulation, + = mild, ++ = moderate, +++ = intense stimulation
↑ = increase, ↑↑ = highly increase, ↓ = decrease, ↔ maintain equal
Dose ranges above are commonly quoted but individual requirements can vary greatly (requiring considerably higher doses) and tachyphylaxis can also occur.

filling pressures and systemic vascular resistance. Their effects are additive to those of the digoxin and are synergistic with sympathomimetic amines. They might be used as an alternative or an adjunct to dobutamine. Amrinone facilitates atrioventricular conduction, causing an acceleration of ventricular rate in patients with atrial fibrillation. Enoximone has more inotropic effects than vasodilation. Prolonged use of these drugs may increase mortality in patients with severe heart failure.

Calcium sensitisation

Levosimendan

Levosimendan is an inodilator working through calcium sensitisation of contractile proteins and opening of ATP-dependent potassium channels. The combination of positive inotropy with anti-ischaemic effects produced by potassium-channel opening offers potential benefits in comparison to currently available intravenous inotropes, which may be harmful in patients with myocardial ischaemia. In patients with heart failure, levosimendan produces

dose-dependent increases in cardiac output and reduced pulmonary artery occlusion pressure. At higher doses, it can induce tachycardia and hypotension. There is some evidence that short-term intravenous treatment with levosimendan might improve the long-term survival of patients with heart failure.

Vasopressors

Metaraminol, phenylephrine and ephedrine

Vasopressors raise blood pressure by acting on α-adrenergic receptors to constrict peripheral vessels; this may reduce splanchnic and peripheral perfusion. By increasing cardiac after-load, they may greatly increase myocardial oxygen consumption. Ephedrine also increases heart rate.

Vasopressin (anti-diuretic hormone)

Vasopressin release from the posterior pituitary is mediated by high serum osmolality or baroreflex. Vasopressin acts through V_1-receptors in the blood vessels (vasoconstriction) and through V_2-receptors in the kidney (anti-diuretic). Under normal conditions anti-diuretic hormone (ADH) regulates the water balance of the body and has little influence on haemodynamics. However, vasopressin is also an important regulator of blood pressure in septic shock, when its stores may be depleted. A continuous infusion of low-dose vasopressin (0.04 units min^{-1}) will increase blood pressure significantly and enable a reduction in the dose of alternative vasopressors such as noradrenaline, without reducing mortality rates.

Further reading

Bangash MN, Kong ML, Pearse RM. Use of inotropes and vasopressors agents in critically ill patients. Br J Pharmacol 2012; 165:2015–2033.

Overgaard CB, Dzavik V. Inotropes and vasopressors: review of physiology and clinical use in cardiovascular disease. Circulation 2008; 118:1047–1056.

Russell JA, Walleys KR, Singer J, et al. Vasopressin versus norepinephrine infusion in patients with septic shock. N Engl J Med 2008; 358:877–887.

Related topics of interest

Liver failure – acute

Key points

- Acute liver failure (ALF) is rare – there are just 400 cases each year in the United Kingdom
- Paracetamol toxicity accounts for 60% of cases of ALF in the UK
- All patients with severe ALF should be referred early to a liver centre
- Those patients who do not require transplantation have a good outcome (80% survival)

Definition

Acute liver failure (ALF) is the abrupt loss of hepatic function, presenting with jaundice, coagulopathy and hepatic encephalopathy, in the absence of pre-existing liver disease, with acuity of onset variously defined as less than 8–26 weeks. It is further sub-classified according to the time between the onset of jaundice and the subsequent onset of encephalopathy, as hyper-acute (0–7 days), acute (8–28 days) and sub-acute (28 days to 12 weeks) [**Table 29**]. This sub-classification has implications for the prognosis and the incidence of cerebral oedema.

Epidemiology

ALF is a rare condition (incidence 1–6 per million); there are approximately 400 cases each year in the United Kingdom and approximately 2500 in the United States. ALF is a distinct entity from acute-on-chronic liver failure in patients with cirrhosis, with important differences in presentation and management.

Pathophysiology

Necrotic injury of liver cells leads to cell rupture and release of cytosolic proteins and liver enzymes. Many synthetic and detoxification mechanisms are impaired, including the transport systems for bilirubin, leading to cholestasis and conjugated hyperbilirubinemia. Loss of Kupffer cell function has a profound effect on clearance of endotoxin, bacteria and inflammatory mediators and is associated with an increased risk of infection and systemic inflammatory response syndrome.

Causes of ALF

The main causes of ALF are shown in **Table 30**.

Paracetamol toxicity is the commonest cause of ALF in the United Kingdom (60%) and United States (40%). Viral hepatitis is the predominant cause of ALF in the developing world, but is an uncommon cause of ALF in the United States and much of Northern Europe, where drug-induced ALF predominates.

Early identification of the cause of ALF is essential, as certain cause-specific interventions are recommended:

- Paracetamol ingestion – *N*-acetylcysteine

Table 29 Sub-classification and typical characteristics of acute liver failure			
Sub-type of acute liver failure	Hyperacute	Acute	Sub-acute
Jaundice to encephalopathy (days)	0–7 days	8–28 days	28 days–12 weeks
Cerebral oedema	Frequent (69%)	Frequent (56%)	In-frequent (14%)
Coagulopathy	+++	++	+
Prognosis without transplantation	Good	Moderate	Poor
Typical cause	Paracetamol, hepatitis A, E	Hepatitis B	Drug-induced (non-paracetamol)

Adapted from O'Grady et al. Acute liver failure: redefining the syndromes. Lancet 1993; 342: 273-75 and Bernal et al. Acute Liver Failure. Lancet 2010; 376: 190–201.

Table 30 Main causes of acute liver failure	
Infective	Hepatitis A, B, C, D, E, seronegative
	Herpes Simplex, cytomegalovirus, Epstein-Barr, varicella
Drug-related	Paracetamol, anti-tuberculous drugs (e.g. isoniazid), anti-convulsants (e.g. phenytoin), antibiotics (e.g. nitrofurantoin), propylthiouracil
Vascular	Ischaemic hepatitis, Budd-Chiari syndrome
Pregnancy-related	Acute fatty liver of pregnancy, HELLP syndrome
Metabolic	Wilson's disease, Reye's syndrome
Toxin-related	*Amanita phalloides*, herbal remedies, *Bacillus cereus*
Miscellaneous	Auto-immune hepatitis, lymphoma, trauma

- Acute fatty liver of pregnancy and HELLP syndrome – delivery of the infant
- Acute Budd – Chiari syndrome – porto-systemic shunt procedure or thrombolysis
- Herpes simplex hepatitis – acyclovir
- Autoimmune hepatitis - methylprednisolone
- Hepatitis B infection – lamivudine;
- Amanita mushroom poisoning – IV penicillin and acetylcysteine

Clinical features

ALF usually presents with malaise, nausea and jaundice. As the liver failure progresses, encephalopathy becomes the characteristic feature.

Encephalopathy is typically classified into grades 1–4:

Grade I: Disordered sleep pattern, altered mood, impaired concentration, mild confusion and asterixis.

Grade II: Drowsy but rousable, disorientation, able to talk but slurred, moderate confusion and marked asterixis.

Grade III: Very drowsy, agitation, aggression, incoherent and marked confusion.

Grade IV: Coma, may respond to painful stimuli (IVa), may not respond to painful stimuli (IVb), sluggish pupil reaction to light, myoclonus, seizures and signs of intra-cranial hypertension (IVc).

Hypotension with high cardiac output and reduced systemic vascular resistance is commonly seen in ALF. Differentiating ALF from septic shock can be difficult.

Investigation and diagnosis

There is no specific diagnostic test for ALF. Extensive investigations are undertaken to assess the cause of the ALF. Bilirubin is elevated and a level > 300 μmol L^{-1} implies severe disease. Plasma AST and ALT are markedly elevated, reflecting hepatocellular damage. The prothrombin time (PT) is elevated and is used as an indicator of the severity of the disease. Other common abnormalities are hypoglycaemia, hyponatraemia, hypomagnesaemia, respiratory alkalosis and metabolic acidosis.

Imaging of the liver (USS or CT) should focus on liver size, demonstration of hepatic vascular flow and evidence of chronic liver disease.

Treatment

All patients with severe ALF should be referred early to a liver centre. Mortality in ALF is attributed mainly to cerebral oedema, multi-organ dysfunction syndrome, and sepsis. Multi-organ support is required to prevent and manage these complications and allow maximum hepatic regeneration. Patients who will not achieve sufficient regeneration need early identification and consideration for emergency liver transplantation.

Management of hepatic encephalopathy and cerebral oedema

Cerebral oedema and raised intracranial pressure (ICP) distinguishes the encephalopathy of ALF from that associated with chronic liver disease; however, cerebral oedema is not universal in ALF encephalopathy. Risk factors for cerebral oedema include high-grade encephalopathy (grades 3 and 4), elevated serum ammonia (greater than 150–200 μmol L^{-1}), hyperacute and acute progression of encephalopathy, infection or systemic inflammatory response syndrome (SIRS), and requirement for vasopressor support or renal replacement therapy (RRT). Cerebral oedema develops in 80% of patients with grade IV encephalopathy and is the cause of death in about 20–25% of patients with ALF.

Neuroimaging is not reliable in diagnosing early intra-cranial hypertension but is valuable to exclude other problems such as intracranial bleeding or stroke.

Management of intracranial hypertension

Many liver centres will place ICP monitors in selected ALF patients with advanced (stage 3 or 4) encephalopathy, but good quality trials showing improvements in survival from ICP monitoring are lacking. Commonly used goals are ICP < 25 mmHg, with a cerebral perfusion pressure (CPP) of 50–80 mmHg.

Intracranial hypertension can be managed with intravenous mannitol 20% or hypertonic saline. Moderate hypothermia (32–34 °C), haemofiltration and albumin dialysis systems (e.g. Molecular Adsorbents Recirculating System) may also have a role in controlling ICP. Steroids do not appear to help.

Controlling ammonia levels

Ammonia levels are elevated in ALF contributing to the pathogenesis of hepatic encephalopathy and cerebral oedema. However, lactulose and non-absorbable antibiotics (e.g. rifaximin and neomycin) do not improve survival or severity of ICP or encephalopathy in ALF.

Intubation and mechanical ventilation

Intubation is normally required once advanced encephalopathy becomes evident, for both airway protection and to help control of ICP. Neurological deterioration can be very rapid. Intubation is required for patients in grade III or IV encephalopathy. Consider elective intubation and ventilation before transfer to a liver unit for patients with grade I–II encephalopathy.

Haemodynamic management

Give careful attention to fluid balance to maintain tissue perfusion. Some centres advocate the avoidance of large volumes of Hartmann's solution to prevent lactate accumulation.

Add noradrenaline to maintain mean arterial pressure above 60–65 mmHg or CPP 50–80 mmHg. Adrenaline is not recommended because of potential detrimental effects on mesenteric and hepatic blood flow. Anti-diuretic hormone analogues (e.g. vasopressin and terlipressin) have also been used successfully in ALF.

Relative adrenal insufficiency occurs in up to 62% of patients with ALF, and corticosteroids (200–300 mg hydrocortisone per day) improve vasopressor responsiveness.

Renal dysfunction

Start RRT early in the course of acute kidney injury to prevent the attendant acidosis and volume overload (exacerbating raised ICP).

Coagulopathy

Severe derangements in coagulation profile are usual. Fresh frozen plasma (FFP) is reserved for invasive procedures or clinically significant bleeding. Prophylactic FFP only briefly reduces INR in ALF patients, does not reduce the risk of significant bleeding or need for transfusion, but obscures the trend of PT which is useful as a prognostic marker.

Recombinant factor VIIa is safe and effective in reversing the coagulopathy in ALF patients, e.g. to facilitate placement of ICP monitors.

Infection

Sepsis is the cause of death in 11% of cases of ALF, and the success of liver transplantation is significantly reduced by systemic infection. Pyrexia, tachycardia and leucocytosis may all be caused by the liver injury alone, and diagnosis of infection requires regular cultures. Fungal infections, in particular *Candida*, may develop in up to one third of patients with ALF.

Prophylactic antibiotics (both intravenous and selective decontamination of the digestive tract) do not improve survival; however, empiric use of antibiotics is often recommended.

Acetylcysteine

Acetylcysteine may improve circulatory dysfunction and impaired oxygen delivery in ALF from all causes, and can improve non-transplanted survival if given early to ALF patients with low-grade (stage I–II) coma.

Liver transplantation

Liver transplantation is the only effective therapy for ALF patients who fail to recover spontaneously.

Multiple prognostic indicators and scoring systems have been devised to predict outcome and the need for transplant in ALF. The King's College Criteria are among the most commonly used (**Table 31**). These criteria exhibit a sensitivity, specificity, positive predictive value, and negative predictive value of 55%, 94%, 87% and 78%, respectively. No current prognostic scoring system reliably identifies all patients requiring liver transplantation and regular discussion with a transplant centre is vital.

Outcome

Outcome data from ALF is dependent on many factors including the cause of the ALF and the availability of transplantation. Overall, those patients who don't require transplantation have good outcome (80% survival). Those who receive a transplant also do well (60–80% survival at one year), but those who meet transplant criteria but do not receive a transplant do poorly (< 10% survival). Advances in critical care management have reduced reported mortality to 33% in some centres. Transplant-free survival is generally highest (50%) for patients with paracetamol overdose, hepatitis A virus, ischaemic hepatitis or pregnancy-related disease.

Table 31 King's College Criteria for increased mortality in acute liver failure	
Paracetamol-induced acute liver failure	Non-paracetamol-induced acute liver failure
Arterial pH <7.3 (after fluid resuscitation)	PT of greater than 100 s (INR > 6.5)
Or all three of:	Or three of the following five criteria:
PT greater than 100 seconds (INR > 6.5)	1. Age < 10 years or > 40 years
Hepatic encephalopathy coma grades 3 and 4	2. ALF caused by non-A, non-B, non-C hepatitis, halothane or other drug aetiology
Serum creatinine greater than 300 µmol L^{-1}	3. Jaundice to encephalopathy > 7 days
	4. PT > 50 s (INR > 3.5)
	5. Serum bilirubin > 300 µmol L^{-1}

Further reading

Bernal W, Auzinger G, Dhawan A, Wendon J. Acute liver failure. Lancet 2010; 376:190–201.

Stravitz RT, Kramer DJ. Management of acute liver failure. Nat Rev Gastroenterol Hepatol 2009; 6:542–553.

Stravitz RT, Kramer AH, Davern T, et al. Intensive care of patients with acute liver failure: Recommendations of the U.S. Acute Liver Failure Study Group. Crit Care Med 2007; 35:2498–2508.

Related topics of interest

Liver failure – chronic

Key points

- Cirrhosis accounts for 2.6% of admissions to UK intensive care units (ICUs) and the incidence of chronic liver disease is increasing
- Patients with chronic liver failure commonly present to the ICU with massive haemorrhage or sepsis
- The mortality rate in patients with cirrhosis and severe sepsis requiring organ support is 65–90%

Epidemiology and Pathophysiology

Cirrhosis is the commonest chronic liver disease (CLD) seen in the intensive care unit (ICU), accounting for 2.6 % of all ICU admissions in the United Kingdom. It is characterised by fibrosis leading to distortion of the hepatic architecture and the formation of regenerative nodules. The incidence of CLD is increasing and while alcohol-related liver disease (ARLD) is still the commonest cause in the United Kingdom, obesity is an increasingly important co-factor. Other causes of CLD include infections (Hepatitis B and C), drugs (methotrexate), autoimmune (primary biliary cirrhosis) and hereditary conditions such as Wilson's disease. CLD often presents late in the disease process with an acute presentation of jaundice, encephalopathy or gastrointestinal bleeding. It is not uncommon for patients to require intensive care before a definitive diagnosis of irreversible liver disease has been made. Whilst CT scanning and ultrasound can help support a diagnosis of cirrhosis, confirmation requires a biopsy. ARLD usually progresses from fatty infiltration (reversible) to cirrhosis (irreversible) with considerable overlap. The clinical presentation can be the same for both groups.

Clinical features

Cardiovascular

Cirrhosis is characterised by a low systemic vascular resistance (caused mainly by splanchnic vasodilation) leading to mild hypotension, tachycardia and a high cardiac output provided that the myocardium is reasonably preserved. A significant proportion may also have cirrhotic cardiomyopathy, which is characterised by a normal or increased cardiac output and contractility at rest, but a blunted response to inotropes or stress. An echocardiogram will give a better assessment of function than cardiac output measurement alone. The right ventricle may be markedly affected if porto-pulmonary hypertension is present.

Nutrition and gastrointestinal function

Malnutrition is very common in this group – all patients are presumed to be Vitamin B and C deficient. Constipation can lead to encephalopathy in otherwise well patients with CLD. Prescribe lactulose early, aiming for 4–5 stools per day. Protein restriction (to avoid encephalopathy) is no longer advocated.

Infection

Whilst gut associated bacteria are common pathogens, these patients are also at high risk of fungal sepsis – consider treating this empirically. Sepsis from pneumonia or spontaneous bacterial peritonitis (SBP) is a common cause of acute decompensation of CLD.

Ascites

Drain ascites if it is the source of infection (SBP) or if it is impeding ventilation. All patients with ascites should have a diagnostic tap to exclude SBP. This is best guided by ultrasound because bowel damage can occur if there are intra-abdominal adhesions. If ascitic drains are placed, leave them for no more than 6 h. Replace each 3 L of drained ascites with 20% albumin 100 mL, to reduce the risk of the post-paracentesis syndrome (CVS and renal dysfunction) after large volume paracentesis.

Electrolytes and renal function

Most patients with severe CLD have muscle wasting and serum urea and creatinine values must interpreted in this context. The urea may be raised secondary to GI bleeding rather than renal dysfunction and the serum creatinine is usually low. A 'normal' creatinine may signify significant renal impairment. The serum sodium is often low in patients with CLD but the whole body sodium is high. Pay careful attention to sodium balance; a low sodium (125-135 mmol L^{-1}) is tolerated. Hypokalaemia secondary to diuretics is common and can worsen encephalopathy.

Alcohol withdrawal

Most patients will require management of alcohol withdrawal. All hospitals should have a local policy. A combination of vitamin replacement and reducing benzodiazepines are usually used.

Common clinical scenarios in patients with CLD presenting to ITU

Massive upper GI bleeding secondary to varices

Portal hypertension in excess of 12 mmHg may provoke variceal bleeding. The first episode of variceal haemorrhage is associated with a mortality rate of 21–50% and the risk of re-bleeding is 50–70%. Most patients with varices have cirrhosis and 40% die of associated medical problems. Most modern therapy involves emergency endoscopy and banding of oesophageal varices or cyanoacrylate glue injection for gastric varices. Balloon tamponade is still used if adequate control cannot be established with endoscopy. Compressive oesophageal stenting has also been used with success. These patients are at high risk of aspiration during and after the procedure and require a definitive airway for protection. They are usually cold, coagulopathic and hypovolaemic. Severe oesophagitis is common after all these procedures – prescribe acid suppression therapy. The protein load will aggravate hepatic encephalopathy. Place a nasogastric tube as soon as possible after the bleeding has been controlled and start lactulose. Give empirical antibiotics (e.g. ciprofloxacin for 5 days) for all CLD patients who have had a variceal bleed. If bleeding is difficult to control, consider a shunt procedure: transjugular intrahepatic portosystemic shunt is the procedure of choice, but may precipitate a severe encephalopathy.

Severe sepsis

Patients with CLD are immunosuppressed and prone to bacterial infections. The commonest causes of infection are SBP and pneumonia. The diagnosis of SBP is established by a positive ascitic fluid bacterial culture and/or an elevated ascitic fluid absolute polymorphonuclear leukocyte count (≥ 250 cells mm^{-3})

Hepatic encephalopathy and low GCS

Occult GI bleeding, constipation, infection, drugs and metabolic derangement can all precipitate an encephalopathy. Patients are not at risk of raised intracranial pressure but require airway protection. Correct electrolyte abnormalities (especially sodium and potassium), exclude and treat infection and manage occult or overt GI bleeding.

Hepatopulmonary syndrome

This is a poorly understood condition that presents with intra-pulmonary shunting and hypoxia in patients with cirrhosis. It is usually worse when the patient is lying down and must be differentiated from pneumonia or pulmonary embolus. It has a very poor prognosis.

Alcoholic hepatitis

The diagnosis is made in a patient with history of significant alcohol intake who develops fever and worsening liver function tests, including elevated bilirubin and aminotransferases. In most cases, the transaminase enzymes are only moderately raised. Patients with hepatitis do not necessarily have cirrhosis. The presenting features range from mild jaundice and raised liver enzymes to severe coagulopathy and encephalopathy. Establishing the diagnosis is important because steroids are given for more severe cases.

Acute kidney injury

Renal dysfunction is common among patients with decompensated cirrhosis. Withdrawing nephrotoxic agents, providing a normal mean arterial pressure for that patient and normalising intravascular volume are the most important therapeutic interventions. The prognosis is very poor if renal replacement therapy is required. In CLD patients in ICU, acute kidney injury (AKI) is most commonly caused by a combination of hypovolaemia and acute tubular necrosis. Hepatorenal syndrome (HRS) is characterised by a low fractional excretion of sodium and a progressive rise in the plasma creatinine concentration in a patient with CLD. The kidneys are histologically normal. Differentiation from pre-renal renal failure is difficult and the diagnosis can be made only when pre-renal causes have been excluded. If patients have failed to respond to the management of pre-renal renal failure, consider a trial treatment with terlipressin and albumin. Some patients with HRS will respond to this but it is used cautiously because it can precipitate gastrointestinal and cardiac ischaemia.

Investigations

An abdominal ultrasound is undertaken to quantify ascites and assess the size and echo pattern of the liver, which may also give an indication of the reversibility of the liver disease. The portal vein is imaged to exclude portal vein thrombosis. Consider endoscopy in intubated patients even if they are not overtly bleeding – many will have varices, which can be treated before they bleed.

Prognosis

The Child-Pugh score (**Table 32**) is used to assess the prognosis of CLD. The MELD score (Model for End-stage Liver Disease) is also used to predict mortality and can be used to provide a priority ranking for liver transplantation. In the United Kingdom, hospital mortality for cirrhotic patients is greater than 50% with little change over recent years. Mortality in patients with cirrhosis and severe sepsis requiring organ support is 65–90%, compared with 33–39% in those without. The prognosis for ICU patients is related to extent of organ failure and not the aetiology of the CLD. Sequential Organ Failure Assessment scores can help to discriminate the survivors from the non-survivors. In CLD patients, renal failure is associated with a poor prognosis regardless of the cause. Unlike patients with many other chronic medical conditions, some of these patients will have reversible disease. Every effort should be made to avoid sepsis in this group (care bundles/airway protection) and if organ function continues to deteriorate despite adequate treatment, consider withdrawal of treatment.

Table 32 Child-Pugh scoring system			
Parameter	Points		
	1	2	3
Ascites	Absent	Slight	Moderate
Bilirubin, umol/L	<34	34–50	>50
Albumin, g/L	>35	28–35	<28
*INR	<1.7	1.71–2.3	>2.3
Encephalopathy	None	Grade 1–2	Grade 3–4
Child Class A: 5–6 points, 1 year survival 100%, 5 year survival 85%.			
Child Class B: 7–9 points, 1 year survival 81%, 5 years survival 57%.			
Child Class C: 10–15 points, 1 year survival 45%, 5 year survival 35%.			

Further reading

Flood S, Bodenham A, Jackson P. Mortality of patients with alcoholic liver disease admitted to critical care: a systematic review. Journal of Intensive Care Society 2012; 13:130–135.

McAvoy N, Thomson E, Wilson ES. Hepatic failure. Anaesth Intensive Care Med 2012; 13:161–165.

O'Brien AJ, Welch CA, Singer M, Harrison DA. Prevalence and outcome of cirrhosis patients admitted to UK intensive care: a comparison against dialysis-dependent chronic renal failure patients. Intensive Care Med 2012; 38:991–1000.

Related topics of interest

Major haemorrhage

Key points

- Major haemorrhage leads to cellular dysfunction, multi-organ failure and disseminated intravascular coagulopathy
- Transfusion of higher ratios of plasma and platelets to blood (e.g. 1:1:1.5) is now advocated
- Permissive hypotension and restricted crystalloid use is also part of the haemostatic resuscitation strategy in trauma

Definition

Massive blood loss in adults is defined as one or more of the following:
- Replacement of total circulating blood volume within 24 h; this corresponds to about 70 mL kg^{-1} of body weight or 5 L in a 70 kg patient
- Replacement of 50% of total circulating blood volume within 3 h
- Need for at least 4 units of red cells (RBCs) within 4 h in the setting of continued major bleeding
- Blood loss exceeding 150 mL min^{-1}
- Need for plasma and platelet replacement

Epidemiology

Massive bleeding may result from trauma (either penetrating or blunt) or as a complication of surgery including gastrointestinal, intra-abdominal, vascular or cardiac operations. It may also occur in obstetrics, patients with hepatic impairment, those with inherited coagulation abnormalities and patients on anticoagulant and antiplatelet treatments.

Pathophysiology

Shock occurs when systemic perfusion does not meet the oxygen and metabolic demands of body tissues. This leads to a cascade of events causing worsening cellular and organ dysfunction.

Cellular respiration within RBCs and skeletal muscle switches from aerobic to anaerobic as a result of impaired oxygen delivery (despite an increase in the oxygen extraction ratio to 50%). This results in only two ATP molecules being generated for each glucose molecule metabolised, compared with 38 during normal aerobic metabolism. Lactic acid is produced as a waste product. Normal cellular functions become disrupted causing impaired homeostasis (e.g. membrane ion channel disruption producing intracellular sodium and calcium accumulation). Cell lysis contributes to hyperkalaemia. The resulting metabolic acidosis shifts the oxyhaemoglobin dissociation curve to the right and impairs enzyme and protein functions. Direct tissue trauma causes the release of inflammatory mediators and cytokines producing further cellular dysfunction.

The worsening metabolic acidosis combined with the haemodynamic changes associated with shock causes organ dysfunction.

Compensatory responses to haemorrhage are categorised into immediate, early and late:
- Immediate – the loss of blood volume is detected by low-pressure stretch receptors in the atria and arterial baroreceptors in the aorta and carotid artery. Efferent responses from the vasomotor centre trigger an increase in catecholamines, which causes arteriolar constriction, venoconstriction and tachycardia
- Early compensatory mechanisms (5–60 min) include movement of fluid from the interstitium to the intravascular space and mobilisation of intracellular fluid
- Long-term compensation to haemorrhage includes:
  - Reduced glomerular filtration rate
  - Salt and water re-absorption (aldosterone and vasopressin)
  - Thirst
  - Increased erythropoiesis

If hypovolaemia is not reversed, progressive decompensation ensues. As compensatory mechanisms fail, acidosis worsens, perfusion decreases and inflammatory mediators are released resulting in fluid and protein loss into the extravascular space. Gastrointestinal mucosal integrity becomes impaired by ischaemia and endotoxins enter the systemic circulation, augmenting the systemic inflammatory response syndrome.

Finally, multiple organ failure ensues in the refractory stage together with disseminated intravascular coagulopathy. At this stage the chances of survival are extremely low.

Clinical features

The clinical features of haemorrhage are divided into four different stages (see **Table 33**). There is wide inter-patient variation in these responses. Age, the presence of co-morbidities, medications and conditions such as pregnancy will impact on the pattern of these classic responses to haemorrhage.

Investigations

Investigations are undertaken concurrently with treatment. Assess the patient using a multidisciplinary systematic approach. Control obvious external haemorrhage, rapidly assess and control the airway (with cervical spine control in trauma cases), breathing, circulation, disability and exposure/environmental factors.

In well organised trauma centres, rapid whole-body computed tomography (CT) may negate the need for initial chest and pelvic radiographs, but the latter will be required if the patient is too unstable for immediate CT. Focused assessment with sonography for trauma (FAST) undertaken in the emergency department will confirm or exclude the presence of free fluid in the peri-hepatic, peri-splenic, hepato-renal, pelvic and pericardial spaces.

Laboratory investigations including urgent full blood count, cross-matching of blood (although group O or group confirmed blood is often issued in these circumstances), clotting screen, fibrinogen level and biochemistry tests are required in any patient who is actively bleeding; however, routine coagulation tests often take too long to provide results to guide transfusion needs. In major centres, point of care testing, including thromboelastography and thromboelastometry, is used to guide blood product transfusion requirements at the 'bedside' and identify abnormal coagulation processes that routine laboratory coagulation tests may not identify.

Surgical control is required for major haemorrhage in operative, post-operative and obstetric cases. Emergency endoscopy is necessary for upper gastrointestinal bleeding.

Treatment

The management of major haemorrhage is divided into supportive measures to establish homeostasis together with specific treatment of its underlying cause.

Activate the hospital's major haemorrhage protocol. Control obvious sources of bleeding using tourniquets, pelvic binding devices, a Minnesota tube in upper GI bleeding and

Table 33 Stages of hypovolaemic shock				
Stage	I	II	III	IV
Blood loss	< 15% < 750 mL	15–30% 750–1500 mL	30–40% 1500–2000 mL	> 40% > 2000 mL
Heart rate (beats min⁻¹)	<100	> 100	> 120	>140
BP	Normal	Decreased pulse pressure (increase in diastolic pressure)	Hypotension	Refractory hypotension
Respiratory rate	Slight increase	Tachypnoea	Moderated tachypnoea	Severe tachypnoea
Urine output (mL h⁻¹)	> 30	20–30	< 20	0–10
Mental state	Normal/anxious	Agitated	Confused	Unconscious

topical haemostatic agents, e.g. QuikClot, HemCon. Give high concentration oxygen and establish large bore intravenous access. In massive haemorrhage, give RBC, fresh frozen plasma (FFP) and platelets early, restrict crystalloid use and consider the use of permissive hypotension (see below). Actively warm the patient, all blood products and fluids. Obtain X-rays, ultrasound and CT scans promptly and consider the need for surgery early. In the operating room, use cell salvage where possible.

Blood product support may be available with 'shock packs' containing a combination of products including RBC, FFP, platelets and cryoprecipitate. Use of higher ratios of FFP and platelets to red blood cells used earlier during massive transfusion may improve outcomes. Give calcium if the plasma ionised calcium value is < 0.9 mmol L^{-1}. The use of tranexamic acid has been associated with reduced mortality and morbidity in bleeding trauma patients provided it is given within 3 h of injury. Until recently, recombinant Factor VII (rFVIIa) was used as part of many massive transfusion protocols where other interventions had failed. Its use has diminished following a randomised controlled trial in seriously injured patients that failed to show improved outcome with rFVIIa. Fibrinogen concentrate (does not need thawing, can be given more rapidly) is an alternative to FFP but is not yet licensed in the United Kingdom.

Damage control resuscitation originated in the military but is now used widely in civilian trauma. Outcomes are improved by preventing hypothermia, acidosis and coagulopathy (the lethal triad) from the point of injury. Haemostatic resuscitation using early and higher ratios of plasma and platelets to blood, limited crystalloid resuscitation and permissive hypotension will help to minimise coagulopathy.

Aggressive fluid resuscitation may lead to clot disruption and a dilutional coagulopathy. Using smaller aliquots of fluid may be appropriate in cases of major haemorrhage together with lower target blood pressures. Blood pressure targets are based on expert-opinion and observational studies in animals and humans: a systolic BP of 80–90 mmHg is suggested in both blunt and penetrating trauma whilst a systolic BP of 100 mmHg is used in patients with haemorrhage and major head injury so that cerebral perfusion is maintained.

Damage control surgery involves an operation of short duration (<60 min) to control haemorrhage, followed by a period of stabilising the patient and restoring normal physiology before definitive surgery is undertaken.

Interventional radiology has a major role in the management of major haemorrhage although is dependant on the availability of an appropriately trained interventional radiologist. Radiologically guided arterial embolisation may prevent the need for surgery in certain cases.

Complications

Invasive ventilatory support, intravascular access techniques, tracheostomy insertion and prolonged ICU stay all carry risks for the major haemorrhage patient. Specific complications include coagulopathy, transfusion-related acute lung injury, acute respiratory distress syndrome, multiple organ failure and sepsis.

Further reading

Jackson K, Nolan J. The role of hypotensive resuscitation in the management of trauma. Journal of Intensive Care Society 2009; 10:109–114.

The Brain Trauma Foundation, The American Association of Neurological Surgeons, The Joint Section on Neurotrauma and Critical Care. Resuscitation of blood pressure and oxygenation. J Neurotrauma 2000; 17:471–478.

Lier H, Bottiger BW, Hinkelbein J, et al. Coagulation management in multiple trauma: a systematic review. Intensive Care Med 2011; 37:572–582.

Thomas D, Wee M, Clyburn P, et al. Blood transfusion and the anaesthetist: management of massive haemorrhage. Anaesthesia 2010; 65:1153–1161.

Shakur H, Roberts I, Bautista R, et al. Effects of tranexamic acid on death, vascular occlusive events, and blood transfusion in trauma patients with significant haemorrhage (CRASH-2): a randomised, placebo-controlled trial. Lancet 2010; 376:23–32.

Related topics of interest

Meningitis and encephalitis

Key points

- Meningitis and encephalitis are life-threatening infections with significant morbidity and mortality if diagnosis is delayed
- Early empirical antibiotic and anti-viral treatments reduce mortality and post infectious complications
- CSF analysis and PCR can modify therapy but lumbar puncture is associated with risk and is should be done selectively
- Dexamethasone should precede or accompany first dose of antibiotics and continue for 4 days, for bacterial meningitis

Meningitis and encephalitis are potentially life-threatening. The aetiology for both can be divided into infective and non-infective processes. Bacteria and viruses can cause both meningitis and encephalitis and opportunistic organisms including protozoa and fungi may cause either in immunocompromised patients. Non-infective processes, such as connective tissue or autoimmune disorders and malignant infiltration can also cause meningo-encephalitis.

Epidemiology

Bacterial meningitis is more common in childhood. The peak incidence of about 1:1000 occurs in children under 1 year of age. The likely causative organism depends upon the age group. Group B streptococci, *Escherichia coli* and *Listeria monocytogenes* are the commonest organisms in neonates. In older children, bacterial meningitis is usually caused by *Neisseria meningitidis* (meningococcus) and *Streptococcus pneumoniae* (pneumococcus). The incidence of *Haemophilus influenzae* meningitis has declined by more than 99% in countries that have adopted an effective immunisation program.

In adults, the most common infecting organisms are meningococci and pneumococci, the latter being more common in elderly patients. A few cases are caused by Gram-negative bacilli and *Listeria* following ingestion of contaminated food such as unpasteurised soft cheeses. Infection with *Listeria* is more common at the extremes of age, pregnancy and in immunocompromised patients. Post-traumatic meningitis is usually caused by pneumococcus, whereas device (CSF drains and shunts)-associated meningitis is usually caused by coagulase-negative staphylococci or *Staphylococcus aureus*. Tuberculous meningitis is more common in children, the elderly, the immunocompromised and the immigrant population.

Encephalitis is also more common in child hood, with an incidence of 0.7–13.8 per 100,000 for all ages. The Herpes simplex virus (HSV) is the most common organism in developed countries. The age of presentation is bimodal with peaks at the extremes of ages in the young and the elderly. HSV-1 is responsible for 90% of cases. Other Herpes viruses such as HSV-2, Varicella Zoster (VZV) and Cytomegalovirus cause infection almost exclusively in the immunocompromised. Enteroviruses (Coxsackie, Echo) are another important group of viruses causing aseptic meningitis and encephalitis. Non-infective encephalitis occurs as a result of antibody mediated processes against voltage-gated potassium channels and N-methyl-D-aspartate antibody receptors, cases of which are increasingly recognised.

Pathology

Meningitis is an intense inflammatory process of the meninges extending into the brain and is usually caused by the presence of bacteria and their fragments within the CSF. The inflammatory reaction causes neuronal damage and death from oedema.

The disease process during encephalitis causes oedema of the brain parenchyma with neuronal cell lysis. In response to this, inflammatory lymphocytes are released. Microglial cells proliferate and surround affected neurons ultimately phagocytosing them. The area of brain involved depends on the causative pathogen, the host's immunocompetence status and other host factors. In viral encephalitis, the virus will replicate and will disseminate via blood stream or via retrograde axonal transport. In autoimmune aetiologies, antibodies directed against normal brain structures play a central role with perivascular and demyelination visible microscopically.

Clinical features

Differentiation between encephalitis and meningitis on clinical signs and symptoms alone remains a challenge with considerable overlap. The classical features of meningism – headache, nuchal rigidity, fever, reduced conscious level are clinical features in both entities. Symptoms of disorientation and focal neurological signs favour encephalitis as a diagnosis but are not specific. Physical findings such as Kernig's (pain on extending the knee from 90° angle when hip is flexed) and Brudzinski's signs (involuntary lifting of knees when head is lifted when supine) – are common in adults but not reliably present in children. Infants with meningitis and raised intracranial pressure (ICP) may have a bulging anterior fontanelle. In tuberculous meningitis, symptoms and signs may develop insidiously over several weeks. A characteristic petechial rash usually accompanies meningococcal meningitis if there is concomitant septicemia.

Investigation

The diagnosis of meningitis/encephalitis is confirmed by examination of CSF obtained by lumbar puncture. If there are signs of raised ICP (e.g. reduced conscious level or papilloedema) or any focal neurology, a CT scan should be performed to look for any complications of the meningitis/encephalitis such as cerebral oedema or to rule out any other differential diagnoses (listed in **Table 34**); however, a CT scan can appear normal in the presence of raised ICP. When there is clinical and/or CT scan evidence of raised ICP, the diagnostic benefits of lumbar puncture should be weighed against the risks, in these circumstances, it may be safer to treat the patient empirically.

The CSF should be sent for immediate gram stain and microscopy to give an initial indication of whether there is an infective cause and what it may be.

Rapid antigen testing and DNA PCR testing of blood to identify the pathogen is available in most centres. *Neisseria meningitidis* samples should be obtained from the patient as soon as possible as early samples are more likely to test positive.

Table X summaries the characteristic CSF patterns seen in patients with CNS infections.

In addition to biochemistry, microscopy and culture all CSF from suspected encephalitis should be sent for HSV, VZV and enterovirus PCR. This will identify 90% of cases. Additional serum and CSF testing may

Table 34 Summary of characteristic CSF patterns in meningitis and encephalitis					
Characteristic	Normal	Bacterial	Viral	TB	Fungal
Opening pressure (cmH$_2$O)	10–20	High	Normal/High	High	Very High
Appearance	Clear	Cloudy	'gin' clear	Cloudy/Yellow	Clear or Cloudy
Cells	<5	100–500,00	5–1000	<500	0–1000
WCC differential	Lymphocytes	Neutrophils	Lymphocytes	Lymphocytes	Lymphocytes
CSF/plasma glucose ratio	50–66%	Low (<50%)	Normal (50–66%)	V Low (<30%)	Normal (50–66%)
Protein (g/L)	<0.45	>1	0.5–1	1–5	0.2–5

Points of caution
1. A raised lymphocyte count is seen in early bacterial meningitis, Listeria monocytogenes, tuberculous and viral meningitis and, importantly, may be seen in partially treated bacterial meningitis. If organisms are not seen on microscopy, culture may take weeks to exclude tuberculosis.
2. In up to 5–15% of suspected encephalitis cases the initial CSF is non diagnostic, in these cases a second sample should be obtained within 48 hours.

be required for atypical presentations and in immunosuppressed patients.

Treatment

Antibiotics and anti-viral therapy should be commenced empirically and given immediately when suspicion of meningitis or encephalitis is raised. The choice of antibiotic is determined by the likely pathogen, the patient's age and local anti-biograms. Microscopy, culture and sensitivity will later confirm the appropriateness of the antibiotic given. Expert microbiological advice should always be sought. In practice, a third-generation cephalosporin such as ceftriaxone is appropriate for adults and children (but not neonates).

Patients over 55 years of age, Neonates, Pregnant women and immunosuppressed patients require additional cover for *Listeria* with either amoxicillin or ampicillin depending on local protocols.

Patients with suspected or proven HSV encephalitis should receive within 6 hours of presentation IV Acyclovir (10 mg kg^{-1}) three times a day. It is important to use reduced dosing in renal impairment and ensure patients are adequately hydrated. Acyclovir should be continued for 14–21 days during which time PCR results will become available.

Unfavourable outcomes in meningitis are thought to be due to inflammation in the sub-arachnoid space. Dexamethasone is recommended to be given before or with the first dose of antibiotic and continued for 4 days, for adult bacterial meningitis is. Steroids are also part of guidelines for the management of meningitis in children and young adults and recommended if it is less than 12 h from the first dose of antibiotics and the LP results show specific markers. If started early, steroids may reduce the incidence of permanent hearing loss in children with *H. influenzae* or pneumococcal meningitis.

The role of steroids in HSV encephalitis is not established. Their use remains controversial and restricted to specialist centres.

Complications

Seizures

Treatment with benzodiazepines, phenytoin or phenobarbital alone or in combination is usually effective. Resistant seizures and status epilepticus may require thiopental or propofol, necessitating intubation.

Raised ICP

This may result from cerebral oedema and/or hydrocephalus, brain abscess, sterile sub-clinical effusion or empyema for which specific neurosurgical treatment may be indicated.

Strategies for the management of raised ICP include:

1. Intubation and ventilation to ensure control of oxygen and CO_2 levels to normal parameters
2. Resuscitation with fluids and use of vasoactive drugs to maintain cerebral perfusion pressure.
3. Nursing in 30° head up to reduce venous pressure and maximise cerebral perfusion.
4. Ensuring normothermia, sometimes requiring active cooling to reduce cerebral metabolic demand.
5. Ensuring normoglycemia avoiding peaks and troughs in serum glucose.
6. Osmotic diuretics such as mannitol may have role in acutely reducing ICP but repeated use in context of impaired blood brain barrier may paradoxycally worsen cerebral odema.

Neurological deficits

Various nerve palsies and learning difficulties may persist in patients recovering from meningitis. Nerve deafness is particularly common.

Prophylaxis

Prophylaxis should be provided to those in extended or close contact with proven infected meningococcal disease. It is not usually considered necessary for contacts of patients with pneumococcal meningitis. Suspected meningitis or meningococcal disease is a notifiable disease. This is essential to trigger contact tracing and chemoprophylaxis. Individuals without functional spleens should receive menigococcal, pneumococcal and Haemophilus vaccination.

Prognosis

With current antibiotic and antiviral regimens and treatment strategies, the mortality of both meningitis and encephalitis the United Kingdom is 10% or less. Approximately 10% of meningitis survivors suffer permanent neurological damage. In patients with encephalitis, the incidence of persistent neurological deficits is considerably higher with personality, memory changes, fatigue and epilepsy affecting as much as one third of patients.

Further reading

Brouwer MC, Thwaites GE, Tunkel AR, van de Beek D. Dilemmas in the diagnosis of acute community-acquired bacterial meningitis. Lancet 2012; 380:1684–1692.

Van de Beek D, Brouwer MC, Thwaites GE, Tunkel AR. Advances in treatment of bacterial meningitis. Lancet 2012; 380:1693–1702.

Solomon T, Michael BD, Smith PE, et al. Management of suspected viral encephalitis in adults – Association of British Neurologists and British infection association National guidelines. J Infect 2012; 64:347–373.

National Institute for Health and Care Excellence (NICE). Bacterial meningitis and meningococcal septicaemia, Clinical Guidence 102. London: NICE, 2010.

Related topics of interest

Meningococcal sepsis

Key points

- Meningococcal septicaemia is a medical emergency with a high mortality. It may affect any age group
- Early antibiotics are essential in suspected cases of meningococcal septicaemia (e.g. ceftriaxone or cefotaxime 2 g IV bd)

Epidemiology

Meningococcal disease can occur in any age group, but rates are highest in infants (related to waning maternal antibodies) and adolescents. Epidemics may occur in adolescents and young adults.

Acquisition of meningococci via respiratory secretions or saliva can lead to colonisation, and in some cases progresses to invasive disease. Host factors, such as absence of protective antibodies, genetic polymorphisms, and immunodeficiency (e.g. HIV and splenectomy) convey susceptibility to invasive disease.

Pathophysiology

Neisseria menigitidis is both a common commensal of the human upper respiratory tract as well as being a virulent pathogen. Meningococci occur as encapsulated or unencapsulated Gram-negative dipplococci, with 13 distinct serotypes. Serogroups B and C most commonly cause disease in industrialised countries, but the incidence of infection with serotype C is reducing since the introduction of vaccination campaigns.

In fulminant meningococcemia, lipooligosccharide (endotoxin) in whole and disintegrated bacteria is abundantly present in plasma and CSF, leading to widespread immune cell activation via cytokines and other inflammatory mediators. This immune activation manifests clinically as the systemic inflammatory response and multi-organ dysfunction syndrome. Excessive activation of the coagulation system and concomitant down-regulation of the fibrinolytic system leads to disseminated intravascular coagulation. Concentrations of natural anticoagulants including protein C and anti-thrombin are reduced.

Clinical features

Meningitis is the most common presentation of invasive meningococcal disease. In this case, the inflammatory response is relatively compartmentalised to the central nervous system.

In contrast, fulminant meningococcal sepsis is characterised by rapid proliferation of organisms in the circulation, with widespread immune activation. Patients present with petichial, rapidly spreading rash (purpura fulminans) and rapidly progressive shock often without clinical signs of meningitis. Death may occur in a matter of hours.

Early meningococcemia presents with a non-specific prodrome of fever, lethargy, headache, anorexia, nausea and vomiting, cold or discoloured extremities, arthralgia and myalgia. These symptoms are similar to those caused by non-threatening viruses, making a confident diagnosis in these early stages difficult. Warning signs of impending/worsening shock requiring urgent intervention include:

- Rapidly progressive rash
- Poor peripheral perfusion: Capillary Refill Time > 4 s, oliguria and/or systolic arterial pressure less than 90 mmHg (hypotension often a late sign)
- Respiratory rate less than 8 or greater than 30 breaths per minute
- Pulse rate less than 40 or greater than 140 beats per minute
- Acidosis: pH less than 7.3 or base excess less than – 5 mmmol/L
- White cell count less than 4×10^3 per μL

Investigations

FBC; U+Es; Blood sugar, LFTs; CRP, Clotting profile. Meningococcal sepsis is often associated with a low white cell count, indicative of the destructive exaggerated immune response.

Arterial or venous blood gases. Elevated lactate is an important indicator of tissue hypoperfusion in septic shock.

Microbiology: Blood culture, throat swab, EDTA blood for PCR. Studies have shown that PCR of blood samples has a higher sensitivity than blood culture.

Do not delay antibiotic administration while awaiting results of investigations.

LP is not indicated in suspected meningococcal septicaemia. It has a low yield, with a high risk of complications.

Diagnosis

Difficulty in early diagnosis, combined with the rapid deterioration seen in fulminant meningococcemia, mean a high index of suspicion is required to make the diagnosis – always consider the possibility of meningococcal disease in the presence of non-specific symptoms such as fever, headache, lethargy and vomiting. In particular, children with non-specific symptoms such as fever and rash require frequent clinical review to detect progressive symptoms.

Treatment

Initial management should follow and ABC approach with particular attention to signs of impending shock. Appropriate intravenous antibiotics (e.g. cefotaxime or ceftriaxone 2 g bd) should be administered without delay. Initial resuscitation should include high flow oxygen and volume resuscitation. Patients should be managed in a critical care area. Frequent assessment of response to resuscitation with invasive monitoring, measurement of urine output, serum lactate and other markers will guide further treatment, including the need for early invasive ventilation, inotropic support and renal replacement therapy.

A role for adjuvant treatments for sepsis such as corticosteroids, vasopressin and immunoglobulin are controversial.

Complications

The exaggerated immune response leads to cardiovascular, pulmonary, renal, adrenal and neurological dysfunction in addition to disseminated intravascular coagulation. Adrenocortical infarction (Waterhouse–Friderichsen syndrome) has been well described in meningococcal sepsis, leading to impaired glucocorticoid and mineralocorticoid production. Thrombotic lesions and vascular complication can lead to loss of digits or limbs leaving survivors significantly handicapped. Mortality may be >40% for patients in shock with multi-organ failure.

Further reading

National Institute for Health and Clinical Excellence (NICE). Bacterial Meningitis and Meningococcal Septicaemia In Children, Clinical Guidence 102. London: NICE, 2010.

Scottish Intercollegiate Guidelines Network (SIGN). Management of Invasive Meningococcal Disease In Children And Young People. Edinburgh: SIGN, 2008.

Heyderman RS. Early Management of suspected bacterial meningitis and meningococcal septicaemia in immunocompetent adults, 2nd edn. J Infect 2005; 50:373–374.

Related topics of interest

- Meningitis and encephalitis (p 217)
- Sepsis – management (p 329)
- Sepsis – pathophysiology (p 333)

Myasthenia gravis

Key points

- Myasthenia gravis is an autoimmune disease in which antibodies are directed against the neuromuscular junction
- Treatment involves cholinesterase inhibitors, immunosuppression and thymectomy in selected patients
- A myasthenic crisis is characterised by life threatening respiratory failure, intubation should be considered if vital capacity falls below 20 mL kg^{-1}

Epidemiology

Myasthenia gravis has an annual incidence of 10–20 new cases per million of the general population per year. Onset is bimodal typically affecting young women aged 20–30 years old and older men aged 60–80 years old.

Pathophysiology

Myasthenia gravis is an autoimmune disease. T-cell dependent immunological attack is directed at the post-synaptic nicotinic acetylcholine receptors in the neuromuscular junction. The number of functional receptors is reduced by antibodies blocking the attachment of acetylcholine and inducing degradation of the receptors. Complement mediated destruction causes loss of the normal convolution of the muscle membrane. Patients with myasthenia gravis typically have 30% of the normal number of functional acetylcholine receptors. The reduced receptor density causes decreased amplitude of post-synaptic action potentials and failure to initiate muscle contraction. Thymic hyperplasia is present in the majority of patients and approximately 10–15% have a thymoma.

Clinical features

Symptoms reflect fluctuating weakness in voluntary muscle exacerbated by exercise and relieved by rest. Ptosis and diplopia are the most common initial symptoms and in 15% the disorder remains confined to the ocular muscles. Weakness is painless and may be localized or widespread. Sensation and reflexes are intact. Respiratory muscles are normally affected only mildly compared to ocular, facial, bulbar and limb muscle groups. Generalised weakness is usually worse proximally but occurs in a varying distribution and is usually asymmetrical.

Investigations

The 'Tensilon test' involves administering intravenous edrophonium, a short acting anticholinesterase, and assessing the response. Resuscitation facilities should be available as profound bradycardia and weakness can be precipitated. Muscle power should improve after 30 s and be sustained for approximately 5 min. Acetylcholine receptor antibodies (Anti-AChR antibodies) or antibodies to muscle specific receptor tyrosine kinase (Anti-MuSK antibodies) are detected in 88–94% of patients with generalised disease. Repetitive nerve stimulation studies and single-fibre electromyography recordings have diagnostic sensitivity of 75% and 95%, respectively. Once the diagnosis is established, a chest computed tomography (CT) or magnetic resonance imaging (MRI) scan should be performed to look for an associated thymoma.

Diagnosis

The initial diagnosis is a clinical one. Serological and electrophysiological studies are used for confirmation. The Tensilon test has a high sensitivity but poor specificity, so false positives limit its usefulness.

Treatment

Long-term treatment utilises anti-cholinesterase agents and chronic immunosuppression with consideration of the need for surgery (thymectomy). Short-term, rapid immunomodulating treatments such as plasmapheresis and intravenous immunoglobulin are used in the critically ill patient.

Anticholinesterase therapy aims to increase neuromuscular transmission by slowing breakdown of acetylcholine at the neuromuscular junction. Pyridostigmine is the most commonly used drug.

Immunosuppression limits disease activity. Corticosteroids are standard therapy but may cause a transient exacerbation when starting treatment. Azathioprine, mycophenolate or ciclosporin is used as adjuncts to steroid treatment.

Thymectomy is indicated in younger patients and those with an associated thymoma. The aim is to induce remission and reduce the requirement for immunosuppressive drugs. Full benefits may take several years to manifest.

Plasmapheresis induces a short-term remission of weakness in patients with a myasthenic crisis or with severe disease before thymectomy. A reduction in circulating autoantibodies leads to a rapid onset but short-term improvement in muscle strength. Intravenous immunoglobulin has indications similar to plasmapheresis and is equally effective but is simpler to administer and has less complications.

Complications

The progression of myasthenia gravis usually peaks within the first 2 years of onset. The most significant complications are the myasthenic crisis and the cholinergic crisis.

Myasthenic crisis

A myasthenic crisis is characterised by disease activity involving respiratory muscle weakness leading to life threatening respiratory failure. Most myasthenic crises occur within the first 5 years of the onset of disease. A myasthenic crisis can be triggered by treatment omission, stress, infection, surgery, pregnancy or drugs. A broad range of drug groups can exacerbate myasthenia including antibiotics: aminoglycosides and fluroquinolones, anticonvulsants: phenytoin and gabapentin, anaesthetic agents: diazepam, ketamine and lidocaine and

other drugs: glucocorticoids, beta-blockers, diuretics and the oral contraceptive pill. A comprehensive medication history should always be taken.

Severe bulbar weakness often accompanies respiratory failure and this predisposes patients to aspiration. Vital capacity and maximal inspiratory force are the most useful measures of respiratory function during a myasthenic crisis, though these need to be interpreted carefully in conjunction with the clinical picture. Vital capacity should be monitored regularly (2–4 h) and the patient admitted to a critical care area if there is concern. Respiratory muscle weakness leads to progressive basal lung collapse and secretion retention increasing the risk of infection. Some patients may fatigue very suddenly, changes in oxygen saturations and blood gas readings are unreliable and may only change after the onset of life-threatening respiratory failure.

Intubation and mechanical ventilation is best performed electively in a controlled manner rather than reacting to respiratory collapse. Intubation should be considered if vital capacity falls to less than 20 mL kg^{-1} or the maximum inspiratory pressure is less than $-30 \text{ cmH}_2\text{O}$. Patients with myasthenia gravis are relatively resistant to depolarising neuromuscular blockers (suxamethonium) requiring higher doses but have an increased tendency to develop dual block. They are extremely sensitive to non-depolarising neuromuscular blocking agents such as atracurium or rocuronium.

Precipitants for the crisis, particularly infection, need to be addressed and plasmapheresis or intravenous immunoglobulin therapy started. Cholinesterase inhibitors are usually withdrawn until a response to treatment is seen and weaning from the ventilator can be commenced. Regular physiotherapy is recommended to reduce the risks of ineffective cough and prolonged ventilation. Plasmapheresis and intravenous immunoglobulin start to work within several days. Steroid therapy is indicated if there is an inadequate response. The timing of weaning from ventilation is dependent on the return of bulbar and respiratory muscle function.

Myasthenic crises are usually associated with prolonged hospitalisation and can carry a mortality rate of 5%.

Cholinergic crisis

During a cholinergic crisis, excess acetylcholinesterase inhibitors cause weakness due to continuous depolarisation of the post-synaptic membrane due to an increased availability of acetylcholine. The presence of excess sweating, salivation, lacrimation, fasciculation, confusion, colic, miotic pupils, bradycardia, hypertension or seizures caused by both excess muscarinic and nicotinic stimulation suggests a cholinergic rather than myasthenic crisis. Cholinergic crises however are rare particularly in patients taking less than 120 mg of pyridostigmine every 3 h. Muscle strength will only improve with edrophonium in a myasthenic rather than cholinergic crisis but this is unreliable and hazardous in this setting and so no longer recommended as a test.

Further reading

Meriggioli MN, Sanders DB. Myasthenia gravis: diagnosis. Semin Neurol 2004; 24:31–39.

Richman DP, Agius MA. Treatment of autoimmune myasthenia gravis. Neurology 2003; 61:1652–1661.

Jani-Acsadi A, Lisak RP. Myasthenic crisis: guidelines for prevention and treatment. J Neurol Sci 2007; 261:127–133.

Related topics of interest

Neurological diseases

Key points

- The identity and stage of a neurological disease may impact on a patient's response to treatment in the intensive care unit (ICU)
- Neurological disease may predispose patients to respiratory compromise
- Drugs used commonly in the ICU may have unpredictable or dangerous effects in patients with underlying neurological disease

Among the wide variety of neurological diseases, this topic will focus on three that are more likely to require treatment on the ICU.

Duchene muscular dystrophy and Becker's muscular dystrophy

Duchene muscular dystrophy (DMD) and Becker's muscular dystrophy (BMD) are X-linked recessive inherited disorders. However, approximately a third of all cases are new mutations.

Epidemiology

DMD occurs in approximately 1 in 3000–3500 live male births.

Pathophysiology

Dystrophin is a protein that binds to muscle cell membranes to anchor muscle cells to the extracellular matrix. Mutations within the Xp21 region (the dystrophin gene) lead to the failure in the production of functional dystrophin in DMD. Mutations leading to defective but partly functioning variants of dystrophin occur in BMD, with reduced dystrophin levels.

DMD is usually apparent by the age of 3–5 years and often causes death by the second or third decade. In BMD, the disorder is less severe, may present much later and has a slower clinical progress. Muscle weakness may only be obvious as a young adult.

Clinical features

Patients have proximal muscle weakness. There is difficulty in standing and running with pseudohypertrophy of the calf muscles. As the disease progresses the patients become severely restricted and wheelchair bound with contractures and scoliosis. Lung function is reduced. Cardiomyopathy and cardiac arrhythmias occur. Death is usually the result of cardiac or respiratory failure.

Investigations

Muscular dystrophy is considered when there is abnormal muscle function in a male, an abnormal creatine kinase (CK) value or raised transaminases. The CK value is significantly elevated (100–200 times normal). Muscle biopsy reveals necrosis, fat and absence of dystrophin. Electromyography (EMG) reveals a myopathic picture. Genetic testing identifies a dystrophin gene mutation.

Diagnosis

If the above investigations are positive the diagnosis is confirmed.

Treatment

Glucocorticoids are used to slow the decline in muscle strength and function.
Musculoskeletal management: Physiotherapy with stretching, positioning and orthoses. Surgical intervention to the lower limbs and spine. Devices to assist and support function.
Respiratory management: Regular vaccinations. Lung recruitment and cough assist techniques. Consideration for non-invasive ventilation.
Cardiac management: Heart failure and arrhythmia drugs and management.
Gastrointestinal management: Prevention and management of constipation. Reflux treatment. Nutritional support. Assessment of swallow.
Pain management.
Psychosocial support: for the patient and family.

Carrier detection is important. Sisters of a patient have a 50% probability of DMD gene carriage. 70% of carriers have an elevated CK, EMG and muscle biopsy abnormalities. Carriers should be offered genetic counselling and advice.

Complications

Cardiac arrhythmias, cardiomyopathy, muscle contractures and respiratory failure develop. Patients are prone to hyperpyrexia and rhabdomyolysis when exposed to depolarising muscle relaxants (DMR) and volatile anaesthetics. Avoid these drugs because the resulting acidosis and hyperkalaemia may cause cardiac arrest. Non-depolarising muscle relaxant (NDMR) action is unpredictable.

Multiple sclerosis

Epidemiology

The prevalence of multiple sclerosis (MS) varies considerably. It occurs more commonly at latitudes that include northern Europe and North America. It rarely occurs at the equator. It has an incidence of 60–100 per 100,000 population in northern Europe. White populations are more commonly affected than asian or black. The median and mean ages of onset are 23.5 and 30, respectively. Females are affected approximately twice as commonly as males. The difference between females and males appears to be increasing.

Pathophysiology

The precise mechanism remains unclear. A widely accepted theory is that MS is initiated by auto-reactive lymphocytes and results in an inflammatory autoimmune disorder. As the disease progresses, microglial activation and chronic neurodegeneration occur. This results in plaques of demyelination which occur at a number of anatomical sites. These include the optic nerves, the periventricular area, the brainstem and its connections to the cerebellum and the corticospinal tracts and posterior columns of the cervical spinal cord. Active disease causes demyelination affecting nerve impulse conduction. Remission halts inflammation and re-myelination may occur.

Clinical features

MS may exhibit a number of different clinical patterns. Relapsing and remitting (80–90% of MS), primary progressive (10–20%), secondary progressive (follows on from relapsing and remitting form) and fulminant MS (<10%). The relapsing and remitting form presents as optic neuropathy, brainstem demyelination and spinal cord lesions.

Investigations

MRI brain and spinal cord is the definitive imaging technique. Multiple plaques are evident and vary from 2 to 20 mm. CSF examination may not be necessary but will reveal oligoclonal IgG bands in 80% of cases. The mononuclear CSF count may be elevated.

Diagnosis

MS requires two or more attacks affecting different parts of the central nervous system. MRI findings aid diagnosis. CSF examination with oligoclonal IgG bands is not specific but may also aid diagnosis.

Treatment

The treatment of MS is tailored to fit the different clinical patterns or the disease activity. Acute exacerbations may be managed with high dose steroids (typically 100 mg methylprednisolone intravenously (IV) for 5 days, followed by dose reduction orally). Consider plasma exchange if neurological symptoms are severe.

Relapsing and remitting MS can be treated with interferon β drugs. High-dose steroids may also be necessary if there is little therapeutic benefit or the disease modifying agents are poorly tolerated.

For secondary progressive MS, monthly intravenous glucocorticoid pulses (typically 1000 mg of methylprednisolone) are used. The addition of intravenous cyclophosphamide may benefit younger patients. Methotrexate, with or without monthly glucocorticoid pulses may benefit some patients but, failing this, interferon may be considered.

Currently, no randomised controlled trials have shown benefit for any treatment of primary progressive MS. Current treatment options are empiric and may include pulsed steroid and additional methotrexate as described for secondary progressive MS.

Complications

MS symptoms are exacerbated by change in temperature, infection, pregnancy, stress, surgery and anaesthesia including the use of local anaesthetic drugs. Non-depolarising muscle relaxants can be used, but depolarising muscle relaxants should be used with caution. Treatment of underlying MS causes immunosuppression, affected patients may be prone to atypical or opportunistic infections.

Motor neurone disease

Motor neurone disease (MND) is a progressive degeneration of upper and lower motor neurones of the spinal cord, the cranial nerve motor nuclei and those in the cerebral cortex. The majority of cases (approximately 90%) occur spontaneously and the remaining 10% are inherited. The mutation is present on chromosome 21q which codes for the free radical scavenging enzyme copper/zinc superoxide dismutase.

Epidemiology

The incidence of the spontaneously occurring form is approximately 2 cases per 100,000 per annum. It usually presents between 50 and 75 years old, with a slight male preponderance over the age of 70.

Pathophysiology

Cortical motor cells degenerate causing axonal loss and gliosis in the corticospinal tract. The resulting gliosis causes bilateral white matter loss. There is spinal cord atrophy, thinning of ventral roots and loss of large myelinated fibres in motor nerves. Muscles supplied by affected nerves display atrophy.

Clinical features

In MND, sensory symptoms are absent. Patients with MND may have clinical features of both upper and lower motor neurone disease. Upper motor neuron findings include weakness, hyperreflexia and spasticity. Lower motor neuron findings include weakness, atrophy or amyotrophy, and fasciculations. Four broad patterns are seen clinically: Progressive muscle atrophy starts with unilateral small muscle wasting of the hand. Bilateral involvement soon becomes apparent. Fasciculation due to spontaneous stimulation of large motor units is common. Cramps but not pain may occur. Wasting and weakness is evident. Reflexes may be lost, present or exaggerated dependent on the site of the predominant lesion. Amyotrophic lateral sclerosis affects the lateral corticospinal tracts causing a progressive spastic tetraparesis. In addition, lower motor neurone signs and fasciculations are present. Progressive bulbar and pseudobulbar palsies cause dysarthria and dysphagia. Primary lateral sclerosis is rare but presents with a progressive tetraparesis and pseudobulbar palsy. 5% of patients develop frontotemporal dementia.

Investigations

EMG and nerve conduction studies can usually identify and confirm MND. There are currently no specific diagnostic tests.

Treatment

MND disease course is variable but survival beyond 3 years is unusual. In rare instances, survival may exceed 10 years. Death is usually caused by pneumonia. Riluzole is used but increases survival by only a few months. Nocturnal non-invasive ventilation prolongs life and improves quality of life. Enteral nutrition is offered, Baclofen is used to aid spasticity. Hyoscine, glycopyrrolate and amitriptyline are used to reduce oral secretions.

Complications

Avoid all neuromuscular blocking drugs when possible or give small doses of non-depolarising relaxants. If ventilated, weaning difficulties are common.

Further reading

Bushby K, Finkel R, Birnkrant DJ, et al. Diagnosis and management of Duchenne muscular dystrophy, part 1: diagnosis, and pharmacological and psychosocial management. Lancet Neurol 2010; 9:77–93.

Bushby K, Finkel R, Birnkrant DJ et al. Diagnosis and management of Duchenne muscular dystrophy, part 2: implementation of multidisciplinary care. Lancet Neurol 2010: 9;177–189.

Compston A, Coles A. Multiple sclerosis. Lancet 2008; 372:1502–1517.

Marsh S, Ross N, Pittard A. Neuromuscular disorders and anaesthesia. Part 1: generic anaesthetic management. Contin Educ Anaesth Crit Care Pain 2011; 11:115–118.

Marsh S, Pittard A. Neuromuscular disorders and anaesthesia. Part 2: specific neuromuscular disorders. Contin Educ Anaesth Crit Care Pain 2011; 11:119–123.

Related topics of interest

- Critical illness polyneuromyopathy (p 122)
- Guillain–Barré syndrome (p 170)
- Myasthenia gravis (p 223)

Nutrition

Key points

- Malnourishment is an important modifiable feature present in up to 50% of critically ill patients
- Precise nutritional requirements vary depending on pre-existing nutritional state, disease, and ability to absorb enteral nutrition
- Results of studies on the use of immunonutrition are inconsistent

Nutritional support for critically ill patients is changing from supportive therapy to an active therapeutic intervention. Many considerations are necessary when planning nutritional requirements, such as pre-existing nutritional status, disease-specific requirements, timing, route, composition of enteral feed and specific immunonutrients, and some of these do not have clear answers at present. However, all critically ill patients need nutritional support, and optimal provision can improve outcomes. Consensus guidelines provided by European, American or Canadian societies are regularly updated.

Recognition of malnutrition

Malnutrition is present in up to 50% of patients on admission to critical care. Malnutrition leads to worse outcomes, via altered immune status and increased susceptibility to infection, duration of ventilation, ICU or hospital stay. Malnutrition can be hard to recognise and is present in cachectic and morbidly obese patients. Diagnostic criteria often vary, and may rely on body mass index (BMI), weight loss, dietary history or biomarkers, all of which may be unreliable or unavailable in the critically ill patient. Chronic malnutrition may initiate the systemic inflammatory response, and vice versa. Observational databases show that a BMI 25–35 is associated with the lowest mortality rates; therefore implying the optimal BMI to survive critical illness is considered overweight or obese.

In addition to pre-disposing malnutrition, intolerance of enteral feeding and unclear nutrition targets lead to protein loss and further muscle wasting, and development of malnutrition within the intensive care unit.

Nutritional requirements

Total energy requirement varies significantly between individuals depending on nutritional status and disease state. It can be measured using indirect calorimetry or estimated using either a nutritional index (e.g. Harris–Benedict and Schofield) or on a simple weight basis: 25–30 kcal kg^{-1} day^{-1} is adequate for most patients. Exceptions include patients with burns, multiple trauma and necrotising pancreatitis who probably have higher requirements. However individual requirements will change with time, being less in the initial resuscitation phase, and increase later during recovery.

Generally 60–70% of enteral feed is given as carbohydrate, 15–30% as fat and 15–20% as protein sources. Recent evidence suggests that a higher protein intake (1.3–2.0 g kg^{-1} day^{-1}) is required to show benefits from targeted nutritional intake in critically ill patients.

The precise requirements for vitamins, minerals and trace elements have yet to be determined. However, failing to include essential components of nutrition, whether administered enterally or parenterally, can result in severe complications, especially when recommencing nutritional support in the severely malnourished. This re-feeding syndrome may manifest as severe electrolyte and fluid shifts associated with metabolic abnormalities. Clinical features are fluid-balance abnormalities, abnormal glucose metabolism, hypophosphataemia, hypomagnesaemia and hypocalcaemia. In addition, thiamine deficiency can occur, producing Wernicke's syndrome. Thiamine 100–300 mg IV should be given to those at risk of re-feeding before feeding is started and repeated daily to reduce this risk.

Timing and route of nutrition provision

Feeding has previously been initiated after initial resuscitation when haemodynamic support requirements are stable, to avoid placing increased stress upon the cardiovascular system and splanchnic circulation. Early enteral nutrition has non-caloric benefits such as maintaining gut integrity, preventing bacterial translocation and immune modulation.

The nasogastric route is most commonly used, but impaired gastric emptying can limit infusion rates. Prokinetics (e.g. erythromycin and metoclopramide) may increase gastric emptying or alternatively, the small bowel can be fed directly via surgical jejunostomy or nasojejunal tubes. These may be placed either endoscopically or blind with the assistance of prokinetic drugs that aid spontaneous passage of nasojejunal tubes through the pylorus. Some newer nasojejunal tubes can be placed blindly with high success rates. Absorption of post-pyloric feed is variable, which may explain a paucity of evidence of benefit for post-pyloric feeding.

If enteral feed is failing then it can be supplemented with parenteral nutrition (PN). European guidelines suggest starting this after 2–3 days of failing enteral nutrition, whereas American guidelines advocate waiting until day 8. Both guidelines were formed from the same evidence base, and consequently practice varies considerably. The recent Early versus Late Parenteral Nutrition in Critically Ill Adults (EPaNIC) study was designed to address this (see below). However parenteral nutrition is recommended when there is obvious malnutrition, or if the gut is unlikely to gain function fully within the first week of admission. Intravenous fat emulsions have replaced glucose as the main energy source because they cause less metabolic derangement. Nitrogen is delivered as amino acids. Most hospitals use parenteral nutrition solutions which have been prepared aseptically in the hospital pharmacy and contain all the requirements for a 24 h period in a single bag. The feeds are non-physiological, hyperosmolar and irritant and are therefore infused into a central vein.

Complications include all those of central venous access. Catheter-related sepsis is reduced by the use of a dedicated lumen, minimising handling of the line and the use of antimicrobial coatings. Subcutaneous tunnelling does not seem to be of benefit. Other complications of parenteral nutrition include gut mucosal atrophy, hyperglycaemia requiring insulin therapy, and hepatobiliary problems, particularly fatty infiltration and intra-hepatic cholestasis. Compared with EN, PN is nutritionally incomplete and dietary deficiencies can occur.

Immunonutrition

Certain nutrients appear to modulate the immune and inflammatory response (immunonutrition). When used in heterogeneous groups of critically ill patients, immunonutrition has not produced better outcomes.

Glutamine is an amino acid that facilitates nitrogen transport and reduces skeletal and intestinal protein catabolism. It is the major fuel for enterocytes and preserves intestinal permeability and function and has been suggested as a beneficial supplement especially in patients with burns or trauma. However the REDOXS trial published in 2013 showed early provision of glutamine or antioxidants did not improve clinical outcomes, and glutamine was associated with an increase in mortality in critically ill patients with multi-organ failure.

Arginine is an amino acid that improves macrophage and natural killer cell cytotoxicity, stimulates T-cell function and modulates nitrogen balance. There is evidence of significant benefit when used before and after major elective surgery (particularly abdominal, head and neck or cardiac surgery), but it causes harm in patients with severe sepsis. In particular, it may be of more benefit in patients receiving omega-3 fatty acids.

Omega-3-polyunsaturated fatty acids derived from fish oil are potent anti-inflammatory agents and immune

Obstetric emergencies – haemorrhage

Key points

- Uterine atony is the commonest cause of major obstetric haemorrhage. Both mechanical and pharmacological management strategies should be employed simultaneously
- All units should have protocols in place for identification and management of obstetric haemorrhage. Regular multidisciplinary team training should be carried out
- Early senior personnel involvement is essential in the management of major obstetric haemorrhage

Epidemiology

The British report of the Centre for Maternal and Child Enquiries 2006–2008 found nine deaths directly due to obstetric haemorrhage (0.39 per 100,000 maternities). These included two cases of placental abruption, two cases of placenta praevia and five cases of postpartum haemorrhage. This is a decline in the incidence of maternal deaths secondary to haemorrhage, with it now the sixth leading cause of direct maternal deaths in the United Kingdom and at its lowest mortality rate since 1985. It is hoped this reflects improvement in the quality and safety of care due to implementation of recommended national guidance, and regular multidisciplinary team skills/drills training.

Obstetric haemorrhage may occur antepartum (APH) or postpartum (PPH). The principles of resuscitation are similar for APH or PPH. The obstetric intervention required will depend upon the cause of the blood loss.

Principles of management of obstetric haemorrhage

The principal goal is successful maternal resuscitation. All foetal issues are secondary to this. The aim is to maintain or restore adequate oxygen delivery to all organs, including the uteroplacental unit.

Antepartum haemorrhage

APH is defined as bleeding from or into the genital tract from the 24th week of gestation and before the birth of the baby. The important causes are placental abruption and placenta praevia.

Placental abruption

Definition: Premature separation of a normally sited placenta from its attachment to the uterus.

Incidence: Occurs in 1–2% of pregnancies. Major abruption occurs in about 0.2% of pregnancies, but may be associated with foetal mortality of 50%. It recurs in 10–15% of pregnancies.

Aetiology: The cause is identified in only the minority of cases. Causes include severe hypertensive disorders, trauma (e.g. road traffic collision and external cephalic version) and sudden reduction in the size of the uterus (e.g. after birth of first twin). Associations include smoking, cocaine abuse, low socioeconomic status, poor nutritional status, advancing age, advancing parity and thrombophilic conditions. These latter factors may be associated with degenerative changes in the basal arteries supplying the placenta or alternative mechanisms of placental ischaemia, which predispose to premature placental separation.

Clinical features: Bleeding may be revealed, concealed or a mixture of the two. If retroplacental haemorrhage of >500 mL occurs, foetal death is likely. If >1000 mL loss, serious maternal sequelae are likely, including shock and disseminated intravascular coagulation (DIC). With increasing placental separation and retroplacental haemorrhage, there is increasing abdominal tenderness, pain and rigidity. The uterine fundus may be higher than expected for gestational age.

modulators. They have significant benefits in other diseases such as rheumatoid arthritis and cardiovascular disease, through a wide range of anti-inflammatory actions. In critically ill patients, they have been studied in patients with acute respiratory distress syndrome, and meta-analyses showed evidence of benefit. However, the recently published OMEGA trial contradicted these results (see below).

Anti-oxidants are a variety of molecules, such as selenium, manganese, vitamins A, C and E. These have varying amounts of supporting evidence but recently there are more emerging studies showing benefit, particularly with selenium.

Recent studies in critical care nutrition

Several recent studies have evaluated a variety of nutritional strategies in critically ill patients.

The TICACOS study aimed to identify whether targeting energy intake to indirect calorimetry measurements was associated with lower mortality, ICU stay or ventilation in comparison with using an estimated requirement of 25 kcal kg^{-1} day^{-1}. The indirect calorimetry group received more calories during their ICU stay, which lead to increased duration of ventilation and ICU stay, but a trend towards reduced mortality. This would suggest that providing more calories may not be as beneficial as previously thought.

The EPaNIC trial compared parenteral nutrition started on either day 3 or day 8 in critically ill patients at risk of malnutrition, in order to meet caloric requirements. Late initiation led to an increased chance of leaving ICU alive (with the same functional status), shortened duration of mechanical ventilation and renal replacement therapy, fewer infections and cholestasis.

The Early PN study assessed whether providing early PN to critically ill adults with relative contraindications to early EN alters outcomes. Early PN for critically ill adults with relative contraindications to early EN, compared with standard care, did not result in a difference in day-60 mortality. The early PN strategy resulted in significantly fewer days of invasive ventilation but no reduction in ICU or hospital stays.

The EDEN-OMEGA trial was a 2 × 2 factorial study in acute lung injury with two aims. Firstly, to assess whether 'trophic' feeding (about 25% of the target) for the first 6 days may alter overall length of mechanical ventilation (EDEN); secondly, whether omega-3 fatty acids and anti-oxidants are beneficial (OMEGA). The EDEN arm recruited 1000 patients, and found no difference in survival between trophic and full feeding in duration of ventilation, ICU stay or mortality. The OMEGA arm recruited 272 patients before being stopped for futility as the patients given omega-3 fatty acids had fewer ventilator-free days and longer ICU stay.

Further reading

Hegazi RA, Wischmeyer PE. Clinical review: Optimizing enteral nutrition for critically ill patients – a simple data-driven formula. Crit Care 2011; 15:234.

Manzanares W, Dhaliwal R, Jiang X, Murch L, Heyland DK. Antioxidant micronutrients in the critically ill: a systematic review and meta-analysis. Crit Care 2012; 16:R66.

Berger MM, Pichard C. Best timing for energy provision during critical illness Crit Care 2012; 16:215.

Related topics of interest

- Diarrhoea (p 133)
- Sepsis and SIRS (p 336)
- Burns (p 64)

Placenta praevia

Definition: Placental implantation partly or wholly in the lower segment of the uterus.

Incidence: Placenta praevia accounts for 0.5–1.0% of pregnancies and is responsible for 15–20% APH.

Grading of placenta praevia:

- Major or complete praevia: if the placenta encroaches onto the cervical os, it is considered a major or complete praevia
- Minor or partial praevia: if the lower segment placenta does not encroach on the cervical os, it is described as minor or partial praevia

The significance of this grading system reflects the increased risk of morbidity and mortality for mother and foetus the more the placenta encroaches upon the os. As the endometrium is less well developed in the lower uterine segment, the placenta morbidly adheres (placenta praevia accreta) causing problems during the third stage when placental separation should occur.

The risk of placenta accreta increases with the number of previous Caesarean deliveries: 9% risk with no previous lower segment Caesarean section (LSCS) up to 40–50% risk with two or more previous LSCS. Placenta increta (where placenta invades myometrium) and percreta (where placental tissue fully penetrates the uterine wall) are rarer and more severe variants.

Aetiology: Implantation low in the uterine cavity increases with age, parity, multiple pregnancy, previous LSCS or termination and smoking.

Clinical features: Painless vaginal bleeding occurs in the latter stages of pregnancy. The onset may be spontaneous or precipitated by coitus, coughing or straining. Any painless bleeding in the second half of pregnancy is placenta praevia until proven otherwise. Definitive diagnosis is by ultrasound scan. If there is a major degree of placenta praevia, Caesarean section will be required for safe delivery. There may be difficulty in delivering the placenta. There is a higher than normal risk of PPH.

Management: Current opinion suggests each woman should be assessed on an individual basis. Pursue conservative management until the foetus is mature. Deliver by LSCS by senior obstetric and anaesthetic personnel. An anterior placenta praevia may be directly under the uterine incision site. Cross-matched blood and blood products should be available. Insert two large-gauge intravenous cannulae and consider invasive arterial blood pressure monitoring. Consider intra-operative cell salvage. Regional anaesthesia is the current preferred technique of choice for elective LSCS delivery, but the mother must be warned of conversion to general anaesthesia. There is insufficient evidence to support one technique over another. Anticipate postpartum haemorrhage.

Primary postpartum haemorrhage

Definition: Bleeding of 500 mL or more from the birth canal in the first 24 h after delivery. Major PPH is blood loss > 1000 mL and severe PPH is blood loss > 2000 mL in the 24 h after delivery.

Incidence: Occurs in approximately 2% of pregnancies.

Aetiology: Commonly categorised by the 'Four T's': Tone (uterine atony), Tissue (retained products of conception), Trauma (genital tract lacerations, uterine rupture) and Thrombin (coagulopathy).

There is increased incidence of PPH if there is a precipitant, prolonged labour, macrosomia, multiple gestation, operative delivery, LSCS, previous PPH, chorioamnionitis and obesity.

Uterine atony

Uterine atony is the most common cause of primary PPH. Prolonged labour (> 12 h), maternal age > 40 years, macrosomic baby (> 4 kg), obesity (BMI > 35), multiple pregnancy and placenta praevia are known risk factors. It is exacerbated by volatile anaesthetics, β-agonists used as tocolytics and magnesium sulphate.

Retained products of conception

Refers to placental and/or foetal tissue that remains in the uterus after a spontaneous or planned abortion, or preterm/term delivery.

Trauma

Uterine rupture: Occurs in multiparous women with large foetus or malpresentation (e.g. brow), injudicious use of oxytocics, operative and other trauma, e.g. external version with uterine scar, vaginal birth after Caesarean. Symptoms include pain and tenderness on abdominal palpation and shock. Contractions decrease and there may be foetal distress. Symptoms are more extreme if the upper segment ruptures. Treatment includes uterine repair or, if necessary, hysterectomy. **Local trauma to the genital tract and pelvis:** May result from LSCS, operative or spontaneous vaginal delivery of a macrosomic or breech baby causing cervical and/or genital tract tears.

Coagulation defect

In obstetric practice, DIC is the commonest cause of failure of blood clotting. Predisposing factors include severe abruption, severe pre-eclampsia, amniotic fluid embolism, sepsis, shock and intrauterine death. Management should include early discussion with a senior haematologist.

Principles of management of PPH

Mechanical: Manoeuvres include ensuring that both the uterus and bladder are empty and bimanual uterine compression.
Pharmacological: Administration in turn of oxytocin, ergometrine, rectal misoprostol (prostaglandin E_1) and intramuscular or intramyometrial injection of carboprost (prostaglandin F_{2a}). Carbetocin, a new synthetic analogue of oxytocin, is attracting interest as an alternative to oxytocin for prophylaxis against uterine atony. It has a longer duration of action than oxytocin (40 min versus 10 min) and reduces the need for further uterotonic therapy in women undergoing elective LSCS.
Surgical: Conservative measures should be initiated sooner rather than later and include intrauterine balloon tamponade and haemostatic brace suturing ('B-Lynch' suture). When PPH is precipitated by retained products of conception (RPOC), treatment includes evacuation of the uterus. If there is placenta accreta, either wholly or in part, there will be no plane of cleavage. Severe haemorrhage may require embolisation or ligation of the uterine or iliac arteries. Hysterectomy may be necessary.

Secondary PPH

Defined as excessive bleeding between the first 24 h postpartum and 12 weeks postnatally, secondary PPH is generally caused by RPOC which act as a nidus for infection and endometritis.
Management: Antibiotics in the first instance. The uterus is friable at this time and care must be taken not to perforate the uterus if surgical evacuation is required.

Further reading

Centre for Maternal and Child Enquiries (CMACE). Saving Mothers' Lives: reviewing maternal deaths to make motherhood safer: 2006–08. The Eighth Report on Confidential Enquiries into Maternal Deaths in the United Kingdom. Brit J Obstet Gynaec 2011; 118:1–203.

Royal College of Obstetricians and Gynaecologists. Antepartum Haemorrhage Green-top Guideline No. 63. London: RCOG, 2011.
Royal College of Obstetricians and Gynaecologists Postpartum Haemorrhage, Prevention and Management Green-top Guideline No. 52. London: RCOG, 2009.

Related topics of interest

- Blood and blood products (p 51)
- Major haemorrhage (p 213)
- Obstetric emergencies – medical (p 236)

Obstetric emergencies – medical

Key points

- Identification and management of sepsis in the peripartum woman is challenging, it is important to have a low threshold of suspicion
- Systolic hypertension above 180 mmHg in the pregnant woman is a medical emergency and must be reduced and controlled urgently
- Experienced senior personnel should be involved early in the management of the acutely unwell peripartum woman

Maternal death statistics in the United Kingdom are taken from 'Saving Mothers Lives', Report of the Centre for Maternal and Child Enquiries 2006–2008 triennium.

Maternal sepsis

Genital tract sepsis is currently the leading cause of direct maternal death in the United Kingdom. Overall mortality rate from sepsis is 1.13 per 100,000 maternities. 50% of deaths are from community-acquired Group A β-haemolytic streptococcal infection, with 5–30% of the population being asymptomatic carriers on skin or in the throat; it is easily spread by person–person contact or droplets. Group A streptococcus causes scarlet fever, streptococcal shock syndrome and necrotising fasciitis. Management of acute sepsis in the pregnant or recently pregnant woman should include current recommendations of the Surviving Sepsis Campaign. Missed opportunities to recognise and aggressively treat sepsis during pregnancy or within 6 weeks post-partum has prompted a call for a national clinical guideline on the identification and management of sepsis in pregnancy, labour and the puerperium.

Pre-eclampsia and eclampsia

Pre-eclampsia and eclampsia are the second commonest cause of direct maternal death (rate 0.83 per 100,000 maternities).

Pre-eclempsia

Pre-eclampsia is pregnancy induced hypertension after 20 weeks of gestation, associated with proteinuria (>0.3 g in 24 h) with or without oedema. It occurs in approximately 10% of maternities, most commonly between 33 and 37 weeks of gestation.

The National Institute for Health and Clinical Excellence defines severe pre-eclampsia as pre-eclampsia with severe hypertension (systolic blood pressure (BP) >160 mmHg, diastolic BP >110 mmHg), and/or with symptoms, and/or biochemical and/or haematological impairment. Clinical features of severe pre-eclampsia (in addition to hypertension and proteinuria) are:

- Severe headache
- Visual disturbance
- Epigastric pain and/or vomiting
- Clonus
- Papilloedema
- Liver tenderness
- Platelet count $< 100 \times 10^9$ L^{-1}
- Abnormal liver enzymes (ALT or AST > 70 IU L^{-1})
- HELLP syndrome

Pre-eclampsia is a multisystem disease with a variable clinical presentation. Placental ischaemia is associated with widespread endothelial damage, which may involve all maternal organ systems. Resolution is usually within 48–72 h of delivery of the placenta. The most common causes of death associated with hypertensive diseases of pregnancy is intracranial haemorrhage and anoxic brain injury secondary to eclamptic seizure induced cardiac arrest. Other causes include liver necrosis and subcapsular haemorrhage, multi-organ failure and complications of acute fatty liver of pregnancy (AFLP).

Eclampsia

Eclampsia is defined as the occurrence of one or more convulsions in a patient with pre-eclampsia. Eclampsia is more common in teenagers and in cases of multiple pregnancy. In the United Kingdom, 44% of eclamptic fits occur after delivery, most commonly within the first 48 h, and up to 4 weeks postpartum. The case fatality rate from eclampsia is 3.1%.

HELLP Syndrome

The haemolysis elevated liver enzymes, low platelets (HELLP) syndrome is a form of severe pre-eclampsia associated with a maternal mortality of up to 24%. HELLP syndrome presents with malaise (90%), epigastric pain (90%) and nausea and vomiting (50%). Physical signs include right upper quadrant tenderness (80%), weight gain and oedema. Blood pressure may be normal and proteinuria may be absent. Resolution of symptoms following delivery may be slow. Studies on the use of corticosteroids have failed to show any clinically important outcomes antenatally or postnatally, and current guidance does not recommend their use.

Management of pre-eclampsia

Key aims are to minimise vasospasm, and improve perfusion of the uterus, placenta and maternal vital organs. The ultimate cure is delivery of the baby and placenta. Systolic hypertension poses the greatest risk of cerebral haemorrhage, >180 mmHg is a medical emergency. Consider invasive arterial blood pressure monitoring and high dependency care.

1. **Antihypertensive agents:** Labetalol, nifedipine or hydralazine is given if the systolic blood pressure (BP) exceeds 150 mmHg, aiming to keep BP < 150/80–100 mmHg.
2. **Clinical assessment:** Foetal growth, proteinuria, uric acid and platelet count are measured.
3. **Steroids:** Give to aid maturation of the foetal lungs if the pregnancy is < 34 weeks. Delivery is ideally delayed for 48 h for maximal benefit.
4. **Magnesium sulphate:** The results of the Collaborative Eclampsia Study and the Magpie Trial support the use of magnesium sulphate as prophylaxis and treatment of eclamptic fits. Load with 4 g over 5 min intravenously, followed by 1 g h^{-1} infusion for 24 h. Recurrent seizures should be treated with further loading of 2–4 g over 5 min. Diazepam, phenytoin or lytic cocktails should not be used as an alternative in eclampsia. Magnesium is a central nervous system depressant, cerebral vasodilator and mild antihypertensive. It increases prostacyclin release by endothelial cells, increases uterine and renal perfusion and decreases platelet aggregation. Conversely, its tocolytic effect may prolong labour and increase blood loss.
5. **Fluid management:** In severe pre-eclampsia, careful fluid management is crucial. Mothers are susceptible to pulmonary oedema due to leaky pulmonary capillaries and low colloid osmotic pressure due to renal protein loss.

Thromboembolism

The incidence of thromboembolism is currently 0.79 per 100,000 maternities. The majority are pulmonary embolism but cerebral vein thrombosis is also reported. Obesity is the most important risk factor.

Amniotic fluid embolism

Amniotic fluid embolism (AFE) causes 0.57 deaths per 100,000 maternities. In the past, mortality from AFE was reported as high as 86%, with 50% dying within the first hour. Current reports suggest a case fatality rate of 16.5%; this may reflect improvements in approaches to resuscitation and maternal collapse.

AFE can occur at any time during pregnancy, following termination of pregnancy or amniocentesis, after closed abdominal trauma, during Caesarean section or artificial rupture of the membranes. Risk factors include: maternal age >35, placental abnormalities (praevia, abruption), Caesarean or instrumental delivery, eclampsia, foetal distress and medical induction/augmentation of labour.

Pathophysiology

This is yet to be determined, but the current theory is that AFE is an immunologic mechanism in susceptible women that is activated on exposure to foetal material. There are similarities between AFE and septic/anaphylactic shock but without mast cell degranulation; studies have shown reduced complement levels.

The haemodynamic changes are biphasic, with initial pulmonary hypertension, hypoxia and right ventricular failure, followed by left ventricular failure.

Clinical features

Typically, there is sudden onset of dyspnoea, cyanosis and hypotension disproportionate to blood loss, followed quickly by cardiorespiratory arrest. Approximately, 20% of women have seizures and up to 83% develop disseminated intravascular coagulation with bleeding from the vagina, surgical incisions and intravenous cannula sites. Management is supportive. Maternal death is caused by sudden cardiac arrest, haemorrhage from coagulopathy or the development of acute respiratory distress syndrome and/or multi-system organ failure after initial survival of the acute event.

Cardiac disease in pregnancy

Deaths from heart disease remain the commonest cause of indirect maternal death (obstetric deaths that occur as a result of a previously diagnosed condition or a condition that develops during the pregnancy which is aggravated by the pregnancy but are deaths that are not directly the result of an obstetric cause), but the commonest cause of death overall. Acquired heart disease is increasing, reflecting the impact of lifestyle factors such as increasing maternal age, obesity and smoking. Deaths from acute myocardial infarction or chronic ischaemic heart disease are reported. Other causes include cardiomyopathy (peripartum, dilated or arrythmogenic right ventricular cardiomyopathies) and aortic dissection. Pre-eclampsia, hypertension and obesity are risk factors.

Cardiac arrest in pregnancy

Hypoxia develops rapidly due to the reduced functional residual capacity and increased oxygen consumption of pregnancy. Caval compression must be avoided and chest compressions performed with a wedge beneath the mother's right hip, or else the gravid uterus displaced manually. Early intubation is essential to prevent aspiration. If spontaneous circulation is not restored rapidly, the foetus should be delivered by immediate Caesarean to minimise aortocaval compression and optimise the chance of maternal survival.

Local anaesthetic toxicity

Typical complaints are circumoral numbness, tinnitus, light-headedness, confusion and a sense of impending doom. Muscle twitching and grand mal convulsion may occur. All these symptoms and signs are exacerbated by acidosis and hypoxia. Central nervous system symptoms usually occur before cardiovascular collapse.

Further reading

Centre for Maternal and Child Enquiries (CMACE). Saving Mothers' Lives: reviewing maternal deaths to make motherhood safer: 2006–2008. The Eighth Report on Confidential Enquiries into Maternal Deaths in the United Kingdom. Brit J Obstet Gynaec 2011; 118:1–203.

National Institute for Health and Clinical Excellence (NICE). Hypertension in pregnancy the management of hypertensive disorders during pregnancy. Clinical Guideline CG107. London: NICE, 2011.

Dedhia JD, Mushambi MC. Amniotic fluid embolism. Contin Educ Anaesth Crit Care Pain 2007; 7:152–156.

Conde-Agudelo A, Romero R. Amniotic fluid embolism: an evidence-based review. Am J Obstet Gynecol 2009; 201:445.e1–13.

Related topics of interest

Oscillation and high-frequency ventilation

Key points

- High-frequency oscillation (HFO) is a lung ventilation strategy with extremely small tidal volumes (1–4 mL kg^{-1}) that facilitates lung recruitment
- It is used as an advanced ventilatory modality in patients with severe hypoxic respiratory failure
- Ventilation and oxygenation are uncoupled in high-frequency oscillation allowing each to be independently optimized
- Lung recruitment allows for improved oxygenation and reduction in inspired fractional oxygen
- HFO allows for effective elimination of CO_2 through combination of mechanisms

Counter-intuitively, in HFO the higher the frequency the lower the minute ventilation; lowering the frequency lowers the $Paco_2$.

Introduction

High-frequency ventilation was first description in by Lunkenheimer in 1972. He described a technique to minimise the cyclical effects of intermittent positive pressure on the cardiovascular system. There are three main techniques to deliver high frequency ventilation i.e. high frequency oscillatory ventilation (HFOV), high frequency positive pressure ventilation (HFPPV) and high-frequency jet ventilation (HFJV).

Definition

HFOV is a form of ventilation characterized by respiratory rate >150 breaths per minute and tidal volumes less than or equal to dead space.

Mechanism of action

The oscillator can be considered as a modified T-piece. The fresh gas flow is called the bias flow and a valve placed on the expiratory limb of the T-piece determines the pressure within the circuit or mean airway pressure (mPaw). The Fio_2 and the mPaw determine oxygenation.

CO_2 control or ventilation is achieved by manipulating the frequency and amplitude by oscillating the inspiratory gas column by via a piston. There are two commercially available HFOV's suitable for adults, the SensorMedics 3100B (for patients weighing > 35 kg) and 'Vision Alpha'. In the SensorMedics ventilator the piston is driven by an electromagnet backwards and forwards much as a loudspeaker cone moves while in the VisionAlpha, it is a rotating electromagnetic valve that drives the piston. The amplitude is controlled by the electromagnet and generates a change in pressure DP superimposed on the mPaw. The DP is adjusted depending on the patients size to produce a visible oscillation of the chest in children or the thighs in adults.

A number of different mechanisms have been postulated to explain the ability of HFO to ventilate patients. These include:

- Taylor dispersion
- Pendelluft theory
- Direct bulk flow to alveolar gas units which are close to the major airways
- Cardiogenic mixing

The frequency used in ventilation in adults is typically in the range of 4–8 Hz. At these frequencies and with a typical DP the VT is <2 mL kg^{-1} avoiding over distension of the lung and the development of VILI.

Clinical application of HFOV

HFOV is often used as a rescue therapy in refractory hypoxic respiratory failure, i.e. failure of oxygenation on despite mechanical ventilation with Fio_2 > than 0.7 with a PEEP > than 15 or failure of ventilation with Vt >6 mL kg^{-1} and PiP >30 cmH$_2$O.

Initiating HFOV

- Familiarise yourself with the machine

- Keep the patient well-sedated and consider neuromuscular paralysis if F_{IO_2} >0.8
- It is important to assess the intravascular volume. If the CVP is < 12 cmH$_2$O, consider administering a 500 mL bolus of a crystalloid or an equivalent colloid

Initial setting on HFOV

- Set F_{IO_2} at 1.0, MAwP at ≥ 5 cmH$_2$O than of conventional ventilation and a bias flow of 20 L min^{-1}
- Frequency of 5 Hz, inspiratory time = 33% and an amplitude (DP) of 60 cmH$_2$O

Oxygenation protocol

- Goals for oxygenation is SpO_2 = 88–92% and PaO_2 ≥ 8 kPa using combination of lowest F_{IO_2} and highest MAwP
- Once the patient is stable on the initial settings, MAwP is increased by 2–3 cmH$_2$O until maximum of 40–45 cmH$_2$O to achieve the target oxygenation
- F_{IO_2} is then reduced by 0.05 every 10–30 to achieve SaO_2 = 88–92%
- Once the F_{IO_2} < 0.6, maintain MAwP at the highest level for 6–12 h, thus ensuring maximum lung recruitment
- Reduce MAwP by 2–3 cmH$_2$O every 2–4 h until at it is back to the initial setting
- If at any time the F_{IO_2} increases >0.6 to maintain SaO_2 88–92%, increase MAwP by 2–3 cmH$_2$O until SaO_2 = 88–92% and F_{IO_2} is reduced to <0.60

Ventilation protocol

The DP is the primary variable to be adjusted and titrated to vibrate the chest wall from the clavicles to the mid-thigh region. DP is subsequently titrated to maintain $PaCO_2$ in the target range as determined clinically.

- If the $PaCO_2$ is >60 mmHg and pH <7.15: increase the power setting to a maximum to increase DP
- If PCO_2 control is still difficult: reduce the frequency by 0.5 to 1 Hz steps to a minimum of 4 Hz, failing which consider deflation of the endotracheal tube cuff
- If the $PaCO_2$ is < 45 mmHg and pH > 45: the DP can reduced to its minimum level of 60 cmH$_2$O and frequency increased to a maximum value of 8–10 Hz

Maintenance

- Patients are maintained on HFOV to facilitate improvement in respiratory failure and clinical condition. During the maintenance phase, the lung recruitment and oxygenation is maintained as described above

Weaning and switching from HFOV to CMV

- Once a decision is taken to wean the patient, the F_{IO_2} is weaned as tolerated, in increments of 0.05–0.1 to a goal of ≤ 0.4, keeping the SaO_2 = 88–93%. Then, the MAWP is weaned by 2 cmH$_2$O to a goal of 22 cmH$_2$O, keeping the SaO_2 = 88–93%
- Switching to CMV was attempted at least once daily if the patient satisfied the above criteria. Frequently, patients can be weaned to a spontaneous mode

Evidence for efficacy

OSCAR (oscillation in ARDS) was a UK-based pragmatic study comparing HFOV with conventional ventilation using a low tidal volume strategy. The authors found no major difference between the two groups with a rate of death from any cause at 28 days was 41.7% in the HFOV group and 41.1% in the usual care control group (P = 0.85 by the chi-square test). OSCILLATE (Oscillation for Acute Respiratory Distress Syndrome Treated Early) trial, compared HFOV strategy with high mean airway pressures with a conventional mechanical-ventilation strategy that used relatively high PEEP levels. The group treated with a HFOV strategy had an in-hospital mortality of 47% as compared with 35% in the control group (relative risk of death with HFOV, 1.33; 95% confidence interval, 1.09–1.64; P = 0.005), leading to a pre-mature termination of the trial.

The average tidal volumes and PEEP applied in the conventional arm of the study OSCAR study was 8.3 mL kg^{-1} and 11.4 cm of H$_2$O as compared to 6.1 mL kg^{-1} and 18 cm of H$_2$O in OSCILLATE. The difference in PEEP can be explained on the basis of the study design, the difference in tidal volume is reflection of a strict adherence to a protocol in OSCILLATE as compared to a pragmatic approach in OSCAR trial.

In OSCAR as compared to OSCILLATE, there was a lower incidence of haemodynamic compromise associated with HFOV, likely due to a lower mean airway pressures used in the OSCAR trial. In both the trials, patients in the HFOV groups received more sedatives and muscle relaxants than did the patients in the

control groups, possibly contributing to the disappointing outcomes.

The results from OSCAR and OSCILLATE raises questions regarding the widespread routine clinical use of HFOV. Importantly, they reinforce possible benefits of a high PEEP and low tidal volume strategy using conventional ventilation. They also seems to suggest that strict adherence to a ventilatory protocol is more likely to deliver greater compliance with a low tidal volume strategy.

Further reading

Sud S, Sud M, Friedrich JO, et al. High frequency oscillation in patients with acute lung injury and acute respiratory distress syndrome (ARDS): systematic review and meta-analysis. Br Med J 2010; 340:c2327.

Derdak S, Mehta S, Stewart TE, et al. High-frequency oscillatory ventilation for acute respiratory distress syndrome in adults. A randomized, controlled trial. Am J Respir Crit Care Med 2002; 166:801–808.

Ferguson ND, Cook DJ, Guyatt GH, et al. High-frequency oscillation in early acute respiratory distress syndrome. N Engl J Med 2013; 368:795–805.

Young D, Lamb SE, Shah S, et al. High-frequency oscillation for acute respiratory distress syndrome. N Engl J Med 2013; 368:806–813.

Related topics of interest

Pancreatitis – acute severe

Key points

- Severe acute pancreatitis is associated with a mortality rate of 10–30%
- Gallstones and alcohol abuse cause 75–85% of cases of acute pancreatitis
- In severe acute pancreatitis, cholecystectomy is delayed until resolution of inflammation and clinical improvement
- Local complications include pancreatic necrosis and the development of pseudocysts and abscesses

Epidemiology

Acute inflammation of the pancreas occurs in 15–42 per 100,000 population. Eighty percentage of cases are mild and resolve without serious morbidity. Twenty percent are severe and are associated with significant systemic inflammatory response, organ failure, and local complications such as pancreatic necrosis or collections (e.g. abscess and pseudocyst). Severe acute pancreatitis (SAP) carries an overall mortality of 10–30%.

Causes

Gallstones and alcohol abuse cause 75–85% of cases of acute pancreatitis. 10–15% of cases have no clear cause ('idiopathic'), but occult gallstones or biliary sludge may be responsible for two-thirds of these. Many other conditions make up the remaining 10% of causes (e.g. drugs, trauma, infections and tumours).

Pathophysiology

Precipitating factors, such as alcohol or passage of a gallstone, lead to the unregulated activation of trypsinogen into trypsin within pancreatic acinar cells. This causes intra-cytoplasmic activation of digestive enzymes such as elastase and phospholipase A2, which damage acinar cells and lead to the development of areas of non-viable pancreatic parenchyma (pancreatic necrosis). The associated release of cytokines and oxygen free radicals and the activation of endothelial cells, complement, coagulation and kallikrein systems combine to produce a systemic inflammatory response syndrome (SIRS) and multi-organ dysfunction.

Clinical features

Abdominal pain radiating to the back, with vomiting and fever are characteristic, but not universal. In severe disease, signs of SIRS are common, and the presence of acute lung injury, pleural effusions, abdominal distension and pain frequently cause respiratory compromise.

SAP commonly runs a biphasic course. An early (1–2 weeks) inflammatory phase of pancreatic and systemic inflammation and multi-organ dysfunction overlaps with a later septic phase (after first week) associated with the development of infection in pancreatic necrosis, local fluid collections or at remote sites.

Investigations

Amylase

Serum amylase values above three times the normal upper limit strongly support the diagnosis of acute pancreatitis. Amylase rises within hours of onset, returning to normal within 3–5 days. Sensitivity approximates 80% on admission, but falls below 30% two days after symptom onset. Moderate elevation of amylase is common in many other surgical and medical conditions.

Lipase

The serum lipase value, where available, is a better diagnostic test for acute pancreatitis as it remains elevated for 8–14 days and still has a sensitivity of 80% 4 days after symptom onset. The combination of both serum amylase and lipase will provide sensitivity and specificity of 90–95% for detecting acute pancreatitis.

Chest X-ray

Chest X-ray (CXR) abnormalities (e.g. pleural effusions and pulmonary infiltrates) are seen in 15% of patients on admission, rising to over 85% by day 5.

Ultrasound scan

Abdominal ultrasound examination is not helpful in diagnosing acute pancreatitis but can be useful for diagnosing gallstones as a cause (sensitivity for gallstones 67%, specificity 100%). Visualisation of the pancreas and of stones in the distal bile duct is often obscured by overlying bowel gas.

Computerised tomography

Contrast-enhanced computerised tomography (CT) is very useful for confirming the diagnosis of acute pancreatitis, for defining the degree of necrosis of the gland, and for detecting local complications (e.g. fluid collections). It should be used on admission if the diagnosis of acute pancreatitis is in doubt, at 48–72 h from onset in patients diagnosed with severe acute pancreatitis, and again at 6–10 days in patients with persisting organ failure, signs of sepsis or clinical deterioration. CT-guided fine needle aspiration can help distinguish sterile from infected necrosis. The sensitivity of CT for detecting gallstones is only 30–50%.

Magnetic resonance imaging

Magnetic resonance imaging visualises the pancreas well, and when combined with magnetic resonance cholangiopancreatography (MRCP), has a higher sensitivity for choledocholithiasis than ultrasound or CT. It can accurately identify ductal gallstones or other obstructing lesions, and aids in identifying patients requiring endoscopic retrograde cholangiopancreatography (ERCP) and sphincterotomy.

Endoscopic ultrasound

Endoscopic ultrasound is more sensitive than abdominal USS or CT and equivalent to ERCP and MRCP for detecting biliary stones. It detects smaller stones or 'biliary sludge' well and may have a role in investigating patients diagnosed with idiopathic pancreatitis.

Diagnosis

The cause of the severe acute pancreatitis should be ascertained. Serum ALT three times upper limit is the best single predictor of biliary aetiology within 48 h of onset, but 20% of patients with gallstone pancreatitis have normal concentrations of liver enzymes. Evidence of co-existent cholangitis or biliary tree obstruction should be sought and warrant consideration for urgent ERCP.

Severity assessment

Early recognition of severe disease is important because it prompts aggressive treatment and appropriate allocation of critical care resources. Several validated severity scoring systems are available which measure various combinations of clinical findings, blood tests and radiological signs. Ranson's criteria (1974 – **Table 35**) and the Imrie (Glasgow) criteria (1985) remain widely used, but do not provide a score until 48 h after admission. The presence of 3–5 Ranson's criteria is common, but correlates poorly with clinical severity or development of necrosis.

Table 35 Ranson's criteria	
At admission	**During initial 48 h**
Age > 55 years	Haematocrit decrease > 10%
White blood count > 16,000 mm^{-3}	Blood urea increase > 1.8 mmol L^{-1}
Glucose > 11 mmol L^{-1}	Serum calcium < 2 mmol L^{-1}
Lactate dehydrogenase > 350 IU L^{-1}	Pao_2 < 8 kPa
Aspartate aminotransferase > 250 U L^{-1}	Base deficit > 4 mmol L^{-1}
	Fluid sequestration > 6 L

However, < 3 Ranson's criteria represents mild disease, and the presence of ≥ 6 criteria correlates well with pancreatic necrosis and increased risk of mortality. The APACHE II system is more reliable but is relatively complex to calculate. Clinical assessment or formal measures of organ dysfunction (e.g. Sequential Organ Failure Assessment scores) correlate well with laboratory-based scoring systems. Systems which grade severity based on CT appearance (e.g. CT severity index – **Table 36**) are relatively easy to perform and correlate well with mortality. Individual factors such as age (particularly > 70 years), obesity (BMI > 30), pleural effusion on CXR and significantly raised CRP (> 150 mg L^{-1} after 3 days) have also been associated with increased severity and worse outcome in severe acute pancreatitis.

Treatment

The treatment of severe acute pancreatitis on intensive care follows the general principles of resuscitation and close monitoring, control of symptoms, nutritional and organ support, and the prevention and treatment of infection.

Nutrition

Attempt to establish enteral nutrition (EN) early in SAP. Bowel rest in SAP is associated with intestinal mucosal atrophy and increased infectious complications and is no longer advocated. Compared with parenteral nutrition (PN), EN in SAP reduces infections, organ failure, need for surgical intervention and mortality. Post-pyloric (naso-jejunal) feeding is ideal since gastric emptying is frequently impaired in SAP, but nasogastric (NG) feeding is probably equivalent if gastric emptying is adequate. Use PN only if enteral nutrition cannot be established.

Prophylactic antibiotics

Infectious complications account for 80% of deaths from SAP, as well as the majority of late-phase complications. The use of prophylactic antibiotics to prevent the development pancreatic (within necrotic tissue or collections) or extra-pancreatic infection is controversial. Randomised controlled trials and meta-analyses have produced conflicting results. A Cochrane Collaboration systematic review in 2010 found no significant benefits from prophylactic antibiotics and most centres and do not currently advocate their use.

Endoscopic retrograde cholangiopancreatography

Early (within 48–72 h) ERCP and endoscopic sphincterotomy are associated with reduced morbidity and mortality in patients with biliary SAP with evidence of co-existent cholangitis or on-going biliary obstruction.

Surgery

The precise role of surgery in acute pancreatitis is controversial and is usually reserved for one or more of the complications discussed below. Cholecystectomy to prevent repeated episodes of gallstone pancreatitis should be considered during admission for mild pancreatitis. In severe acute pancreatitis, cholecystectomy should be delayed until resolution of inflammation and clinical improvement (ideally within 6 weeks).

Table 36 CT severity index			
CT crade	**Points**	**Necrosis score**	**Points**
Normal appearance	0	0%	0
Pancreatic oedema and enlargement	1	< 30%	2
Pancreatic or peri-pancreatic inflammation	2	30–50%	4
1 peri-pancreatic fluid collection	3	> 50%	6
> 1 peri-pancreatic fluid collection	4		
Max total score = 10 Score ≥ 7 predicts high morbidity and mortality			

Complications

Local complications include pancreatic necrosis, the development of a pseudocyst and abscess formation.

Pancreatic necrosis

Non-viable areas of pancreatic parenchyma are detected by lack of enhancement on contrast-enhanced CT scan. When necrosis remains sterile, mortality is usually low (approx. 10%) and treatment should be conservative as early surgical debridement increases mortality. Late drainage (> 2–3 weeks) of sterile necrosis remains controversial, but may be considered for persistent or progressive organ failure.

Necrosis becomes secondarily infected (typically after the second week) in 40–70% of cases, and is associated with a substantial morbidity and mortality. USS or CT-guided needle aspiration of pancreatic tissues confirms the diagnosis with a sensitivity of 83–96% and specificity of 93%. When infection is proven, debridement and/ or drainage is usually required. Surgical options include open necrosectomy with post-op irrigation, or serial laparotomies, but minimally invasive techniques such as laparoscopic and retroperitoneal approaches, trans-gastric/duodenal endoscopic drainage and radiologically guided percutaneous drainage are being increasingly adopted in specialist centres.

Pseudocyst

A pseudocyst is a collection of pancreatic secretions enclosed by a wall of granulation tissue that results from pancreatic duct leakage. Pseudocysts usually require 4 weeks for maturation of the cyst wall and complicate acute pancreatitis in fewer than 5% of cases. Drainage is required if the pseudocyst becomes infected, causes persistent pain, continues to enlarge, or compresses adjacent organs (e.g. causing gastric outlet obstruction or obstructive jaundice).

Further reading

Pezilli R, Zerbi A, Di Carlo V, et al. Practical guidelines for acute pancreatitis. Pancreatology 2010; 10:523–535.

Haas B, Nathans A. Surgical indications in acute pancreatitis. Curr Opin Crit Care 2010; 16:153–158.

Frossard JL, Steer ML, Pastor CM. Acute pancreatitis. Lancet 2008; 371:143–152.

Brisinda G, Vanella S, Crocco A, et al. Severe acute pancreatitis: advances and insights in assessment of severity and management. Eur J Gastroenterol Hepatol 2011; 23:541–551.

Villatoro E, Mulla M, Larvin M. Antibiotic therapy for prophylaxis against infection of pancreatic necrosis in acute pancreatitis. Cochrane Database of Syst Rev 2010:CD002941.

Related topics of interest

• Sepsis and SIRS (p 336)

Pandemic influenza

Key points

- Influenza occurs in distinct outbreaks of varying extent every year. The epidemiologic pattern reflects the changing nature of the antigenic properties
- Clinical presentation of uncomplicated influenza virus infection includes fever, headache, myalgia and malaise and features of respiratory illness with cough sore throat and rhinitis
- Viral isolation or detection of viral proteins or viral RNA in respiratory tract secretions is essential for diagnosis and influences decisions regarding infection control, prophylaxis and treatment
- Confirmed or suspected influenza infection require treatment with a neuraminidase inhibitor (e.g. oseltamivir and zanamivir)
- Annual seasonal influenza vaccine (multi-strain and currently including H1N1 2009) is recommended to for any person aged 6 months and over who wishes to reduce the likelihood of becoming ill with influenza

Introduction

The World Health Organization currently defines a pandemic as the worldwide spread of a new disease. An influenza pandemic occurs when a new influenza virus emerges and spreads around the world, and most people do not have immunity.

Influenza occurs in distinct outbreaks of varying extent every year. The epidemiology reflects the changing nature of the antigenic properties of influenza viruses and the pathogenicity depends on transmissibility of the virus and susceptibility of the population.

Influenza A virus has a remarkable ability to undergo periodic changes in the antigenic characteristics of the envelope glycoproteins, hemagglutinin and neuraminidase. Influenza hemagglutinin is a surface glycoprotein that binds to sialic acid residues on respiratory epithelial cell surface glycoproteins and is necessary for the initiation of infection.

Neuraminidase cleaves these links and liberates the new virions; it also counteracts hemagglutinin-mediated self-aggregation entrapment in respiratory secretions.

Among influenza A viruses that infect humans, three major subtypes of hemagglutinins (H1, H2 and H3) and two subtypes of neuraminidases (N1 and N2) have been described. Influenza B viruses have a lesser propensity for antigenic changes, and only antigenic drifts in the hemagglutinin have been described.

Pandemics over the past 100 years and antigen shifts

1918: Extensive pandemic (swine influenza or Spanish influenza), associated with the emergence of antigenic shifts in both the hemagglutinin (H1) and the neuraminidase (N1) of influenza A. May have been responsible for more than 50 million deaths.
1957: Shift to H2 and N2 resulted in a severe pandemic.
1968: Antigenic shift involved only the hemagglutinin (from H2N2 to H3N2); the resulting pandemic was less extensive than that seen in 1957.
1977: Emerged from a shift to H1N1 affecting primarily young individuals who lacked pre-existing immunity to H1N1 (i.e. those born after H1N1 viruses had last circulated from 1918 to 1957).
March 2009: Novel H1N1 human-swine-avian virus in March 2009 associated with a pandemic. Was responsible for more than 6000 deaths.
July 2011: H3N2 variant influenza associated with mild illness.

Case definitions

Influenza-like illness (ILI) is defined as fever (temperature of 100 °F [37.8 °C] or greater) with cough or sore throat in the absence of a known cause other than influenza.

A confirmed case of pandemic H1N1 influenza A is defined as an individual with an ILI with laboratory-confirmed H1N1 influenza A virus detection by real-time reverse transcriptase (rRT)-PCR or culture.

Definitions of illness severity

- **Mild or uncomplicated illness:** Characterised by fever, cough, sore throat, rhinorrhea, muscle pain, headache, chills, malaise and sometimes diarrhoea and vomiting, but no shortness of breath and little change in chronic health conditions
- **Progressive illness:** Typical symptoms plus signs or symptoms of respiratory or cardiopulmonary insufficiency, central nervous system impairment, severe dehydration or exacerbations of chronic conditions
- **Severe or complicated illness:** Severe or complicated illness is characterised by signs of respiratory failure or encephalopathy, complications of hypotension, myocarditis, rhabdomyolysis or invasive secondary bacterial infection based on laboratory testing or clinical signs

Predictors of outcome

- Older age
- Presence of pre-existing conditions
- Requirement for mechanical ventilation

Diagnostic assays

- rRT-PCR is the most sensitive and specific test for the diagnosis of pandemic influenza A virus infection
- Isolation of pandemic H1N1 influenza A virus using culture is also diagnostic, but culture is usually too slow to help guide clinical management
- A negative viral culture does not exclude pandemic H1N1 influenza A infection
- **Rapid antigen tests:** Certain rapid influenza antigen tests that are commercially available can distinguish between influenza A and B viruses, but cannot distinguish among different subtypes of influenza A.
- **Immunofluorescent antibody testing:** Direct or indirect immunofluorescent

antibody testing (DFA or IFA) can distinguish between influenza A and B, but does not distinguish among different influenza A subtypes.

Treatment

- During the 2009 to 2010 H1N1 influenza A pandemic a neuraminidase inhibitor (orally inhaled zanamivir or oral oseltamivir) was recommended
- Zanamivir was the preferred agent for patients with oseltamivir-resistant pandemic H1N1 infuenza A infection
- Antiviral therapy was recommended for individuals with suspected or confirmed pandemic H1N1 influenza A infection who were severely ill or who had risk factors for complications (e.g. pregnancy, age <5 or >65 years, severe immunocompromise)
- Several studies during the pandemic suggest treatment with a neuraminidase inhibitor (most commonly oseltamivir) reduced disease severity and mortality in hospitalised patients
- Post exposure prophylaxis was recommended for in adults and children with close contact with a confirmed or suspected case and in those who were either at increased risk for influenza complications or who were health care workers or emergency medical personnel

ICU management and referral guidelines for severe hypoxic respiratory failure

Hypoxic respiratory failure fulfilling ARDS criteria:

- ARDS: Non-cardiogenic pulmonary oedema of recognised aetiology, i.e. influenza.
- PCWP < 18 mmHg or assumed LA pressure <18 mmHg. Consider ECHO
- Bilateral infiltrates on CXR. **Consider CT chest** to exclude PE, pneumothorax, etc.
- P/F ratio < 200 mmHg (26.7 kPa). Measure and document P/F ratios

- High-risk groups for H1N1:
  1. **Peri-partum**
  2. **Obesity**
  3. **Chronic lung disease**
  4. **Immuno-compromise**

Non-ventilatory management

Microbiology
    Respiratory Samples
        Nasopharyngeal swab
        NBL or BAL
    Blood cultures
Anti-microbial
    IV antibiotics: Beta-lactam and Macrolide
    for a possible community acquired
    pneumonia
    Oral oseltamivir
Aerosol precautions for all clinical staff

Ventilatory management

0–48 h

- Measure and monitor P/F ratio
- Sedate
- Paralyse for first 24–48 h, especially if severe respiratory failure
  Review daily thereafter
- Controlled mode of ventilation
- Oxygenation (see **Figure 11**)
  i. Oxygenation
  (a) Aim for a Pao_2 8–9 kPa,
      Fio_2 and PEEP titration as per ARDS protocol.
      Reduce Fio_2 if Pao_2 > 9 kPa.
  (b) Accept, Pao_2 7–8 kPa, if Fio_2 > 0.8 and no significant evidence of organ hypoperfusion and no significant history of cardiovascular disease.
  (c) If, Pao_2 <8 kPa on Fio_2 > 0.8, consider chest X-ray to rule out a pneumothorax and treat as appropriate.

If in doubt, early referral to respiratory centre

  ii. Ventilation (CO_2 elimination, see **Figure 69.1**)
  (a) Measure patients height and calculate ideal body weight (IBW).
  (b) Tidal volume 4–6 mL kg^{-1} and plateau pressure < 30 cmH_2O.
      To achieve the above, accept pH> 7.25 regardless of $Paco_2$.

Aim for the lowest possible tidal volume and plateau pressure, as long as the pH> 7.25.
  (c) If tidal volume is > 6 mL kg^{-1} and/or plateau pressure > 30 cm of H_2O and pH < 7.25.
Consider, increasing sedation and paralysis.
Bolus and/or infusion of $NaHCO_3$.
Accepting pH >7.2, regardless of pCO_2, if the patient is haemodynamically stable.

If in doubt, early referral to respiratory centre

Day 3 onwards

Ventilatory management: Principles similar to that as described for the first 24 h

Special considerations:

1. **Persistent fever may reflect:**
   Co-infection esp. Streptococcal infections
       Review cultures
       Review antibiotics
       Chest X-ray and/or ultrasound thorax to rule out a pleural effusion (empyema)
   Persistent viraemia
       Review dose of oseltamivir
       Discuss with microbiology/virology team
       Resistance to oseltamivir is reported.
       Patients failing to respond should be considered for iv zanamivir.
   Thromboembolic disease especially if associated with refractory hypoxia
       Doppler legs, if possible CT pulmonary angiogram
       Consider anticoagulation
   Other causes: e.g. **line sepsis**

2. **Refractory hypoxia and cardiovascular instability may reflect:**
   Thromboembolic disease
   Myocarditis
       Check ECG
       2D echocardiogram
       Cardiology review
   Biventricular failure including pulmonary hypertension
   Check **ECG**
   2D echocardiogram
   Cardiology review

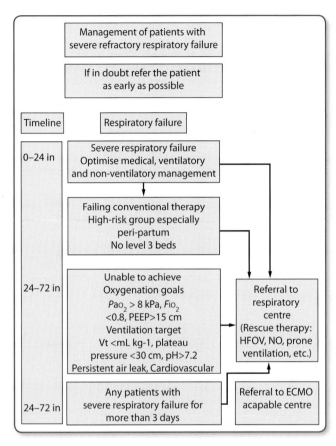

Figure 11 Management of patients with severe refractory respiratory failure.

3. **Fluid management**

Aim for a neutral or a negative fluid balance after the initial resuscitation Consider using diuretics or renal replacement therapy.

If in doubt, early referral to respiratory centre

Referral to respiratory centre

Indications for referral to respiratory centre:

1. Age: >16 years, if less liaise with regional PICU centre
2. Oxygenation

First 24 h

- Unable to achieve a Pao_2 > 8 kPa, with PEEP > 15 cm of H_2O and/or Fio_2> 0.8. Subsequently (days 2–7)
- Unable to maintain a Pao_2 > 8 kPa, with PEEP > 15 cm of H_2O and/or Fio_2> 0.8.
3. Respiratory acidosis

First 24 h

- Unable to maintain tidal volume <6 mL kg^{-1} and plateau pressure <30 cm of H_2O and pH >7.2 (if haemodynamically stable) or 7.25 (if haemodynamically unstable). Subsequently (days 2–7)
- Uncompensated respiratory acidosis with a pH <7.2 despite optimum treatment for greater than 48 h of conventional treatment (may include treatment with $NaHCO_3$ or CVVH).
4. Associated respiratory complication. i.e. bronchopleural fistula, uncontrolled air leak, etc.
5. Associated cardiovascular complication: biventricular failure, moderate-severe pulmonary hypertension.
6. Associated high risks, e.g. pregnancy, haematological malignancy and immunosuppressed.
7. Worsening/evolving multi-organ failure.

Further reading

Centers for Disease Control and Prevention (CDC). Update: novel influenza A (H1N1) virus infections – worldwide, May 6, 2009. MMWR Morb Mortal Wkly Rep 2009; 58:453.

Dawood FS, Jain S, Finelli L, et al. Emergence of a novel swine-origin influenza A (H1N1) virus in humans. N Engl J Med 2009; 360:2605–2615.

Webb SA, Pettilä V, Seppelt I, et al. Critical care services and 2009 H1N1 influenza in Australia and New Zealand. N Engl J Med 2009; 361:1925–1934.

Related topics of interest

- Acute respiratory distress syndrome (ARDS) – treatment (p 11)
- Extracorporeal membrane oxygenation (p 147)
- Respiratory support – invasive (p 306)

Patient safety

Key points

- Interventions to improve patient safety can effect outcomes even more than disease specific therapies.
- Creating a patient safety culture is of paramount importance when delivering quality improvement interventions.
- Many intensive care organisations have declared a major focus on improving patient safety, in collaboration with quality improvement organisations such as the Institute for Healthcare Improvement.

Quality, safety and error

Improving patient outcomes is the goal of every member of the critical care multi-disciplinary team. Every year there are many thousands of articles published suggesting new approaches and interventions aimed at this goal. Many research efforts focus on discrete therapeutic interventions, but it has proven difficult to show improvement in 'real world' outcomes that are important to patients. A more effective means of improving outcome may be identified through investigating the processes of care and finding methods of reducing avoidable harm.

Quality of care

The quality of healthcare is composed of three domains: patient experience, patient outcome and patient safety. A patient safety incident can be defined as any healthcare event that is unexpected, unintended and undesired and that could have or did cause harm to patients. An error in a healthcare process might be due to an omission (potential or actual harm from the failure to do something) or a commission (potential or actual harm from doing the wrong thing). In order for harm to occur it is often necessary for several errors to occur in sequence. Active errors are dynamic and limited to the incident itself (e.g. misidentification of potassium chloride as sodium chloride solution), while latent errors are systematic and potentially common to several situations (e.g. failure to store potassium chloride and sodium chloride ampoules separately).

In the United States (US), errors in healthcare processes cause between 50,000 to 100,000 deaths each year. Critically ill patients are at particular risk of harm from medical error, as they are exposed to highly invasive treatments, which can cause serious complications, frequently receive parenteral medications and are commonly unable to participate in their own care because of the nature of their illness.

Risk factors

Observational studies on European intensive care units (ICUs) indicate that 1% of the studied population suffer death or permanent harm as a result of a medication errors alone. Increasing frequency and severity of organ failure, increasing levels of critical care support, the number of patients per nurse, the number of parenteral medications and the use of any intravenous medication were all risk factors for harmful errors. Conversely, the use of basic monitoring, a critical incident reporting system, routine handover protocols at nursing shift changes and an increased ratio of patient turnover to the size of the unit were protective.

Quality improvement

Over recent years there have been concerted efforts to reduce the incidence of medical errors and to reduce the harm associated with them. In the US, the Institute for Healthcare Improvement (IHI) delivered the '5 Million Lives' campaign from 2006–2008, which led to similar programmes in the United Kingdom, Europe and Australia. Until it was abolished, the National Patient Safety Agency (NPSA) had been collating patient safety incidents across the United Kingdom and publishing quarterly data summaries, enabling an overview of patterns and trends to be developed. The NPSA in collaboration with the Health Foundation and the NHS Institute for Innovation and Improvement ran the Patient Safety First campaign, which focused on the implementation of five interventions: leadership for safety, reducing harm from deterioration, reducing harm from high-risk medicines and reducing harm in perioperative care and reducing harm in critical care. The Clinical Excellence Commission has been doing similar work in Australia.

Care bundles

A care bundle is a group of best practices around a disease process or medical intervention, each of which is beneficial but which result in substantially greater improvement when applied together. The bundle typically contains 4–5 interventions, but does not seek to be a comprehensive list of best practice. Crucially, for the bundle to be most effective all the interventions must be executed together, in an all-or-none strategy. Compliance with all parts of the bundle must be assessed and can be used as part of continuous audit activity to ensure that appropriate standards of care are being delivered.

Matching Michigan

Central venous catheter-related blood stream infections (CRBSIs) are an important complication of critical care. Intensive care units across the state of Michigan collaborated in a targeted safety improvement programme, which reduced the incidence of CRBSIs by 90% and reduced deaths by around 10%. The same group demonstrated similar improvements in the rate of ventilator-associated pneumonia (VAP) and has shown that the improvements can be sustained over a prolonged period. This experience has been replicated in the United Kingdom and in Australia.

Critical care bundles

Two particular care bundles for reducing harm in critical care have been described: a central line bundle and a ventilator care bundle. The details of these are given in Table 37. Daily recording of compliance with each part of the bundle is mandatory, as is recording the time between episodes of VAP and CRBSIs.

Promoting the safer ICU

The improvements demonstrated in Michigan were not all attributable to the implementation of care bundles. Just as important was engendering a culture of patient safety awareness within each unit and within each organisation. This empowered all members of the critical care team to speak up about safety concerns, and also involved regular measurement of outcomes and feedback of infection rates to staff and managers.

Encouraging a blame-free environment and utilising critical incident reporting enables improvements to be measured and makes it easier to identify where focused intervention may be beneficial. Despite

Bundle	Element
Ventilator care bundle	Elevation of the head of the bed
	Daily sedation interruption and assessment of readiness to extubate
	Peptic ulcer disease prophylaxis
	Venous thromboembolism prophylaxis
Central line bundle	Hand hygiene
	Maximum barrier precautions
	Chlorhexidine skin antisepsis
	Optimal catheter site selection
	Daily review of line necessity and prompt removal

Table 37 The elements of the Patient Safety First ventilator care bundle and central line bundle

this, numerous studies have shown that despite individual acceptance of particular interventions it is difficult to deliver best practice to every patient. For example, lung-protective ventilation strategies incorporating tidal volume limitation decrease mortality and ventilator associated lung injury, yet observational studies show it is delivered in less than 30% of cases.

In 2009, a group of intensive care and patient safety organisations released the Declaration of Vienna, which pledged to improve the knowledge and understanding of the causes of failures in patient safety, develop and promote criteria to assess safety in ICU and work to translate this understanding into improvements in quality of care.

Further reading

Berenholtz S, Pronovost P, Lipsett P, et al. Eliminating catheter-related bloodstream infections in the intensive care unit. Crit Care Med 2004; 32:2014–2020.

Moreno R, Rhodes A, Donchin Y. Patient safety in intensive care medicine: the Declaration of Vienna. Intensive Care Med 2009; 35:1667–1672.

Bion J, Richardson A, Hibbert P, et al. 'Matching Michigan': a 2-year stepped interventional programme to minimise central venous catheter-blood stream infections in intensive care units in England. Br Med J quality & safety 2013; 22:110–123.

Related topics of interest

Pituitary disease

Key points

- Derangement of pituitary function occurs in all critically ill patients
- Distinguishing between 'adaptive' endocrine changes and what is pathological in critical illness is difficult
- Many of the tests developed for assessment of endocrine function in outpatients are difficult to interpret on the intensive care unit

Anatomy and physiology

The pituitary gland is situated in the sella turcica, in the base of the skull. Although it weighs less than 1 g (500–900 mg) and has a volume of less than 1 cm³ (15 × 10 × 6 mm), it plays a critical role in normal homeostatic function. It is divided into the anterior and posterior pituitary, both of which lie outside the blood-brain-barrier. The anterior pituitary makes up around 2/3 of the gland and secretes the majority of the hormones (see **Table 38**).

The anterior pituitary is regulated by hypothalamic-tropic hormones, which reach it via the portal venous system. The posterior pituitary is directly regulated by the hypothalamus. Hypothalamic nerves project directly to the posterior pituitary and synapse with the cells within it. Most of the anterior pituitary hormones work via a negative feedback mechanism (**Figure 12**). The exception is during the mid menstrual cycle – when high levels of oestradiol cause luteinizing hormone (LH) release. This subsequently causes release of the ova.

The pituitary in intensive care patients

Virtually all patients in intensive care will have significant abnormalities of pituitary hormone secretion. The majority of these will be adaptive; that is, that they are a normal response to an abnormal situation.

In the majority of patients, cortisol levels rise in response to illness. This is adrenocorticotrophic hormone (ACTH) driven initially, but in later stages, it is driven by some other factors.

Circulating levels of testosterone fall in the first few days of critical illness, despite normal levels of the pituitary produced gonadotropins. The gonadotropin levels fall after a few days of critical illness leading to further testosterone deficiency.

The 'sick euthyroid syndrome' is well-recognised and is characterised by a fall in the levels of T3 and a rise in the levels of reverseT3 (rT3). Both thyroid stimulating hormone (TSH) and T4 rise initially and then fall (although T4 can fall acutely).

There is no consistent change in growth hormone (GH) levels after surgery and in critical illness. Rises, falls and normal levels have all been seen.

Traumatic brain injury and subarachnoid haemorrhage

Since most patients with traumatic brain injury (TBI) and subarachnoid haemorrhage (SAH) are critically ill, distinguishing which

Table 38 Pituitary hormones	
Anterior pituitary hormones	**Posterior pituitary hormones**
Adrenocorticotrophic hormone (ACTH)	Anti-diuretic hormone (ADH)
Thyroid stimulating hormone (TSH)	Oxytocin
Follicle stimulating hormone (FSH)/Luteinizing hormone (LH)	
Growth hormone (GH)	
Prolactin	
β-melanocyte stimulating (MSH)	
Endorphins/encephalins	

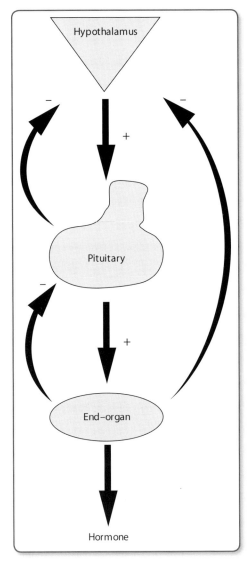

Figure 12 Schematic of the hypothalamic – anterior pituitary feedback system.

Labels within figure: Hypothalamus, Pituitary, End–organ, Hormone

there appears to be no correlation between initial adrenal function and that at 6 months.

Over 80% of patients will have a reduction in levels of their gonadotropins with secondary gonadal failure after TBI and >50% will have hyperprolactinaemia. The thyroid profile after TBI is essentially that of the 'sick euthyroid' syndrome. There is little evidence to guide practice with regard to GH.

Diabetes insipidus (DI) is much more common in TBI, whereas Syndrome of Inappropriate Anti-Diuretic Hormone (SIADH) is seen more often in SAH. DI occurs in 25–50% of TBI episodes, but significantly less (<5%) in SAH. It is associated with a higher severity of injury, more cerebral oedema and a higher mortality. DI can persist permanently after TBI. SIADH is almost always transient after TBI and is usually seen in the first 2 days after the injury, although it can occur up to 2 weeks afterwards.

Panhypopituitarism

Panhypopituitarism does not occur until at least 75% of the cells of the anterior pituitary have been destroyed. Complete loss of hormone secretion does not occur until >90% of the cells are non-functional. The indolent nature of this means that those with reduced pituitary function can remain unsuspected for many years and only become apparent with an intercurrent illness. In those who are susceptible, the stress of surgery and critical illness can lead to a panhypopituitary state.

The commonest cause for panhypopituitarism is iatrogenic following pituitary surgery. 'Sheehans syndrome' (hypotension during childbirth causing pituitary infarction) is the most common after that. Causes of panhypopituitarism are outlined in **Table 39**. Symptoms of a hypopituitary state include hypotension, hypoglycaemia and coma.

Pituitary insufficiency should be considered in those patients with a history of past pituitary surgery, pituitary adenoma, peripartum haemorrhage with failure of lactation or restart of menstruation, loss of menstruation, libido and hair and impotence.

changes are adaptive and which are as a result of direct pituitary damage is difficult. There is a reasonable amount of evidence that both cortisol and ACTH rise immediately after the injury, although following this, rates of relative adrenal insufficiency are higher in those with TBI than in the general intensive care population. Quite how many of these patients will go on to have long term problems still needs to be elucidated, but

Table 39 Causes of panhypopituitarism
Mass lesions – pituitary/hypothalamic
Pituitary surgery
Radiotherapy
Infiltration – sarcoid/mastocytosis/haemochromatosis
Infarction
Apoplexy
Trauma (base of skull fracture)
Empty sella syndrome
Infection (TB)

As with most emergencies, treatment occurs in parallel with investigation and is general and supportive. Specific measures for panhypopituitarism are:
- Blood for Cortisol, ACTH, Prolactin, Thyroid, LH, FSH and GH
- IV fluids to restore circulating volume
- IV Hydrocortisone – many of its vascular tone effects are mediated by extracellular receptors and have effects rapidly. Fluids and hydrocortisone are the life-saving measures
- Intravenous T3 after starting hydrocortisone can be considered although it is currently unclear whether this improves outcomes
- Look for precipitating cause (usually an infection)
- Short synacthen test and LH / thyrotropin releasing hormone (TRH) tests can be done together if the patient is relatively well before treatment
- CT/MRI of pituitary
- Early endocrinology consultation
  - Long term, patients will require hydrocortisone, thyroxine, sex hormones and possibly GH

Pituitary tumours

Primary pituitary tumours are almost always benign and account for around 10% of primary intracranial neoplasms. They may be derived from any hormone producing cell and most are adenomas. Carcinomas are very rare.

The symptoms of pituitary tumours are either those of hormone hyper- or hypo-secretion or those of mass effects. The presentation is dependent on tumour size and cell type. Microadenomas are <1 cm in diameter and present with symptoms of hormone excess, for example Cushing's disease. Macroadenomas are >1 cm in diameter and usually present with mass effects, most usually visual field defects and headache. Later presenting larger tumours may present with hydrocephalus (due to obstruction of the IVth ventricle), hypopituitarism (due to compression ischaemia of the pituitary) or as an incidental finding on CT scanning.

Table 40 details the different types of anterior adenoma tumours. Posterior pituitary tumours are vanishingly rare due to the limited capacity of these cells for mitotic division. Most ADH secreting tumours are not primarily intracranial, but from extra-cranial sites, such as the bronchus.

Multiple endocrine neoplasia

The multiple endocrine neoplasia (MEN) is a group of neoplastic syndromes that involve both benign and malignant tumours of the endocrine glands. They receive disproportionate attention for their low prevalence because they allow understanding of the pathways that regulate their constituent tumours. They are all inherited in an

Table 40 Different types of anterior adenoma tumours				
Type of adenoma	**Incidence**	**Signs and symptoms**	**Management**	**Other information**
Prolactinoma	22–73% of pituitary adenomas	Galactorrhea, menstrual disturbance, erectile dysfunction and gynaecomastia.	Dopamine agonists reduce prolactin levels, improve symptoms (including visual field defects) and shrink the tumour by up to 70%. Surgery is reserved for those who fail to respond to medical therapy and women seeking fertility.	F:M 10:1 before the age of 50. Equal thereafter. Prolactin levels correlate with tumour size.
Non-functioning adenomas	30–39% pituitary adenomas	Some large tumours cause hormone hypersecretion (usually prolactin) or hypopituitarism by compression.	Unless there are mass effects, they are usually treated conservatively with annual MRI scans and visual field tests.	Male preponderance.
Somatotropinoma (GH secreting)	15–21% of pituitary adenomas	Gigantism in children. Acromegaly in adults: large hands and feet, prognathism, deepening voice, hypertension, insulin resistance and sleep apnoea.	Medical treatment: Dopamine agonists (cabergoline), somatostatin antagonists (octreotide) and GH-receptor antagonists (pegvisomant). Radiation therapy – including gamma knife surgery. Almost all will be hypopituitary after 15 years. Surgery is final therapeutic option.	Diagnosed by MRI brain and elevated GH and IGF-1 (insulin like growth factor-1) levels. IGF-1 correlates more closely with disease severity. 25% of GH tumours also secrete prolactin.
Corticotropinoma (ACTH secreting)	5–11% of pituitary adenomas	Present with Cushing's features: moon face, thin skin, hypertension, hirsutism, obesity, buffalo hump, muscle weakness, diabetes.	Medical therapy includes metyrapone and ketoconazole. Tumours are treated by trans-sphenoidal surgery. Radiation therapy for those with minimal surgical response.	Responsible for 70% of those with Cushing's syndrome.
Thyrotropinoma (TSH secreting)	< 1% of pituitary adenomas	Usually present with thyrotoxicosis or mass effect. Raised TSH and T4.	First line of treatment is neurosurgical.	Up to 15% co-secrete: usually GH or prolactin, but sometimes gonadotropins.

autosomal dominant fashion and occur in characteristic patterns divided as below:

MEN I
- Parathyroid adenoma/hyperplasia
- Pancreatic islet cell tumour
- Pituitary adenoma
- *Small bowel tumours*
- *Differentiated thyroid carcinoma*
- *Non-functioning adrenal adenomas*
- *Lipomas*

Those in *italics* are rare.

MEN IIa
- Medullary thyroid carcinoma
- Phaeochromocytoma
- Parathyroid hyperplasia

MEN IIb
- Medullary thyroid carcinoma
- Phaeochromocytoma
- Marfanoid features, multiple neuromas, neurofibromas and GI ganglioneuromas

FMTC
- Familial medullary thyroid carcinoma

Further reading

Melmed S, Polonsky KS, Reed Larson P, et al. Williams Textbook of Endocrinology, 12th edn. Philadelphia: Elsevier Saunders, 2011.

Hannon MJ, Sherlock M, Thompson CJ. Pituitary dysfunction following traumatic brain injury or subarachnoid haemorrhage - in "Endocrine Management in the Intensive Care Unit". Best Pract Res Clin Endocrinol Metab 2011; 25:783–798.

Lleva RR, Inzucchi SE. Diagnosis and management of pituitary adenomas. Curr Opin Oncol 2011; 23:53–60.

Related topics of interest

- Adrenal disease (p 14)
- Thyroid gland disorders (p 365)

Pleural disease

Key points

- On a chest radiograph signs of pleural disease are often subtle – a high index of suspicion is required
- In the presence of an effusion, use ultrasound before any pleural procedure
- If disease is non-resolving, discuss early with surgeons

Epidemiology

Pleural disease is common in the ICU and ranges from small effusions requiring no intervention to life-threatening tension pneumothorax requiring immediate treatment.

Pneumothorax

Pneumothoraces are divided into primary (no underlying lung disease) or secondary (presence of underlying lung disease). Secondary pneumothoraces can be spontaneous, iatrogenic or secondary to trauma.

Pleural effusion

Pleural effusions are present on >60% of chest radiographs in ICU and have many causes. The majority are transudates (pleural fluid protein <30 g L^{-1}) secondary to a combination of cardiac, renal or hepatic failure plus hypoalbuminaemia. The more common causes of an exudate are infection, malignancy and post-surgery (thoracic or upper gastrointestinal).

A haemothorax occurs when the pleural fluid haematocrit is >50% of the peripheral blood haematocrit.

Empyema

Causes of pleural infection include pneumonia, iatrogenic causes (e.g. chest drain insertion), oesophageal rupture or spread of infection from other sites, e.g. mediastinitis.

The bacteria involved depend on the underlying cause and whether the infection is community or hospital acquired. Methicillin-resistant *Staphylococcus aureus* is the commonest cause of nosocomial infections. Gram-negative organisms such as pseudomonas account for the majority of the remainder. Streptococcal species are the most commonly cultured from community acquired pneumonias. If DNA amplification is used, anaerobes are identified in up to 76% of cases. No organisms are cultured in about 40% of cases of empyemas.

Clinical features

Pneumothorax

The clinical features vary depending on whether the patient is ventilated and if it is a simple or tension pneumothorax. Symptoms include increasing dyspnoea and pleuritic chest pain. Examination may reveal hyper-resonance to percussion and reduced chest wall movement of the affected side, tachycardia and surgical emphysema. The trachea deviates towards a simple pneumothorax but away from a tension pneumothorax.

In a ventilated patient the signs may not be so classical. There is increasing difficulty maintaining adequate ventilation with increasing peak airway pressures, reduced tidal volumes and worsening hypoxia. A tension pneumothorax leads to increasing cardiorespiratory compromise and cardiac arrest.

Pleural effusions

Examination findings include decreased air entry, stony dullness to percussion and reduced chest wall movement. As the effusion increases in size it can lead to signs of respiratory compromise.

Empyema

This is suspected in anyone with a pleural effusion and signs of sepsis with no known cause or a lack of response to treatment of a known source.

Consider empyema in a patient with pneumonia who has ongoing sepsis or a failure of the C-reactive protein to reduce by 50% after 3 days.

Haemothorax

Haemodynamic compromise occurs earlier and with smaller volume than other effusions. Suspect haemothorax in anyone with a history of trauma or in any patient with an effusion or haemodynamic compromise following thoracic procedures.

Investigations

Chest radiograph

This is the first line investigation unless a tension pneumothorax is suspected when it is treated immediately based on clinical suspicion.

In ventilated supine patients, a pneumothorax can be difficult to see on a chest radiograph and can be confused with bullae or skin folds. Signs of a pneumothorax on a supine film include the deep sulcus sign (where the costophrenic angle is abnormally deepened), hyperlucent hemithorax, increased basal lucency, depressed diaphragm, clear or sharp heart border and the double hemidiaphragm sign.

In a supine patient with an effusion, there may simply be diffuse increased shadowing of the affected side rather than a classic fluid level.

Ultrasound

This is far superior to chest radiography for detecting effusions, especially if they are small or if there is also consolidation.

It is recommended before any intervention for pleural fluid, particularly in ventilated patients, as it reduces the incidence of complications such as pneumothoraces.

It provides additional information, e.g. the presence of septa.

Computed tomography

This provides diagnostic information about the underlying cause, e.g. malignancy or trauma.

It can detect small pneumothoraces and helps to differentiate between a large bulla and a pneumothorax. Consider obtaining a computed tomography (CT) scan in the presence of known bullous disease prior to intervention if the patient's condition allows.

CT helps to differentiate between a pleural and pulmonary collection.

Pleural aspiration

This is unnecessary in all patients with an effusion but should be performed in suspected pleural infection or when there is diagnostic uncertainty. Send a 50 ml sample for protein, glucose, LDH, MC+S, AFB's, cytology and pH.

Treatment

Pneumothorax

Small, asymptomatic pneumothoraces can often be monitored. High-flow oxygen increases the pleural air reabsorption rate. Traditionally, a chest drain was inserted if the pneumothorax was greater than 2 cm when measured at the hilum. It is now accepted that in asymptomatic patients with a primary pneumothorax, a patient can be treated conservatively with larger pneumothoraces.

A chest drain is usually required in patients undergoing mechanical ventilation or if they are secondary pneumothoraces.

Do not clamp chest drains routinely and never remove or clamp a chest drain if bubbling because this risks a tension pneumothorax.

If a tension pneumothorax is suspected in conjunction with significant haemodynamic compromise, decompress with a cannula in the second intercostal space at the mid-clavicular line and then insert a chest drain.

Effusions

Transudative effusions rarely require intervention. Even if a large effusion is drained there is often little improvement in oxygenation, but sometimes weaning is facilitated.

Management of an exudative effusion will depend on the cause and size of the effusion. An empyema will need draining whereas a simple parapneumonic effusion could be managed conservatively if small but, if large, may need draining to facilitate weaning.

Empyema

Treatment includes draining the infected fluid, targeted antibiotics and careful evaluation of nutritional requirements. Antibiotics should reflect the high level of penicillin resistant organisms and include anaerobic cover. In hospital-acquired infections, cover MRSA as well as anaerobes and gram negative and positive aerobes.

There is no agreement on the optimum timing of surgery – it will depend to some degree on availability. Discuss with a surgeon if there are ongoing signs of sepsis and a persistent collection at 5–7 days. If the cause is iatrogenic, following surgery or oesophageal rupture obtain a surgical review immediately.

Surgical options include rib resection and drainage (which can be performed under local anaesthetic), video-assisted thorascopic surgery and thoracotomy and decortication.

The use of fibrinolytic drugs is controversial. British Thoracic Society guidelines recommend their use in large, loculated fluid collections resistant to chest tube drainage where thoracic surgery is not suitable or available.

Assume a bronchopleural fistula (BPF) in anyone with an empyema who has undergone recent thoracic surgery. Isolate the lung before applying positive ventilation so that soiling of the unaffected lung is prevented; otherwise, ventilation may be very difficult and a tension pneumothorax may result. Even if there is no BPF at the time of intubation, any suture line is likely to be extremely fragile and susceptible to rupture with ventilation.

Size of chest drain

There is no consensus on the optimal drain size. Trials of chest drains in pleural infections showed increased complications and no benefit with larger drains. There is good evidence that small drains lead to good outcomes but require regular flushing.

Large-bore drains (>28 Fr) are recommended for a haemothorax, thick pus, a large air leak, worsening surgical emphysema or complicated effusions, e.g. hydropneumothorax.

Seldinger drains are potentially dangerous if used when there is insufficient air or fluid in the pleural space. Consider blunt dissection if ultrasound is not used to guide insertion or if there is any concern about the underlying lung e.g. presence of tethering or bullous disease.

Complications

Complications of chest drain insertion include penetration of major organs, such as lung, liver or spleen, damage of major blood vessels, pleural infection and surgical emphysema.

In the presence of an effusion these risks are greatly reduced by using real time ultrasound.

Further reading

Davies HE, Davies RJ, Davies CW. Management of pleural infection in adults: British Thoracic Society pleural guidelines 2010. Thorax 2010; 65:ii41–53.
Walters J, Foley NM, Molyneux M. Pus in the thorax: management of empyema and lung abscess. Contin Educ Anaesth Crit Care Pain 2011; 11:229–233.

Bateman K, Maskell N. Pleural Disease. In: Hughes M, Black R (Eds). Advanced Respiratory Critical Care (Oxford Specialist Handbooks in Critical Care) 1st edn. Oxford: Oxford University Press, 2011:481–492.

Related topics of interest

Pneumonia – community acquired

Key points

- The incidence of community-acquired pneumonia (CAP) is 5–11 per 1000 adults; one third of these will require hospital admission and, of these, 5–10% will require ICU admission
- *Streptococcus pneumoniae* is the commonest cause of CAP – it is isolated in about 30% of cases
- Severity of CAP is assessed using the CURB-65 score

Epidemiology

Community-acquired infection is an infection that occurs in a patient who has not been hospitalised in the preceding 2 weeks or one that occurred within 48 h of admission to hospital. The incidence of community-acquired pneumonia (CAP) is 5–11 per 1000 adults. About two-thirds will be treated at home and the remaining third are admitted to hospital – 5–10% of the latter will require admission to an intensive care unit (ICU). The mortality is 5–15% among those requiring hospital admission and 35–50% for those admitted to an ICU. Community-acquired pneumonia occurs more commonly in those over 65, smokers, and those with other non-respiratory illnesses.

Streptococcus pneumoniae is the commonest cause of CAP – it is isolated in about 30% of cases. No organism is isolated in one-third of cases. Pathogens causing adult CAP in the United Kingdom are listed in **Table 41**. Among patients admitted to an ICU, *Legionella* is the second commonest cause of CAP.

H. influenzae is the commonest cause of bacterial exacerbation of chronic obstructive pulmonary disease. The possibility of *S. aureus* should be considered during an influenza epidemic, particularly if there is radiological evidence of cavitation. Mycoplasma is commonly associated with cough, sore throat, nausea, diarrhoea, headache and myalgia. Generally, clinical and radiological features are not sensitive or specific enough to predict the microbial aetiology.

Viral pneumonia is most commonly caused by influenza virus and can occur in pandemics.

Table 41 Pathogens causing adult community acquired pneumonia in the United Kingdom by site of care (%)			
	Community	Hospital	Critical care unit
Streptococcus pneumoniae	36.0	39.0	21.6
Haemophilus influenzae	10.2	5.2	3.8
Legionella species	0.4	3.6	17.8
Staphylococcus aureus	0.8	1.9	8.7
Gram-negative enteric bacilli	1.3	1.0	1.6
Mycoplasma pneumoniae	1.3	10.8	2.7
Chlamydophila pneumoniae	?	13.1	?
Viral (mainly influenza A and B)	13.1	9.1	5.4

Adapted from: The British Thoracic Society. Guidelines for the management of community-acquired pneumonia in adults: update 2009. Thorax 2009; 64 (suppl III): iii1–ii55.

Clinical features and initial management

The features of CAP in hospital patients are:
- Cough and new focal chest signs
- At least one systemic feature of sweating, shivers, malaise and/or fever of at least 38 °C
- New shadowing on chest X-ray with no other explanation
- Patient presents with above features as primary reason for hospital admission

Initial assessment and management follows standard ABCDE principles. Oxygen is given to maintain arterial oxygen saturation > 92%. Look for signs of respiratory distress, listen for focal chest signs, assess the circulation to identify evidence of shock, and document conscious level. The British Thoracic Society recommends use of the CURB-65 score to assess severity.

CURB-65

One point is given for each of:
- **Confusion**: new onset confusion (mini-mental test ≤ 8)
- **Urea**: raised > 7 mmol L^{-1}
- **Respiratory rate**: raised ≥ 30 min^{-1}
- **Blood pressure**: systolic blood pressure < 90 mmHg and/or diastolic blood pressure ≤ 60 mmHg
- **65**: age ≥ 65 years

A CURB-65 score of 0–1 indicates CAP of low severity with associated mortality of < 3%; a score of 2 indicates moderate severity with a mortality risk of 9%; a score 3–5 indicates high severity with a risk of death of 15–40%. Patients with a CURB-65 score of 4 or 5 should be referred to ICU.

Investigations and diagnosis

Investigations should be undertaken to assess severity and identify aetiology.
- Chest X-ray – consolidation (patchy or lobar)
- Arterial blood gas analysis and lactate
- Full blood count – neutrophilia or neutropaenia
- C-reactive protein
- Urea, electrolytes and liver function tests

- Sputum Gram stain, culture and sensitivity. The presence of Gram-positive diplococci implies pneumococcal infection
- Urine antigen test. Antigens of *S. pneumoniae* and *Legionella* spp. can be detected in urine, sputum or blood even in patients who have already received antibiotics. The test for *Legionella* has a sensitivity of 80% and a specificity of > 95%. The sensitivity for pneumococcal urinary antigen in defining invasive pneumococcal disease is 60–90% with specificity close to 100%
- Blood culture, ideally before the first dose of antibiotic. They are positive in about 10–20% of cases
- Paired serology testing (on admission and 7–10 days later) is available for influenza A and B viruses, respiratory syncytial virus, adenovirus, *C. burnetti*, *C. psittaci*, *M. pneumoniae* and *L. pneumophila*, but does not often provide diagnostic changes early enough to be clinically useful
- Polymerase chain reaction (PCR) is now used to diagnose *Mycoplasma pneumonia*, *Chlamydophilia* species and several respiratory viruses. Nasopharyngeal asoirates or swabs are suitable initial samples for PCR testing for viruses but endotracheal or bronchoscopic aspirates have higher yields in patients with CAP
- In intubated patients, bronchoscopy enables sampling by bronchoalveolar lavage. Bronchoscopy will also enable the diagnosis of any underlying lung disease such as a bronchial tumour

Treatment
Antibiotics

Antibiotics should be given to treat severe CAP as soon as possible and certainly within 4 h of admission to hospital. The infecting organism is usually unknown when treatment is initiated. Empirical therapy should always cover *S. pneumoniae*. Penicillin-resistant pneumococci are increasing worldwide, although less so in the United Kingdom.
- Initial antibiotic therapy comprises a broad-spectrum β-lactamase stable

antibiotic together with a macrolide, e.g. co-amoxiclav 1.2 g 8 h IV with clarithromycin 500 mg 12 h IV. Antibiotic treatment is continued for 7–10 days and then reviewed

- If the patient is allergic to penicillin, give either a third-generation cephalosporin (e.g. cefotaxime or ceftriaxone) or vancomycin, together with clarithromycin
- If *Legionella* is confirmed, combine clarithromycin with rifampicin or ciprofloxacin and give for 14–21 days
- Antibiotics given for pneumonia caused by *Staphylococcus aureus* (flucloxacillin) or for Gram-negative enteric bacilli are continued for 14–21 days
- Methacillin resistant *Staphylococcus aureus* (MRSA) is a rare cause of CAP although it is becoming more common in nursing homes. MRSA pneumonia is treated with linezolid 600 mg 12 h IV
- Patients admitted to ICU with severe CAP and who have influenza identified in nasopharyngeal aspirate are given oseltamivir 75–150 mg twice daily for 5 days, although there is little evidence for its efficacy in critically ill patients

Ventilation

Non-invasive ventilation (NIV) and continuous positive airways pressure may produce transient improvement in oxygenation but most patients in whom this is attempted eventually require intubation. For this reason, if a trial of NIV is to undertaken it should be attempted only in an ICU where, if necessary, intubation can be achieved rapidly.

Circulation

Septic shock is common in severe CAP and will require optimal fluid loading and use of vasopressors with or without inotropes. Although steroids are not given to treat severe CAP, for patients requiring more than 0.025 mcg kg^{-1} min^{-1} noradrenaline, it is reasonable to add hydrocortisone 50 mg qds, which may enable reduction of the vasopressor dose.

Complications

- Parapneumonic effusions develop in 40–60% of patients with bacterial CAP. The BTS recommends early thoracocentesis in all patients with a parapneumonic effusion. Pleural drainage is required for empyema (cloudy fluid, frank pus or organisms on Gram stain) or if the pleural fluid is clear but has a pH < 7.2. Frank pus or a loculated effusion may require surgical drainage
- Lung abscesses can occur in debilitated patients
- Metastatic infection resulting in meningitis, endocarditis and septic arthritis can occur with *S. aureus* or *S. pneumonia*

Further reading

Lim WS1, Baudouin SV, George RC, et al. BTS guidelines for the management of community-acquired pneumonia in adults: update 2009. Thorax 2009; 64:iii1–55.

van der Poll T, Opal SM. Pathogenesis, treatment, and prevention of pneumococcal pneumonia. Lancet 2009; 374:1543–1556.

Bautista E, Chotpitayasunondh T, Gao Z, et al. Clinical aspects of pandemic 2009 influenza A (H1N1) virus infection. N Engl J Med 2010; 362:1708–1719.

Related topics of interest

Pneumonia – hospital acquired

Key points

- Ventilator associated pneumonia (VAP) accounts for more than 80% of hospital acquired pneumonia episodes in the ICU
- Use of clinical criteria alone for diagnosis produces 30–35% false negative results and 20–25% false positive results. The addition of microbiological criteria improves diagnostic accuracy considerably
- VAP can be prevented by reducing colonisation of the gastrointestinal tract and oropharynx, prevention of aspiration, and by limiting the duration of mechanical ventilation

Epidemiology

Nosocomial infection is defined as an infection occurring more than 48 h after hospital admission, or within 48 h of discharge. Hospital acquired (nosocomial) pneumonia (HAP) accounts for 15% of all hospital-acquired infections and 31% of infections acquired in the ICU. The incidence of HAP is 5–15 episodes per 1000 hospital admissions. More than 80% of HAP episodes in the ICU occur in intubated patients undergoing mechanical ventilation – ventilator associated pneumonia (VAP). Ventilator associated pneumonia occurs in 9–27% of mechanically ventilated patients, representing five cases per 1000 ventilator days.

Pathophysiology

The aetiology of HAP is influenced significantly by the patient's length of stay in hospital. The early onset (< 5 days) HAP is likely to be caused by potentially pathogenic micro-organisms (PPM) that were carried by the patient at the time of hospital admission, e.g. *Streptococcus pneumoniae*, *Haemophilus influenzae* and *Staphylococcus aureus*.
In health, an intact mucosal lining, mucus, normal gastrointestinal motility, secretory IgA, and resident anaerobes inhibit colonisation of the gastrointestinal tract by aerobic bacteria. In the critically ill, impairment of these protective mechanisms promotes colonisation of the gastrointestinal tract by aerobic Gram-negative bacteria (e.g. *E. coli*, *Psuedomonas aeruginosa*, *Klebsiella* spp. and *Proteus* spp.), *S. aureus* (including MRSA) and yeasts (e.g. *Candida* spp.). Secondary endogenous infection is caused by PPMs acquired in the critical care unit. These multi-drug resistant pathogens are a significant cause of late onset (> 5 days) HAP. Other risk factors for development of multi-drug resistant HAP are:

- Antimicrobial therapy in the last 30 days
- Immunosuppressive disease or therapy
- Hospitalisation for > 2 days in the last 90 days
- Residence in a nursing home
- Chronic haemodialysis

Intubation and mechanical ventilation increase the risk of HAP by up to 20 times. Factors contributing to the development of VAP include:

- The tracheal tube bypasses the protective upper airway reflexes, prevents coughing and promotes microaspiration of oropharyngeal secretions contaminated with aerobic Gram-negative bacteria that pool above the tracheal tube cuff. Folds in the tracheal tube cuff enable secretions to travel down the airway
- A bacterial biofilm forms on the inside of the tracheal tube and is pushed into the lower airways during positive pressure ventilation
- The supine position increases the risk of micro-aspiration. Risk of aspiration may be increased with enteral feeding but the latter is generally considered to provide advantages that outweigh this risk
- Opiates, high F_{IO_2}, inadequate humidification, and tracheal suctioning impair mucociliary transport
- A gastric pH > 4.0 encourages colonisation by Gram-negative organisms. Thus H_2-blockers and proton pump inhibitors may contribute to VAP
- Patients over the age of 70 years and those with chronic lung disease are more likely to develop VAP

The main organisms causing VAP are listed in **Table 42**.

Table 42 Causes of ventilator acquired pneumonia (VAP) (868 micro-organisms isolated from 685 VAP episodes among intensive care unit patients in France 1997-2008)	
Micro-organism	*n* (%)
Gram positive	244 (28.1)
Streptococcus pneumonia	45 (5.2)
Staphylococcus aureus	84 (9.7)
Methicillin susceptible	49 (5.6)
Methicillin resistant	32 (3.7)
Coagulase-negative staphylococci	7 (0.8)
Enterococci	27 (3.1)
Streptococcus, other	
Gram negative	554 (63.8)
Haemophilus influenzae	63 (7.3)
Enterobacteriaceae	66 (7.6)
Escherichia coli	38 (4.4)
Klebsiella sp.	37 (4.3)
Enterobacter sp.	16 (1.8)
Citrobacter freundii	21 (2.4)
Serratia marcescens	14 (1.6)
Proteus mirabilis	13 (1.5)
Morganella morganii	227 (26.2)
Pseudomonas aeruginosa	24 (8.2)
Acinetobacter sp.	35 (4.0)
Stenotrophomonas maltophilia	
Other	70 (8.1)
Data from Bekaert M et al.	

Diagnosis

The diagnosis of HAP should be suspected in any patient with new or progressive infiltrates on chest X-ray, plus two or more of the following:
- Purulent tracheal secretions
- Blood leucocytosis or leucopaenia
- Temperature greater than 38.3 °C

Diagnosis of VAP is particularly challenging because other conditions that are common in the critically ill can mimic VAP, e.g. pulmonary oedema and acute respiratory distress syndrome. Use of clinical criteria alone for diagnosis produces 30–35% false negative results and 20–25% false positive results. For this reason, ideally, samples should be obtained from the lower respiratory tract before antibiotics are started. Samples can be obtained invasively [bronchoalveolar lavage (BAL) or protected specimen brushing (PSB)] or non-invasively (simple tracheal aspirates). Invasively obtained samples are analysed quantitatively with diagnostic thresholds of 10^3 colony forming units (cfu) mL^{-1} for PSB and 10^4 cfu mL^{-1} for BAL. The protected mini-BAL technique combines attributes from the PSB and BAL techniques. Tracheal aspirates can be analysed quantitatively or qualitatively. A randomised trial of BAL and quantitative culture versus non-quantitative culture of tracheal aspirates for the diagnosis of VAP showed no difference in the primary outcome.

Treatment

If there is high clinical suspicion of HAP antibiotics should be started promptly but, ideally, microbiological sample should be obtained first. Choice of antibiotics are directed by local guidelines that will have been written with knowledge of local microbiological data. For example: for severe HAP in patients hospitalised for less than 5 days and who have had no previous antibiotics, co-amoxiclav is suitable; for patients hospitalised for 5 days or more or

who have been given antibiotics previously, piperacillin-tazobactam (with vancomycin if MRSA is suspected) would be appropriate. In all cases, if the patient has evidence of generalised sepsis, a dose of gentamicin 5 mg kg^{-1} may also be beneficial.

Prevention of ventilator-associated pneumonia

There are three main ways of preventing VAP: reduce colonisation of the gastrointestinal tract and oropharynx by Gram negative organisms; prevent aspiration; and limit the duration of mechanical ventilation. The Institute for Healthcare Improvement (IHI) has developed a ventilator bundle comprising five elements – three of these target VAP while the other two address prevention of stress ulcers and thromboembolic disease:

- Elevation of the head of the bed to 45°
- Daily sedation holds and assessment for potential extubation
- Daily oral care with chlorhexidine
- Stress ulcer prophylaxis with proton pump inhibitors or H$_2$-receptor antagonists
- Anticoagulants and/or compression devices

Selective decontamination of the digestive tract involves oral and gastric administration of non-absorbable antibiotics and administration of intravenous antibiotics. Numerous studies have shown that this strategy reduces the incidence of VAP and at least one high quality study has shown reduced mortality, although only after risk-adjustment. However, unproven concerns about selecting out antibiotic resistant organisms have prevented the strategy from being used widely in the United Kingdom. Oral decontamination with chlorhexidine reduces the VAP rate (a meta-analysis of 11 studies showed a relative risk of 0.61; 95% CI 0.45–0.82) and this is used widely as part of the IHI ventilator bundle. The use of silver-coated tracheal tubes reduces bacterial colonisation and the VAP rate but does not reduce mortality.

Nursing patients in the 45° head up position reduces the risk of regurgitation and aspiration of gastric contents. Sub-glottic drainage using specially designed tracheal tubes and tracheostomy tubes halves the risk of VAP in patients expected to need ventilation for more than 72 h. A tracheal tube with a modified cuff, with fewer and narrower longitudinal folds when inflated, has been shown to reduce the risk of VAP. Reduction of the duration of ventilation by minimising the use of sedation and use of weaning protocols should reduce the risk of VAP.

Further reading

Hunter JD. Ventilator associated pneumonia. Br Med J 2012; 344:e3325.

Bekaert M, Timsit J-F, Vansteelandt S et al. Attributable mortality of ventilator-associated pneumonia. Am J Respir Crit Care Med 2011;184:1133–1139.

O'Grady NP, Murray PR, Ames N. Preventing ventilator-associated pneumonia: does the evidence support the practice? J Am Med Assoc 2012; 307:2534–2539.

Related topics of interest

Post-resuscitation care

Key points

- Most patients resuscitated after a prolonged period of cardiac arrest will develop the post cardiac arrest syndrome
- All survivors of out-of-hospital cardiac arrest should be considered for urgent coronary angiography unless the cause of cardiac arrest was clearly non-cardiac or continued treatment is considered futile
- Several interventions may impact on neurological outcome; the most significant of these is targeted temperature management
- In patients remaining comatose after resuscitation from cardiac arrest, prediction of the final outcome in the first few days may be unreliable

Epidemiology

Post-cardiac arrest patients account for about 6% of the bed days on intensive care units (ICUs) in the United Kingdom (UK). Approximately 30–40% of patients admitted to an ICU after cardiac arrest will survive to be discharged from hospital and of these approximately 80% will function independently ('good' neurological outcome).

Pathophysiology – the post cardiac arrest syndrome

Systemic ischaemia during cardiac arrest and the subsequent reperfusion response after return of spontaneous circulation (ROSC) causes the post cardiac arrest syndrome (PCAS); its severity is determined by the cause and duration of cardiac arrest, and has four main domains (**Table 43**).

All components of the PCAS must be addressed if outcome is to be optimised and post cardiac arrest care begins immediately after ROSC has been achieved, irrespective of location. An 'ABCDE' (Airway, Breathing, Circulation, Disability and Exposure) systems approach is used to identify and treat physiological abnormalities and organ injury.

Airway and breathing with controlled reoxygenation

After ROSC has been achieved, patients who remain comatose or agitated with a decreased conscious level, and those with breathing difficulties will require sedation, tracheal intubation and mechanical ventilation. Increasing evidence suggests that hyperoxaemia after ROSC is harmful and worsens outcomes. Current guidelines recommend that the inspired oxygen concentration immediately after ROSC be adjusted to achieve normal arterial oxygen saturation (94–98%) when measured by pulse oximetry or arterial blood gas analysis. Ventilation is adjusted to achieve normocarbia and monitored using end-tidal CO_2 with waveform capnography, and arterial blood gases. Avoid hyperventilation, which may cause cerebral ischaemia.

Circulation

About 80% of sudden out-of-hospital cardiac arrests (OHCAs) are caused by coronary artery disease. Early reperfusion therapy is indicated for ST elevation myocardial infarction (STEMI) and this is achieved most effectively with primary percutaneous intervention (PCI) as long as a first medical

Table 43 Key components of the post cardiac arrest syndrome	
Key component	
Post-cardiac arrest brain injury	This manifests as coma and seizures
Post-cardiac-arrest myocardial dysfunction	This can be severe and usually recovers after 48–72 h
Systemic ischaemia/reperfusion response	Tissue reperfusion can cause programmed cell death (apoptosis) effecting all organ systems
Persisting precipitating pathology	Coronary artery disease is the commonest precipitating cause after OHCA

contact-to-balloon time of less than 90 min can be achieved; if not, fibrinolysis (thrombolysis) may be preferable. Consider immediate coronary artery angiography in all OHCA patients without an obvious non-cardiac cause of arrest regardless of electrocardiogram (ECG) changes. This is because the early post-resuscitation 12-lead ECG is less reliable for diagnosing acute coronary occlusion than it is in non-arrest patients. About 25% of patients without an obvious non-cardiac cause for their cardiac arrest and no evidence of STEMI on their initial 12-lead ECG will have a coronary lesion on angiography that is amenable to stenting.

After cardiac arrest, reversible myocardial dysfunction is common and may cause haemodynamic instability and arrhythmias. The severity increases with the duration of the arrest and in those with pre-existing myocardial dysfunction. Echocardiography shows typically global impairment with both systolic and diastolic dysfunction. Although systematic vascular resistance (SVR) may be high initially, the release of inflammatory cytokines associated with the PCAS will then result in a low SVR. Treatment with fluids, inotropes and vasopressors is guided by blood pressure, heart rate, urine output, and rate of plasma lactate clearance, central venous oxygen saturations, and cardiac output monitoring. In patients with severe cardiogenic shock intra-aortic balloon counter-pulsation may be used. There are no proven evidence-based targets for post cardiac arrest patients, although the use of a goal directed protocol may improve outcomes.

Patients who survive a cardiac arrest caused by ventricular fibrillation/pulseless ventricular tachycardia (VF/pVT) and who have no evidence of a disease that can be effectively treated (e.g. coronary revascularisation) should be considered for an implantable cardioverter-defibrillator before leaving hospital.

Brain (disability)

Neurological injury (leading to withdrawal of care) is the cause of death in about two-thirds of OHCAs and a quarter of in-hospital cardiac arrests admitted to ICU. Aneurysmal subarachnoid haemorrhage is a potential cause of OHCA and should be excluded in comatose victims with ROSC because thrombolysis will be contraindicated.

Targeted temperature management

Pyrexia associated with a systemic inflammatory response is common in the first 72 h after cardiac arrest, and is associated with worse outcome. Mild hypothermia improves outcome after a period of global cerebral hypoxia-ischaemia. Cooling suppresses many of the pathways associated with ischemiae-reperfusion injury, including apoptosis (programmed cell death) and the harmful release of excitatory amino acids and free radicals.

Indications for post-arrest cooling

Animal studies have shown that cooling after ROSC improves neurological outcome. Two randomised studies showed improved neurological outcome at hospital discharge or at 6 months in comatose patients after out-of-hospital VF cardiac arrest. Cooling was initiated within hours after ROSC and a target temperature of 32–34 °C was maintained for 12–24 h. The use of hypothermia for non-shockable rhythms and after in-hospital cardiac arrest is supported only by observational data. Despite this, many centres use hypothermia irrespective of initial cardiac arrest rhythm or location. The targeted temperature management (TTM) study randomised patients with ROSC after OHCA to TTM at either 33 °C or 36 °C – there was no difference in all cause mortality, the primary end point, between the two groups.

Cooling techniques

Targeted temperature management comprises induction of hypothermia, maintenance at 32–34 °C, re-warming while preventing hyperthermia. Following the recent TTM trial, this target may be revised. Infusion of 30 mL kg^{-1} of 4 °C 0.9% sodium chloride or Hartmann's solution decreases core temperature by approximately 1.5 °C and this fluid was thought to be well tolerated even in patients with post-cardiac arrest myocardial dysfunction. In contrast, a recent large study of prehospital cooling with cold 0.9% sodium chloride showed that it increased the incidence of pulmonary oedema and the risk of re-arrest during transport to hospital.

Following induction with cold IV fluids, ice packs and/or wet towels can be used to maintain hypothermia but fluctuations in temperature are common when using techniques that do not include temperature feedback control and automatic temperature regulation. Several cooling devices (surface and intravascular) that include temperature feedback control are available. Intravascular cooling systems provide tight temperature control via a cooling catheter in a large vein (usually femoral) but they produce no better neurological outcome than the external cooling systems. Initial cooling is facilitated by concomitant neuromuscular blockade with sedation to prevent shivering. By starting cooling in the pre-hospital phase, it is possible to achieve the target temperature more rapidly but this has not been shown to improve outcome.

The optimal duration of induced hypothermia is unknown. Although current guidelines suggest 12–24 h, some experts are using longer periods of hypothermia (at least 24 h and sometimes up to 72 h) especially when there has been a long duration of cardiac arrest. Rewarming should be controlled at 0.25–0.5 °C per hour and potentially harmful rebound hyperthermia avoided. The complications of therapeutic hypothermia are listed in **Table 44**; many of these are normal physiological responses to mild hypothermia.

Sedation

Patients are sedated during treatment with therapeutic hypothermia because this reduces oxygen consumption, prevents shivering and facilitates cooling. Short-acting sedatives and opioids (e.g. propofol, alfentanil and remifentanil) will enable earlier neurological assessment after re-warming. Clearance of many drugs is reduced by about one-third at 34°C and this must be considered carefully before making decisions about prognosis.

Cerebral perfusion

Auto-regulation of cerebral blood flow is impaired after cardiac arrest and cerebral perfusion is dependent on an adequate blood pressure. Brain oedema can occur transiently after ROSC following asphyxial cardiac arrest but sustained intracranial hypertension is rare. Aim to maintain a normal mean arterial pressure for that particular patient.

Control of seizures

Seizures or myoclonus or both occur in about 24% of those who remain comatose and are cooled after cardiac arrest. Ideally,

Table 44 Complications associated with therapeutic hypothermia	
Shivering	Reduced with sedation, neuromuscular blockers and magnesium
Dysrhythmias	Bradycardia is the most common
Diuresis	May cause hypovolaemia and electrolyte abnormalities
Electrolyte abnormalities	Hypophosphataemia; hypokalaemia; hypomagnesaemia; hypocalcaemia.
Decreased insulin sensitivity and insulin secretion	Hyperglycaemia
Impaired coagulation and increased bleeding	
Impairment of the immune system	Increased infection rates, e.g. pneumonia
Increased plasma amylase concentration	
Reduced drug clearance	Clearance of sedative and neuromuscular blocking drugs is reduced by up to 30% at a temperature of 34 °C

continuous EEG monitoring is used in patients receiving neuromuscular blocking drugs to ensure seizures are not missed. Seizures are associated with a fourfold increase in mortality, but good neurological recovery has been documented in 17% of those with seizures. Seizures should be treated with benzodiazepines, phenytoin, sodium valproate, propofol or a barbiturate. Clonazepam is most effective for treating myoclonus, but sodium valproate, levetiracetam and propofol may also be effective; phenytoin is often ineffective.

Glucose control

Both hyperglycaemia and hypoglycaemia after ROSC are associated with a poor neurological outcome. Based on the available data and expert consensus, following ROSC, blood glucose should be maintained between 4–10 mmol L^{-1}.

Prognostication

Predicting outcome in patients remaining comatose after cardiac arrest is problematic. The implementation of therapeutic hypothermia has invalidated standard guidelines that suggested, e.g. that a GCS motor score of 1 or 2 on day 3 after cardiac arrest reliably predicted a poor outcome. This may reflect a direct effect of hypothermia on the progress of neurological recovery and/or the residual effects of sedatives and opioids, which tend to be used in larger doses and take longer to clear after hypothermia, confounding neurological assessment. Several studies have shown that a GCS motor score of 1 or 2 on day 3

is highly unreliable as a predictor of poor outcome in patients who have been cooled. The absence of EEG background reactivity to a stimulus (e.g. tracheal suction) and bilateral absence of N20 responses on somatosensory evoked potentials are strong predictors of a poor outcome but these tests are often unavailable. The current consensus is that a multimodal approach should be used for prognostication in comatose patients after cardiac arrest; ideally, this means a combination of neurological examination and electrophysiological investigations. Concerns about delayed clearance of sedation have led some experts to suggest that prognostication should be delayed until 72 h after return to normothermia.

Organ donation

Up to 16% of patients who achieve sustained ROSC after cardiac arrest fulfil criteria for brain death and can be considered for organ donation. Transplant outcomes for organs from donors who have suffered a cardiac arrest are similar to those achieved with organs from other beating-heart donors.

Cardiac-arrest centres

Post-cardiac-arrest patients may have improved outcomes if they are cared for in a hospital that offers a comprehensive package of care that includes PCI, therapeutic hypothermia and neurological service. Although this has yet to be proven in prospective trials the regionalisation of cardiac-arrest care is already being implemented in many areas.

Further reading

Nolan JP, Laver SR, Welch CA, et al. Outcome following admission to UK intensive care units after cardiac arrest: a secondary analysis of the ICNARC Case Mix Programme Database. Anaesthesia 2007; 62:1207–1216.

Nolan JP, Neumar RW, Adrie C, et al. Post-cardiac arrest syndrome: epidemiology, pathophysiology, treatment, and prognostication. A Scientific Statement from the International Liaison Committee on Resuscitation; the American

Heart Association Emergency Cardiovascular
Care Committee; the Council on Cardiovascular
Surgery and Anesthesia; the Council on
Cardiopulmonary, Perioperative, and Critical
Care; the Council on Clinical Cardiology;
the Council on Stroke. Resuscitation 2008;
79:350–379.

Holzer M. Targeted temperature management for
comatose survivors of cardiac arrest. N Engl J
Med 2010; 363:1256–1264.
Nielsen N, Wetterslev J, Cronberg T, et al. Targeted
temperature management at 33°C versus
36°C after cardiac arrest. N Engl J Med 2013;
369:2197–2206.

Related topics of interest

- Acute coronary syndrome (p 4)
- Cardiac arrhythmias (p 77)
- Cardiopulmonary resuscitation (p 100)
- Seizures – status epilepticus (p 323)

Potassium

Key points

- Potassium is the main intracellular cation
- Potassium regulates the resting membrane potential, which makes it vital at the cellular level
- Disorders of potassium homeostasis can cause severe cardiac dysrhythmias

Introduction

Potassium is the major intracellular cation that provides osmotic pressure, regulates acid-base balance, establishes the resting membrane potential of excitable tissues (particularly myocardial) and affects metabolism.

Homeostasis

Potassium is absorbed by diffusion from the gastrointestinal tract. Total body potassium is approximately 50 mmol kg^{-1}, of which only 2% is extracellular. The normal extracellular concentration ranges from 3.5 to 5.0 mmol L^{-1}; the intracellular concentration is 150 mmol L^{-1}. The average daily requirement for potassium is 1 mmol kg^{-1}. Large changes in total body potassium can occur without significant effect on plasma concentration. It is renally excreted and dependent on urinary flow, sodium reabsorption and acid–base balance. Potassium entry into cells is regulated by the sodium-potassium-adenosine triphosphatase (Na-K-ATPase) pump. Regulation is influenced by aldosterone, insulin, catecholamines, β-adrenergic agonists, osmolality and bicarbonate. Extracellular potassium is controlled by acid–base status, osmolality, mineralocorticoids, glucocorticoids and insulin. Homeostatic mechanisms are altered in the critically ill, precipitating the need for emergent treatment and monitoring.

Hypokalaemia

Defined as a serum potassium of <3.5 mmol L^{-1} and is severe if below <2.5 mmol L^{-1}.

Causes

Hypokalaemia can be acute or chronic. Acute causes include increased renal or gastrointestinal losses and movement of potassium from extracellular to intracellular fluid. Chronic causes include dietary insufficiency, malabsorption or endocrine disorders resulting in decreased total body potassium.

Gastrointestinal loss

Diarrhoea, vomiting, fistula loss, laxative abuse, ureterosigmoidostomy and colonic mucus-secreting neoplasms.

Renal loss

Drugs (diuretics, acetazolamide, corticosteroids, carbapenems and amphotericin), hyperaldosteronism, Cushing's syndrome, renal tubular acidosis, diuretic phase of acute kidney injury, hypomagnesaemia and Bartters's/Gitelman's syndrome.

Potassium shift

Drugs (β-agonists, phosphodiesterase inhibitors, caffeine, insulin), metabolic alkalosis, refeeding syndrome, hypothermia.

Clinical features

Mild hypokalaemia is often asymptomatic; diagnosis is made on blood analysis. It is associated with increased morbidity in those with cardiovascular disease. Severe hypokalaemia may cause generalised weakness, cramps, nausea, vomiting, ileus and constipation with loss of tendon reflexes or ascending paralysis. Blood pressure may be increased secondary to sodium retention. Loss of hydrogen ions in exchange for potassium leads to a metabolic alkalosis. Profound hypokalaemia may cause ventilatory failure, atrial tachycardias, supraventricular tachycardia (especially with digoxin therapy), ventricular tachycardias (classically 'torsades de pointes') and cardiac arrest and even coma. ECG changes may be non-specific with a prolonged PR interval, U waves, depressed ST segments and flattened or inverted T waves. Prolonged hypokalaemia can result in the development of nephrogenic diabetes insipidus.

Management

Confirm that the serum potassium value is correct. Stop giving potassium-wasting drugs and ensure that potassium therapy accounts for both maintenance and replacement requirements.

Intravenous or oral potassium will correct hypokalaemia. Oral potassium supplementation is safer as it is slower to enter the circulation, but may cause gastrointestinal symptoms. Intravenous potassium can be administered with maintenance fluids, parenteral nutrition or via a central venous catheter (CVC) with ECG monitoring.

Potassium chloride is given by intravenous infusion at 10 mmol h^{-1} peripherally or 20 mmol h^{-1} via a CVC to avoid the irritant effect on peripheral veins. Adjust the rate according to repeated measurements every 1–4 h. Do not exceed 40 mmol h^{-1} so that the risk of precipitating ventricular fibrillation (VF) is minimised. In profound hypokalaemia (< 2.5 mmol L^{-1}), potassium can be given more rapidly via a CVC. Reduce initial therapy by 50% if renal impairment is present. Potassium phosphate can be used to provide both potassium and phosphate replacement. If renal tubular acidosis is present, potassium citrate or acetate is preferred. Correct any hypomagnesaemia concomitantly.

Hyperkalaemia

Hyperkalaemia is defined as a serum potassium of greater than 5.5 mmol L^{-1}. The European Resuscitation Council Guidelines categorise hyperkalaemia into mild (5.5–5.9 mmol L^{-1}), moderate (6.0–6.4 mmol L^{-1}) and severe (≥ 6.5 mmol L^{-1}). Most patients will be asymptomatic until the potassium is over 6.0 mmol L^{-1}.

Causes

True hyperkalaemia may be caused by extracellular shifts, excessive intake or impaired elimination.

Impaired renal excretion

Acute renal impairment, chronic kidney disease, drugs (potassium-sparing diuretics, angiotensin-converting-enzyme inhibitors, angiotensin II receptor blockers, non-steroidal anti-inflammatory drugs, trimethoprim and cyclosporin), steroid deficiency (Addison's disease or hypoaldosteronism).

Potassium shift from cells

This occurs in metabolic acidosis, insulin deficiency, hyperosmolality, haemolysis, massive blood transfusion, tumour lysis syndrome, tissue injury, e.g. trauma, rhabdomyolysis, reperfusion injury, malignant hyperpyrexia, post cardiac arrest, drugs (suxamethonium, especially in patients with neurological disease or denervation, digoxin overdose and beta-blockers).

Other

Excess potassium intake, spurious sampling, thrombocythaemia, leucocytosis and variants of hyperkalaemic periodic paralysis.

Clinical features

Symptoms are related to changes in muscle and cardiac function and include nausea, vomiting, paraesthesia, weakness, flaccid paralysis, hypotension and arrhythmias. Arrhythmias are related to the rate of rise rather than the absolute value. Other metabolic disturbances can affect the signs and symptoms of hyperkalaemia. ECG changes include peaked T waves, prolonged PR interval, widened QRS complex, absent P waves and slurring of ST segments eventually leading to a sine wave (potassium > 7.0 mmol L^{-1}) and VF.

Management

After ensuring that the serum potassium value is correct, take a thorough history and examine the patient. Treatment is directed at the underlying cause. In asymptomatic patients, stop all potassium-containing fluids or potassium-sparing drugs. Record a 12-lead ECG urgently for any symptomatic patient with serum potassium > 6.0 mmol L^{-1}. The presence of ECG changes requires immediate treatment. The UK Renal Association recommends a five-step strategy:

- **Protect the myocardium**
  Intravenous calcium increases cardiac electrical conduction velocity and improves contractility in those with ECG changes. Give calcium chloride 10% 10 mL (or calcium gluconate 10% 30 mL) and repeat after 5–10 min if the effect is inadequate
- **Shift potassium intracellularly**
  If moderate or severe hyperkalaemia, start an infusion of 50 mL of intravenous 50% glucose with 10 units soluble insulin. This is most effective in lowering serum potassium – concentrations start to decrease within 15 min. Give nebulised salbutamol 10–20 mg as adjunctive therapy for moderate or severe hyperkalaemia – this increases the efficacy of the insulin-glucose infusion. Intravenous sodium bicarbonate has minimal effect and is considered only for patients with severe acidosis. There is little evidence to support this practice
- **Remove potassium from body**
  Ion exchange resins, e.g. calcium resonium enhance elimination, though this method is not appropriate acutely. It can be considered in the non-urgent management of mild or moderate hyperkalaemia. Haemodialysis or haemofiltration (at an effluent volume ≥ 20 mL kg^{-1} h^{-1}) removes potassium and corrects acidosis effectively
- **Monitoring**
  Measure serum potassium to assess for rebound hyperkalaemia and effectiveness of treatment. For symptomatic patients with moderate and severe hyperkalaemia, monitor the 3-lead ECG continuously. Monitor blood glucose regularly if infusing insulin and glucose
- **Prevention**
  After acute treatment, take measures to prevent recurrence and arrange appropriate follow up
- Consider referral to the critical care unit for patients with severe hyperkalaemia, those who are not responding or are unstable, and those likely to require renal replacement therapy.

Further reading

Weisberg LS. Management of severe hyperkalaemia. Crit Care Med 2008; 36: 3246–3251.

Alfonzo A, Soar J, Nolan J, et al. Treatment of acute hyperkalaemia in adults. Petersfield; The Renal Association, 2012.

Kellum J, Lameire N, Aspelin P, et al. Kidney disease improving global outcomes (KDIGO). KDIGO clinical practice guideline for acute kidney injury. 2012; 1:1-138.

Related topics of interest

Pre-hospital care

Key points

- Pre-hospital care is part of the continuum of patient care
- Appropriate and timely intervention reduces mortality and morbidity
- Good pre-hospital care is about the marriage of resource and requirement

Introduction

Healthcare is a continuum from onset of illness or injury through to recovery and rehabilitation. Trauma is particularly relevant as it remains the leading cause of death in the first four decades of life and the fourth most common cause of death in the Western world. The first hours after major trauma are critical and good decision-making and appropriate skilled interventions can make a major difference to mortality and morbidity.

Historically, civilian pre-hospital care consisted of simple mechanisms to deliver patients to the nearest hospital. This has evolved over time and now optimal pre-hospital care ensures the delivery of the right care to the right patient at the right time. This can be accomplished by a combination of effective treatment at scene and rapid transfer of patients to the most appropriate destination.

In the United Kingdom, doctor involvement has traditionally been delivered as a voluntary service mainly by general practitioners and other practitioners through schemes such as the British Association for Immediate Care (BASICS). The 2007 NCEPOD (National Confidential Enquiry into Patient Outcome and Death) report 'Trauma: who cares?' recommended further development of doctor delivered pre-hospital care. Pre-hospital emergency medicine is now a recognised medical subspecialty within the UK.

Advanced pre-hospital interventions

Sedation, analgesia and anaesthesia

Paramedics have a limited formulary so pre-hospital doctors are able to provide a greater range of drugs to the patient, although weight, space and stability necessitate some restrictions. Pre-hospital patients can be haemodynamically unstable and both etomidate and ketamine provide good cardiovascular stability for induction of anaesthesia. Ketamine is especially versatile as it also provides dissociative sedative and analgesia. Morphine and midazolam are usually used for maintenance of anaesthesia. Conventional neuromuscular blocking drugs are used. Advanced analgesic techniques such as nerve blocks can be performed.

Airway management

Paramedics are trained to use basic airway manoeuvres and adjuncts as well as supra-glottic airway devices and, in some cases, oral intubation in obtunded patients. Doctors can provide drug-assisted intubation (rapid sequence induction and intubation). Pre-hospital anaesthesia should be performed to the same standard as in-hospital with full monitoring including the use of waveform capnography and the presence of a trained assistant.

Circulatory control

Uncontrolled haemorrhage remains a leading cause of pre-hospital death after military and civilian trauma. The military have developed advanced haemostatic control techniques for catastrophic haemorrhage, which are now used in civilian practice.

Intraosseous (IO) access devices (e.g. EZ-IO, FAST and BIG) facilitate vascular access in severely shocked patients. IO access is reliable in all age groups and can save valuable time in the initial resuscitation. Recommended access sites are the tibia, humeral head or sternum.

Arterial tourniquets are applied to limbs in cases of life-threatening bleeding. The most common tourniquet in use is the CAT (Combat Application Tourniquet). Arterial tourniquets are marked with the time they were placed and time of application and location are handed over to the receiving team. Minimise the ischaemic time by applying for a maximum of 1.5–2 h. When releasing the tourniquet, treat both the potential on-going haemorrhage and reperfusion injury caused by the return of toxic products of ischaemia and muscle damage, most importantly H^+, K^+ and lactate.

Haemostatic dressings may be used to promote clotting. These dressings reduce mortality in animal ex-sanguination models and have been widely used in recent conflicts by the US and UK armed forces.

Surgical procedures

It is not possible to carry a large range of equipment or achieve sterility in the pre-hospital arena, therefore only immediately lifesaving surgical procedures can be performed. A surgical airway is performed when oral intubation is impossible. Thoracostomies are performed for relief of a significant haemopneumothorax and a formal intercostal drain is sited (in a different incision) after arrival at the receiving hospital. Clamshell thoracotomies can be used to relieve pericardial tamponade caused by penetrating trauma when cardiac arrest has occurred within the last 10 min.

Delivering the right resources to the patient

Pre-hospital care often requires the co-ordinated efforts of multiple resources including, but not limited to, the emergency services (ambulance, fire and police) and other agencies such as mountain rescue or the coastguard.

The use of helicopters is often thought to be of most benefit in transferring patients to hospital quickly, but has a more important role in rapidly delivering a critical care team (a relatively scarce resource) to critically ill patients over a large geographic area. Interventions include stabilisation of acutely unwell patients, simple diagnostic investigations, early treatment and decision-making processes based on an understanding of the underlying patient pathology and resources available locally and nationally.

Technological advances in equipment such as ultrasound probes and screens that fit into a large pocket or small bag have already been developed. These enable diagnostic procedures such as basic echocardiography, assessment for pneumothorax and haemothorax and lung consolidation, fluid within the abdomen and measurement of elevated intracranial pressure at scene in a non-invasive manner.

Delivering the patient to the right resources

Increasing tertiary specialisation has meant that it is often best to bypass the nearest hospital and delivering directly to a regional facility; this enables appropriate treatment to be given more rapidly and eliminates the need for secondary transfer.

The future of pre-hospital care

Increasingly sophisticated algorithms and decision-making processes will enable the timely dispatch of skilled critical care teams to the most unwell patients. High-speed data networks and smart phones make it possible for experienced personnel to view pre-hospital scenes live and to guide the practitioners at the scene. There will be further technological advances in resuscitation equipment: portable extracorporeal membrane oxygenation devices have already been used in the pre-hospital environment in cases of severe hypothermia and drowning. Although never likely to be common, it is a powerful demonstration of the ability to bring the hospital to the patient.

Further reading

Cowan GM, Burton F, Newton A. Prehospital anaesthesia: a survey of current practice in the UK. Emerg Med J 2012; 29:136–140.

Filanovsky Y, Miller P, Kao J. Myth: Ketamine should not be used as an induction agent for intubation in patients with head injury. Can J Res E Med 2010; 12:154–157.

National Confidential Enquiry into Patient Outcome and Death (NCEPOD). Trauma: who cares? London; NCEPOD, 2007.

Related topics of interest

• Airway management in an emergency (p 21)
• Major haemorrhage (p 213)
• Transport of the critically ill (p 377)

Pulmonary function tests

Key points

Pulmonary function tests:
- Aid decision making in pre-operative evaluation
- Allow the clinician to monitor response to treatment
- Direct on-going mechanical ventilation strategies

Indications

Pulmonary function tests (PFTs) have a role in selected patients undergoing intermediate or major procedures or to quantify disease progression or response to treatment during critical care admission.

Pre-operative assessment

- Basic pulmonary function testing should be performed in all preoperative patients with significant dyspnoea on mild or moderate exertion to help establish a diagnosis and achieve optimal disease management. PFTs and baseline arterial blood gas analysis should be performed in patients undergoing elective thoracotomy to assist surgical decision making and assess post-operative recovery or in any patient with dyspnoea on minimal exertion. Dyspnoea can be graded according to the American anaesthetist Dr Michael Roizen's classification – **Table 45**

Monitoring disease progression or response to treatment during critical care admission

- PFTs can be used to monitor severity of disease states for example a forced vital capacity (FVC) of less than 1 L in a patient presenting with acute weakness can help to delineate when mechanical ventilation is needed

Many of the commonly performed PFTs are expressed as a percentage of the predicted value based on large studies of healthy subjects matched for age, sex, height and ethnicity. The commonly used PFTs are discussed below.

Spirometry and diffusing capacity

Spirometry is the most commonly performed PFT and produces a graph of volume against time. The patient inspires maximally and then exhales as rapidly as possible. The values measured are the forced expiratory volume in 1 s (FEV1), the FVC and the ratio of these two volumes (FEV1/FVC). An FEV1/FVC <70% demonstrates airway obstruction such as asthma or chronic obstructive pulmonary disease whereas a ratio >80% demonstrates a restrictive problem such as pulmonary fibrosis. (see **Figure 13**).

When FEV1/FVC<70% then FEV1 can be compared to predicted values and used to classify the degree of airways obstruction. (see **Table 46**).

Diffusing capacity is calculated using uptake of dilute carbon monoxide (CO) from a single breath held for 10 s. CO is used because its uptake is diffusion limited and is unaffected by changes in perfusion. Diffusing capacity is referred to as DLCO (diffusion capacity of the lung for carbon monoxide). At rest the normal value is 25 mL min^{-1} $mmHg^{-1}$.

Table 45 Roizen's classification of dyspnoea	
Grade	Level of dyspnoea
0	No dyspnoea while walking on the level at normal pace
I	'I am able to walk as far as I like providing I take my time'
II	Specific street blocks limitation – 'I have to stop for a while after one or two blocks'
III	Dyspnoea on mild exertion – 'I have to stop and rest going from the kitchen to the bathroom'
IV	Dyspnoea at rest

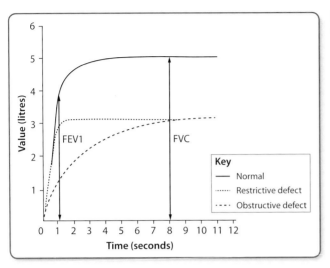

Figure 13 Normal, restrictive and obstructive spirometry.

Table 46 Classifying obstructive lung disease	
FEV1 as % of predicted value	**Stage**
>80%	Mild
50–79%	Moderate
30–49%	Severe
<30%	Very severe

It is dependent upon two components: the transfer coefficient of CO and alveolar volume. The transfer coefficient is reduced by diseases which increase the thickness of the alveolar capillary membrane such as fibrosing alveolitis or congestive heart failure. Alveolar volume may be reduced by lung resection, respiratory muscle weakness or bronchiectasis. Severity of diffusion limitation can be classified according to the % of predicted value (see **Table 47**).

Both of these tests have a particular role in the preoperative assessment of patients with lung cancer for potential resection. Predictive post-resection values of 40% used to be the cut-off for offering surgical resection but in the most recent guidelines from the British Thoracic Society, this has been revised and it is now recommended that this high risk group of patients be offered surgery as long as they are appraised of the risks of significant post-operative dyspnoea.

Flow-volume loops

These loops are produced by plotting flow against volume when a patient takes a maximal inspiration followed by a maximal expiration. They are useful pre-operatively because they can demonstrate obstructive

Table 47 Classifying diffusion limitation	
DLCO as a % of predicted value	**Severity of diffusion limitation**
60% lower limit of normal	Mild
40–60%	Moderate
<40%	Severe

and restrictive airway defects and they also show characteristic patterns when there is intra-thoracic (e.g. tumour) or extra-thoracic airway obstruction (e.g. tracheal stenosis).

In **Figures 14** and **15** shown below, it is important to note that the inspiratory limb of the loop is that portion below the x axis and that the lung volume decreases from left to right along the 'x' axis. This situation is sometimes reversed when the loop is shown on mechanical ventilators.

Cardiopulmonary exercise testing

Since the early 1990s cardiopulmonary exercise testing (CPET) has been used to identify patients who may benefit from post-operative care in a high dependency setting. CPET combines cardiac, pulmonary and circulatory assessment in one relatively safe test. A metabolic cart and an exercise bike are connected via a computer which regulates cycle resistance and monitors the patients vital signs, gas exchange, work rate, 12 lead ECG and ST segments. A nine panel plot is produced which is used to produce a variety of data.

Clinically, the most useful data has proven to be the anaerobic threshold, the onset of anaerobic metabolism signifying inadequate oxygen delivery. The value of < 11 mL kg^{-1}

min^{-1} has been used successfully to stratify patients post-operatively to critical care. AT is unusual in that it is an effort independent variable and easily reproducible.

Peak oxygen uptake (VO$_2$ max) correlates with outcome in oesophagectomy, hepatic transplantation, thoracic and vascular surgery. However, CPET is costly, and the less expensive 6-min-walk tests and incremental shuttle walk test both correlate well with VO$_2$ max. CPET has the additional advantage that it can delineate the cause of dyspnoea in patients who have normal PFTs and cardiac echocardiography.

Other investigations

Patients undergoing major surgery with respiratory symptoms or signs should have a chest radiograph performed – abnormalities predict post-operative respiratory failure. Computerised tomography scans may rarely be performed pre-operatively to assess bullous disease and evaluate lung parenchyma for fibrotic change both of which may impair post-operative recovery. Patients with dyspnoea at rest or mild exertion undergoing intermediate or high-risk surgery should have baseline arterial blood gas analysis performed as a predictor of post-operative pulmonary complications.

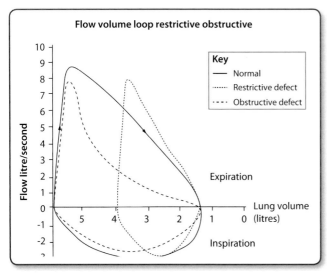

Figure 14 Flow-volume loops showing restrictive and obstructive defects.

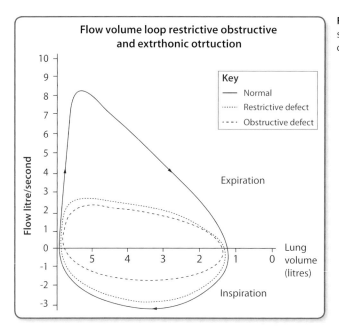

Figure 15 Flow-volume loops showing intra- and extra-thoracic obstruction.

Further reading

Liang BM, Lam DC, Feng YL. Clinical applications of lung function tests: A revisit. Respirology 2012; 17:611–619.

Lim E, Baldwin D, Beckles M, et al. Guidelines on the radical management of patients with lung cancer. Thorax 2010; 65:iii1–27.

Agnew N. Preoperative cardiopulmonary exercise testing. Contin Educ Anaesth Crit Care Pain 2010; 10:33–37.

Related topics of interest

- Asthma (p 47)
- Chronic obstructive pulmonary disease (p 112)

- Respiratory support – invasive (p 306)
- Respiratory support – non-invasive techniques (p 311)

Quality indicators

Key points

- Quality of care has become increasingly important in critical care in the last decade
- Quality indicators can be broadly divided into three domains – structure, process or outcome
- Individual units should develop quality indicators specific to their practice as well as using national quality indicators

Background

In 2000, the UK Department of Health (DH) commissioned a paper entitled 'Comprehensive Critical Care' which reviewed adult critical care services. This document acknowledged the need for an increased critical care bed base and started to focus attention on patient centred care, i.e. care defined by patient need regardless of location. The division between high dependency beds and intensive care beds was discouraged and patient treatment was to be determined by their dependency (**Table 48**).

In 2005, a critical care stakeholder forum was commissioned by the DH and the document 'Quality Critical Care – Beyond Comprehensive Critical Care' was published. This placed a far greater emphasis on quality outcomes rather than quantity.
The Intensive Care Society (ICS) has published a list of quality indicators based on the following criteria:

- Evidence based
- Relatively easy to collect
- Measurable frequently and used to drive improvement

- Sufficiently sophisticated to adjust for varying levels of risk in the studied population

These quality indicators were grouped into one of three domains: structure, process or outcome.

The intensive care national audit and research centre (ICNARC) in the United Kingdom and the Australian and New Zealand Intensive Care Society Centre for Outcome and Resource Evaluation (ANZICS CORE) run audits of case-mix that allows participating units to submit data which are validated, analysed and used to generate a data analysis report each quarter. This report enables units to see how they compare with units of a similar size and case-mix, and assists with local performance management. Some of the quality indicators listed below are collected by ICNARC. At present 94% of adult intensive care units in England, Wales and Northern Ireland contribute data to ICNARC.

Structural-based quality indicators

1. Continuous availability of a trained intensivist – patients do better in closed units – those that are managed by intensive care clinicians; they also do better when individual clinicians manage the unit for several days at a time.
2. Nurse:Patient ratio – a ratio of 1:1 nursing for level 3 patients and 1:2 for level 2 patients is associated with higher quality care and fewer health-care associated infections.

Table 48 Defining levels of support in critically ill and recuperating patients	
Level 0	Patients whose needs can be met on a general ward in an acute hospital.
Level 1	Patients at risk of deteriorating or who have recently been discharged from a critical care unit. Can be looked after in an acute ward with additional advice from critical care team.
Level 2	Patients requiring single organ support, or post-operative care or who are stepping down from Level 3.
Level 3	Patients requiring advanced respiratory support alone or basic respiratory support with support of at least 2 other organ systems.

3. Appropriate isolation of patients with infections – patients infected with methicillin resistant *Staphylococcus aureus* (MRSA), vancomycin resistant *Enterococcus, Clostridium difficile* (CD), or bacteria producing extended spectrum β-lactamases should be cared for in single rooms or cohorted.

4. Days of 100% bed occupancy – if a unit is full, it cannot accept further referrals, this will increase the number of non-clinical transfers which exposes patients to unnecessary risk. Patients who are cared for in full units are at greater risk of infection.

5. Use of a daily goals sheet – explicit, visible recording of daily goals agreed at the ward round improves communication and reduces length of stay.

6. Multi-disciplinary ward rounds – improve communication and may reduce drug errors.

7. Structured handover – a formally recognised time period for handover of patients between day and night teams improves communication.

Process-based quality indicators

1. Hand hygiene compliance – an important marker of good infection control practice.

2. Presence of an end-of-life care pathway – recognition of the importance of high quality care for critical care patients who are dying.

3. Early enteral nutrition – preserves the gastrointestinal (GI) tract and may reduce infections caused by translocation. Patients who are haemodynamically unstable or have impaired perfusion to their GI tract are not included in this measure.

4. Patients readmitted to the unit within 48 h of discharge – patients should be well enough upon discharge to be cared for on a general ward. The need for rapid readmission suggests untimely discharge.

5. Proportion of overnight discharges – discharging patients to medical wards overnight is not in that patient's best interest. Hospitals run with fewer ward staff at night time leading to a less effective handover and an association with increased morbidity and mortality.

6. Participation in a quality improvement programme – involvement in such a local or network based programme reflects a unit focussed on delivering high-quality care and driven to improve.

Outcome-based quality indicators

1. Number of non-clinical transfers – this reflects either a lack of capacity or poor planned discharge practices, both reduce the quality of care that patients receive.

2. Regular review of morbidity and mortality – important for discussion of difficult cases and to raise awareness of critical illness, these meetings can be used to promote change based on previous experiences.

3. Unit-based bacteraemias – patients who develop a bacteraemia more than 48 h following admission to critical care may have acquired that bacteraemia nosocomially which may reflect poor infection control practices.

4. Unit acquired MRSA infection – there is clearly an infection control deficiency if patients acquire MRSA infections following admission to critical care.

5. Catheter-related blood stream infections (CRBSIs) – CRBSIs may indicate poor infection control techniques and rates should be regularly audited.

6. Unit acquired CD or MRSA infection rates – as with the previous three quality indicators acquisition of these infections reflect possible infection control deficiencies.

7. Standardised mortality ratio – regular review of the observed versus expected mortality may provide an early indication of deficiencies in quality of care.

Further reading

Harper SJ, Penden C. ICS quality indicators, 2010. www.ics.ac.uk. Accessed 30/6/2013.

Critical Care Stakeholder Forum (CCSF). Quality Critical Care, Beyond 'Comprehensive Critical Care'. London: CCSF, 2005.

Gawande A. Better: A Surgeons Notes on Performance. New York: Picador, 2008.

The Faculty of Intensive Care Medicine (FICM) and the Intensive Care Society (ICS). Core Standards for Intensive Care Units. London: FICM, 2013.

Related topics of interest

Quality of life after ICU

Key points

- The Short Form-36 and EuroQol-5-Dimension questionnaires are the most commonly used tools to assess quality of life after critical illness
- A quarter of patients will need assistance with activities of daily living 6 months after discharge from ICU
- Chronic pain, decreased mobility, anxiety and depression often affect patients after discharge. Good communication between hospital and primary care will help to optimise rehabilitation

Introduction

The quality of life regained after surviving a period of treatment on an intensive care unit (ICU) is of considerable importance to the patient and their family. Anticipation of the eventual quality of life likely to be achieved by a patient influences greatly the clinician's admission and management decisions, yet this outcome is relatively under studied and difficult to predict for individual patients. Approximately 140,000 patients are treated in critical care units each year in the United Kingdom and therefore outcomes beyond mortality alone have important implications for society as well as the patients and their families. It is essential to know if gains in life expectancy are achieved without the burden of an unacceptable quality of life.

Measuring quality of life

Several scales are available to measure health-related quality of life, some disease specific and others generic, allowing their application across the ICU population.

The Short Form-36 (SF-36) is a 36-point questionnaire that reliably measures health related quality of life after critical illness. Questions cover domains including: physical functioning, physical and emotional role, bodily pain, general health, vitality, social functioning and mental health. It is common for there to be a deficit in all domain scores after critical illness compared to that of a matched general population.

The EuroQol-5-Dimension (EQ-5D) questionnaire assesses five domains: mobility, self-care, usual activities, pain/discomfort and anxiety/depression. Scores are assigned for moderate or severe problems.

Limitations common to outcome research include: losses to follow up, recall bias – having only a retrospective recall of quality of life prior to critical illness – and response shift – where patient perception of ill health improves over time living with ill health. There may be important differences between responders and non-responders that influence results.

Systematic review of quality of life studies is problematic because of methodological differences in trial designs, patient populations and follow up times; however, patients with acute respiratory distress syndrome, severe sepsis, severe trauma and prolonged mechanical ventilation appear to have the worst reduction in quality of life. Older patients are often more accepting of disability. Factors such as age and length of ICU or hospital stay do not reflect in general quality of life after discharge.

Care requirement

A study of 293 patients from 22 UK hospitals found 25% needed assistance with activities of daily living 6 months after discharge and 22% at 12 months. Of those needing assistance at 12 months, 26% needed over 50 h of assistance per week; 13% had required some assistance prior to their admission. Family members provide the majority of care and this has substantial impact on the caregiver's options for paid employment and household income.

In a study of patients that underwent prolonged ventilation (> 21 days without tracheostomy or >4 days with tracheostomy), 56% survived to 1 year but only 9% of these survivors had good functional status and 33% good quality of life as assessed by surrogates.

Chronic pain

In the UK study above, 73% of patients reported moderate or severe pain at 6 months, compared with 51% at admission. In a single centre study of 404 patients, 44% reported chronic pain at 6 months, most commonly in the shoulder (22%). Severe sepsis and older age were independent risk factors for developing chronic pain. The shoulder is thought to be susceptible to loss of muscle tone during illness, immobility from central venous catheter or ventilation tubing positioning and potential strain during rolling.

Mobility

Recovery of mobility depends on age, previous level of fitness, severity and duration of illness and may take several months to reach pre-admission levels. Critical illness polyneuropathy, (an axonal peripheral neuropathy) and critical illness myopathy, (a primary myopathy that is not secondary to muscle denervation), occur in 46% of patients who have prolonged mechanical ventilation, sepsis or multiple organ failure. The limb and diaphragm weakness can persist months to years after the episode of critical illness, resulting in a third of affected patients not recovering to spontaneous ventilation or walking independently. Critical illness myopathy has a better outcome than critical illness polyneuropathy.

Tracheostomy

Late complications of tracheostomy include tracheal stenosis, granulation tissue, tracheomalacia, tracheo-innominate and tracheoesophageal fistula. The latter two are very rare. Most patients will have a degree of tracheal narrowing after prolonged mechanical ventilation, but only 3–12% will have clinically important stenosis that requires intervention. Facial scaring from tracheal tube ties and tethering of skin at tracheostomy sites can also cause significant distress.

Appetite

Alterations in taste and fatigue may contribute to loss of appetite after critical illness but most taste changes return to normal after a few weeks.

Sleep

Disruption to circadian rhythm occurs commonly during hospital admission and frequently persists beyond discharge. This can be exacerbated by nightmares, hallucinations and anxiety.

Anxiety/depression/post-traumatic stress disorder

In the UK study above, 46% of ICU patients reported moderate or extreme anxiety or depression at 6 months, 44% at 12 months after critical illness compared with 30% at admission.

Post-traumatic stress disorder (PTSD) is a severe anxiety disorder involving persistent re-experiencing of the trigger event, avoiding stimuli associated with the trauma and flattening of emotional responsiveness that persists for longer than a month and impairs social function. Rates of PTSD in ICU survivors vary between 9% and 27%. Risk factors include use of benzodiazepines, duration of sedation and delirium during the ICU admission.

National Institute of Health and Care Excellence Guidance

Rehabilitation after critical illness guidance was published in 2009 with the aim of optimising recovery and preventing physical and non-physical morbidity. Key recommendations include short- and medium-term rehabilitation goals, use of a self directed rehabilitation manual, ensuring good communication between hospital and community/primary care and undertaking functional reassessment at 2–3 months after discharge from ICU.

Follow-up clinics

In 2006, 30% of UK ICUs ran a follow-up clinic, of which only 47 (59%) were funded. The PRaCTICaL study, a UK multi-centre RCT, did not identify a benefit of nurse led follow-up clinics on quality of life in the first 12 months after critical illness, but which patients to target and what is the best follow up intervention are important unanswered questions.

Further reading

Oeyen SG1, Vandijck DM, Benoit DD, Annemans L, Decruyenaere JM. Quality of life after intensive care: a systematic review of the literature. Crit Care Med 2010; 38:2386–2400.

Griffiths J, Hatch R, Bishop J, et al. An exploration of social and economic outcome and associated health-related quality of life after critical illness in general intensive care unit survivors: a 12-month follow-up study. Crit Care 2013; 17:R100.

Cox CE, Martinu T, Sathy SJ, et al. Expectations and outcomes of prolonged mechanical ventilation. Crit Care Med 2009; 37: 2888–2894.

Latanico N, Bolton CF. Critical illness polyneuropathy and myopathy: a major cause of muscle weakness and paralysis. Lancet Neurol 2011; 10:931–941.

Epstein S. Late complications of tracheostomy. Respir Care 2005; 50:542–549.

Wade D1, Hardy R, Howell D, Mythen M. Identifying clinical and acute psychological risk factors for PTSD after critical care: a systematic review. Minerva Anaesthesiol 2013;79:944–963.

National Institute for Health and Clinical Excellence (NICE). Rehabilitation after critical illness, clinical guideline 83. London: NICE, 2009.

Cuthbertson BH1, Rattray J, Campbell MK, et al. The PRaCTICaL study of nurse led, intensive care follow-up programmes for improving long term outcomes from critical illness: a pragmatic randomised controlled trial. Br Med J 2009; 339:b3723.

Related topics of interest

- Critical illness polyneuromyopathy (p 122)
- Tracheostomy (p 368)

Radiology for critical care

Key points

- Modern imaging techniques assist diagnosis and increase therapeutic options
- Imaging confers risks and benefits that must be assessed on an individual patient basis
- Excellent communication between critical care and radiology teams is essential to ensure that the correct investigation is performed and the result reported and acted upon in a timely manner

Imaging for critically ill patients

Imaging modalities from plain radiographs through to magnetic resonance (MR) imaging have much to offer critically ill patients. Electronic storage of images is now standard and enables rapid review of all previous imaging for every patient.

Plain films

The plain chest radiograph (CXR) is the most commonly requested imaging investigation in critical care. A recent meta-analysis demonstrated that stopping non-selective imaging in all ventilated patients does not increase the risk of adverse outcome; thus, routine, daily CXRs in ventilated critically ill patients are unnecessary.

Portable CXRs performed on critical care are usually taken as anterior-posterior projections because the patient is unable to stand for a posterior-anterior (PA) film (**Figure 16**).

CXRs are reported in a systematic manner; it is unimportant which of the numerous described methods is chosen as long as a comprehensive approach is adopted. Assess the following on each CXR:

- Confirm correct patient identity
- Is inspiration adequate? The diaphragm should be crossed by the anterior portion of the 5th to 7th rib in the mid-clavicular line
- Rotation – the thoracic spinous processes should be equidistant from the medial clavicular heads
- Penetration – thoracic vertebrae should be just visible behind the heart

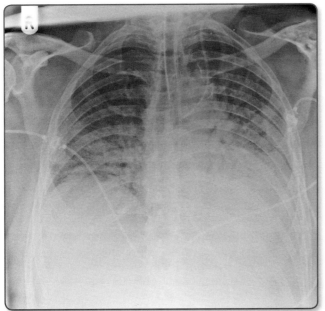

Figure 16 CXR showing diffuse bilateral infiltrates consistent with pulmonary oedema, left internal jugular central line, nasogastric tube and tracheal tube (should be withdrawn by 2 cm).

- Heart – the heart border should be clearly visible
- Diaphragm – should be well-defined and dome shaped with clear costo-phrenic angles. The right diaphragm is usually higher than the left
- Hila – composed of the pulmonary arteries and veins, left is usually higher than right, the reverse suggests significant pathology
- Bones – useful landmarks for assessing inspiration and rotation. Assess for fractures or metastatic lesions
- Lungs – divided into upper, middle and lower zones
- Mediastinum – should be less than 8 mm at level of aortic arch on a PA film
- Tracheal tube – tip should lie 4 cm above the carina
- Central venous catheter – should lie within superior vena cava and not within right atrium. Exclude pneumothorax or increased mediastinal width following placement
- Nasogastric tube – tip should be visible below level of diaphragm
- Intercostal drains – confirm placement within the thoracic cage
- Intra-aortic balloon pump – tip should be visible just above left main bronchus

Lateral decubitus CXR can differentiate pleural fluid from other causes of opacification and may reveal free intra-peritoneal air if the patient is placed in the left lateral position.

Occasionally it is necessary to perform plain radiographs of the abdomen, facial bones or extremities on critical care but better results are achieved by transferring the patient to the radiology department when stable.

Plain radiographs are now rarely used for imaging the spine – computerised tomography (CT) or MR scanning are the investigations of choice.

Ultrasonography

Ultrasound (US) does not expose the patient to ionising radiation and can be performed within the critical care unit. It can be used to diagnose pneumothoraces and to assess fluid status, myocardial function and lung recruitment. The addition of Doppler enables imaging of vascular inflow and outflow to limbs and organs. US can also be used to facilitate drainage of pleural, abdominal and pelvic collections and should be used when inserting central venous catheters.

Focussed assessment with sonography for trauma (FAST) scanning, looking for free fluid in the pericardium, peritoneum or pelvis, is advocated in many centres for those patients who are admitted to hospital with abdominal trauma and are either hypotensive or have impaired consciousness.

Cross-sectional imaging

Cross-sectional imaging includes CT and MR scanning. Both require transfer of the patient and often extended time periods in remote sites. It is essential that the patient is stable, appropriately monitored and accompanied by trained personnel.

With the advent of multi-slice (now up to 512 slices) CT, images can be acquired rapidly at high resolution and reformatted to provide 3D reconstructions with great detail.

In spinal disease, CT is invaluable in evaluating the bony integrity of the cervical spine in multiply-injured patients. Thoracic CT provides detailed information about airway anatomy, effusions and empyema and the distribution of collapse and consolidation that can be used to direct ventilatory strategies.

Within the abdomen, intestinal obstruction can be diagnosed accurately and often the radiologist can identify a transition point. CT can also identify the site of perforations and their subsequent complications such as abscess formation and enable pre-operative surgical planning. Ischaemic bowel cannot be excluded by a normal CT scan but early visible signs include bowel wall thickening, pneumatosis and ascites.

CT scanning exposes the patient to a significant dose of radiation that has unpredictable (stochastic) and predictable (deterministic) effects such as malignancy and pulmonary fibrosis respectively.

Table 49 Radiation exposure from plain film and CT scanning			
Investigation	Effective radiation dose (milli-Sieverts)	Equivalent number of CXRs	Equivalent period of background radiation
CXR	0.02	1	3 days
CT head	2.3	115	1 year
CT thorax	8	400	3.6 years
CT abdomen	10	500	4.5 years

A 20-year-old woman undergoing a CT pulmonary angiogram has a 68% greater risk for developing breast cancer by age 35 than a 20 year old without this exposure (**Table 49**).

IV contrast can cause renal, cardiac and neurological toxicity and rarely anaphylaxis. The toxic effects of contrast can be mediated by adequate intravenous fluid administration.

MR is excellent for imaging the brain and spinal cord but as with CT there are drawbacks, MR can cause malfunctioning of implantable devices but newer MR compatible implants are becoming available.

MR contrast is Gadolinium based, in patients with a low glomerular filtration rate there is a risk of the rare but potentially fatal condition nephrogenic systemic fibrosis developing.

Other considerations with MR:
- Use of 100% inspired O_2 concentration can alter CSF appearance – tell the radiographer
- Acoustic noise – if greater than 80 dB people in the scan room should wear ear protection
- A pre-scan safety questionnaire is completed to highlight safety issues
- Magnetic field strength may be up to 3 tesla

Further reading

Raoof S, Feigin D, Sung A, et al. Interpretation of plain chest roentgenogram. Chest 2012; 141:545–558.

Sarma A, Heilbrun M, Conner K, et al. Radiation and chest CT scan examinations. What do we know? Chest 2012; 142:750–760.

Oba Y, Zaza T. Abandoning daily routine chest radiography in the intensive care unit: meta-analysis. Radiology 2010; 255:386–395.

Related topics of interest

Rapid response systems

Key points

- 'The most sophisticated intensive care often becomes unnecessarily expensive terminal care when the pre-ICU system fails'... Peter Safar
- Many cardiac arrests, deaths and ICU admissions are preventable
- All hospitals should have systems to identify and intervene when patients are deteriorating

The mortality rate following in-hospital cardiac arrest is high with <20% survival at 1 year. Adverse events such as cardiac arrest, unexpected death and unanticipated ICU admission are common and occur in 4–17% of admissions. Analyses of such events show that many are predictable and preventable. Up to 80% of patients with in-hospital cardiac arrest have changes in vital signs within 8 hours before arrest and up to 41% of admissions to ICUs are potentially avoidable. To prevent these avoidable adverse events hospitals should provide:

1. Care for patients at risk of clinical deterioration in appropriate areas (e.g. CCU, high dependency unit), with the level of care matched to patient needs.
2. Regular observations with a documented plan for vital signs monitoring and frequency of measurement according to the needs of the patient.
3. A track-and-trigger system (using 'calling criteria' or early warning system) to identify patients who are critically ill and who need escalation of care (e.g. National Early Warning Score (NEWS).
4. A charting system that enables the regular measurement and recording of vital signs including pulse, blood pressure, respiratory rate, conscious level, temperature and pulse oximetry (SpO_2) and early warning scores (e.g. observation chart for the NEWS).
5. A specific policy that requires a clinical response to abnormal physiology, based on the track-and-trigger system which includes specific responsibilities of staff.
6. An identified response to critical illness which may include an outreach service or resuscitation team [e.g., Medical Emergency Team (MET), Rapid Response Team]. This service must be available at all times and include staff with the appropriate resuscitation skills.
7. Training in the recognition, monitoring and management of the critically ill patients, and advice on management while awaiting the arrival of more experienced staff.
8. Staff of all disciplines who are empowered to call for help when they identify a patient at risk of deterioration or cardiac arrest. Staff should be trained in the use of structured communication tools to ensure effective handover of information.
9. Ways to identify patients for whom intensive care interventions and cardiopulmonary resuscitation are inappropriate, and patients who do not want these interventions. A do-not-attempt resuscitation (DNAR) policy, based on national guidance, should be in place.
10. Audit of the performance indicators of: cardiac arrest, 'false arrest', unexpected deaths and unanticipated ICU admissions. Audit should also include antecedents and the clinical response to these events to assess preventability and opportunities for improvement.

The MET system was introduced at Liverpool Hospital, Sydney in 1990 using simple criteria to call an advanced life support team to the patient's bedside, and was incorporated in a New South Wales State-wide initiative called 'Between the Flags' in 2009. Since 1990 many different track-and-trigger systems have been developed and in 2012, the NHS introduced NEWS supported by the Royal College of Physicians, which, with the Royal College of Nursing and the National Outreach Forum, has developed an online training programme. The aim is that the score and rapid response systems be adopted as soon as possible across the whole NHS.

Studies suggest these systems are associated with fewer unanticipated critical care unit admissions, better documentation of DNAR decisions and a reduced incidence of and mortality from unexpected cardiac arrest in hospital.

Further reading

Jones DA, DeVita MA, Bellomo R. Rapid-response teams. N Engl J Med 2011; 365:139–146.

Hillman K1, Parr M, Flabouris A, Bishop G, Stewart A. Redefining in-hospital resuscitation: the concept of the medical emergency team. Resuscitation 2001; 48:105–110.

Deakin CD1, Nolan JP, Soar J. European Resuscitation Council Guidelines for Resuscitation 2010 Section 4. Adult advanced life support. Resuscitation 2010; 81:1305–1352.

National Early Warning Score (NEWS). www.rcplondon.ac.uk/resources/national-early-warning-score-news.

Related topics of interest

- Cardiopulmonary resuscitation (p 100)

Refractory hypoxaemia

Key points

- Refractory hypoxaemia affects less than 10% of patients with respiratory failure; however, it is associated with a mortality rate of greater than 50–60%
- A low-tidal-volume ventilatory strategy is the cornerstone of management
- Several rescue therapies are available for the management of hypoxic respiratory failure, but none improve survival

Definition

There is no standard definition for refractory hypoxaemia. In most reports, it is defined as one or more of the following:

- a PaO_2/FIO_2 (PF) ratio of < 100 mmHg
- inability to maintain Pplat <30 cmH$_2$O despite a tidal volume of 4 mL kg^{-1} ideal body weight (IBW)
- the development of barotrauma
- an oxygenation index (OI) = [(FIO_2 × mean airway pressure)/PaO_2)] of >30

Epidemiology

Refractory hypoxaemia affects less than 10% of patients with respiratory failure; however, it is associated with a mortality rate of greater than 50–60%.

Identifying patients at risk of developing refractory respiratory failure

Among patients with acute respiratory distress syndrome (ARDS) receiving lung protective ventilation (LPV), an improvement in oxygenation within 24 h is associated with a mortality rate of 13–23%. Patients with little improvement in PF ratio after 24 h of LPV have a significantly higher mortality of 53–68%.

Management

The principles of management include:
1. Diagnosing the underlying cause and early institution of appropriate treatment.
2. Management of respiratory failure: ventilatory and non-ventilatory strategies.
3. Good supportive management including and prevention of harm.

Diagnosis and appropriate treatment

Initial empiric therapy is with broad spectrum antibiotics. Send sputum and blood for culture and urine for atypical serology. Once a diagnosis is made, start targeted therapy as soon as possible. If the patient presents with abdominal symptoms, request an X-ray abdomen and serum amylase, etc.

If oxygenation continues to get worse, repeat all the microbiology investigations, perform a bronchoscopic alveolar lavage, and obtain a computerised tomography (CT) scan of the chest including a pulmonary angiogram, and/or a CT abdomen.

Good supportive management

This includes early enteral nutrition, deep vein thrombosis prophylaxis, stress ulcer prophylaxis, attention to oral hygiene, 30° head elevation, meticulous attention to central and peripheral catheters, sedation breaks with trial of spontaneous breathing, etc.

Management of respiratory failure

Ventilatory management

Lung protective strategy
Use small tidal volumes (limiting tidal volumes and pressures) and adequate levels of PEEP. Consider accepting a higher-than-normal $PaCO_2$ (permissive hypercapnia) and lower-than-normal PaO_2 (permissive hypoxemia).

High PEEP strategy
High PEEP results in alveolar recruitment, reduction in the shunt fraction, improvement in PaO_2 and reduction in FIO_2. Three large high-PEEP studies (ALVEOLI, LOV and EXPRESS study) demonstrated a reduction in refractory hypoxaemia and reduction in

the use of rescue therapy but did not report a reduction in mortality.

Rescue therapy

Use of rescue therapies is controversial. Thus far, none has been shown to reduce mortality when studied in large heterogeneous populations of patients with ARDS. However, some rescue therapies improve oxygenation, which may be an important short-term goal in the small, but significant, minority of patients deteriorating with hypoxaemic respiratory failure.

Lung recruitment manoeuvres:
A recruitment manoeuvre temporary increases the transpulmonary pressure, which reopens collapsed alveoli and improves gas exchange. There are several recruitments manoeuvres but an example is a sustained high inflation pressure of 30–50 cmH$_2$O for 20–40 s.

High-frequency oscillation ventilation:
High-frequency oscillation ventilation may improve oxygenation in patients with refractory hypoxemia; however, there is insufficient evidence to recommend it as routine therapy.

Airway pressure release ventilation: During airway pressure release ventilation (APRV), patients can breathe spontaneously while receiving high airway pressure with an intermittent release in pressure. A high airway pressure facilitates alveolar recruitment, thus improving oxygenation and enabling FIO$_2$ to be titrated. The timing and duration of the pressure release, i.e. low airway pressure, as well as the patient's spontaneous breathing, determine alveolar ventilation (PaCO$_2$). The ventilator driven tidal volume depends on lung compliance, airway resistance and the duration and timing of the pressure-release manoeuvre. It is essential that the patients are lightly sedated to enable spontaneous ventilation.

The potential benefits of improved oxygenation and reduced need for sedation make APRV an attractive ventilator mode. However, without randomised controlled trials (RCTs) demonstrating improved patient outcomes, its routine use is not recommended.

Prone ventilation: CT scans of patients with ARDS performed in the supine position show a predominantly dorsal area of consolidation (in the dependent regions). When these patients are turned prone the consolidation moves to ventral areas. In the supine position pleural pressure is highest in the dorsal regions, which causes atelectasis and reduces tidal volumes. This is due to the superimposed weight of the heart and mediastinum, the weight of the non-dependent lung, and transmitted intra-abdominal pressure. On turning prone ventilation is distributed more uniformly because the mediastinum and heart exert their weight on a smaller volume of lung tissue and the alveoli in the dorsal part of the lung are optimally inflated. Thus, there is an anatomical and physiological advantage in adopting the prone position; indeed, within the mammalian kingdom only the sloth has a predominantly supine lifestyle.

Regional perfusion in the lung also explains the advantages of prone positioning. In both the supine and prone positions, perfusion is highest in the dorsal region of the lung. Thus, the prone position improves ventilation/perfusion (V/Q) ratios in the dorsal region of the lung and this improves oxygenation. Other explanations for the actions of prone positioning include a freeing of secretions by the action of turning and improved drainage of secretions in the prone position.

A 2013 French randomised controlled trial showed a survival advantage for prone (for at least 16 h a day) versus supine ventilation in patients with severe ARDS (P:F ratio <150): 28-day mortality was 16.0% in the prone group and 32.8% in the supine group ($P < 0.001$).

Non-ventilatory strategy

i.   Neuromuscular blocking drugs
ii. Fluid management
iii. Corticosteroids
iv. Extracorporeal membrane oxygenation (ECMO)
v.   Enhanced nutrition

Neuromuscular blocking drugs:
Neuromuscular blocking drugs are used

commonly to promote patient-ventilator synchrony and improve oxygenation. A large RCT studied patients with Pao_2/Fio_2 ratio < 150 mmHg and ventilated with low tidal volumes. Addition of a neuromuscular blocking drug compared with deep sedation for 48 h resulted in sustained improvements in oxygenation, with average increases in Pao_2/Fio_2 ratio of 25–75% on day 1 and up to 50–140% on day 5. Unfortunately, use of neuromuscular blocking drugs, particularly by continuous infusion, increases the risk of prolonged weakness.

Fluid management: In a large RCT, a conservative fluid management strategy resulted in less extra-vascular lung water, shorter duration of mechanical ventilation, and shorter ICU length of stay. In another multi-centre RCT, conservative fluid management improved oxygenation modestly, averaging a 15% increase in P/F ratio over 7 days compared with an 8% increase with liberal fluid management ($P < 0.07$).

The ideal fluid-management strategy remains to be defined. However, a conservative approach that uses diuresis, along with albumin for hypoproteinemic patients, may improve oxygenation and haemodynamic status.

Corticosteroid therapy: The role of corticosteroids in the management of ARDS and ALI has been controversial. A recent international consensus on the use of steroids in ARDS concluded that moderate-dose glucocorticoids should be considered in the treatment of patients with early severe ARDS and before day 14 for patients with unresolving ARDS. This was a weak recommendation supported by evidence of only moderate quality.

Enhanced nutrition: There is some evidence that the use of an enhanced nutritional product rich in antioxidants and supplemented with v-3 fatty acids, such as eicosapentaenoic acid and g-linoleic acid, can improve oxygenation and other ICU outcomes. However, there is insufficient evidence for routine use of these therapies.

ECMO: see topic on extracorporeal membrane oxygenation.

Further reading

Ventilation with lower tidal volumes as compared with traditional tidal volumes for acute lung injury and the acute respiratory distress syndrome. The Acute Respiratory Distress Syndrome Network. N Eng J Med 2000;342:1301–1308.

UK Expert Group. Management of Severe Refractory Hypoxia in Critical Care in the UK in 2010. Kent; UK Expert Group, 2010.

Esan A, Hess DR, Raoof S et al. Sever hypoxemic respiratory failure: part 1--ventilatory strategies. Chest 2010:137(5):1203-1216.

Related topics of interest

Renal – acute kidney injury

Key points

- The Kidney Disease Improving Global Outcomes (K-DIGO) group has produced a unifying definition of acute kidney injury (AKI) based on the increase in serum and creatinine and/or urine volume
- On the day of admission to the intensive care unit, the incidence of AKI may be as high as 36%
- The cause of AKI is pre-renal in 85% of cases
- Early and aggressive application of preventative strategies may restore renal function and prevent the need for renal replacement therapy

Definition

Acute kidney injury (AKI) has replaced the term acute renal failure. The Acute Dialysis Quality Initiative proposed the RIFLE (risk, injury, failure, loss and end stage) classification. The RIFLE classification included three levels of severity (risk, injury and failure) and two outcomes (loss of function and end-stage kidney disease). The Acute Kidney Injury Network (AKIN) simplified this further by dropping the term 'failure' and the two outcomes and defining AKI in three stages based on serum creatinine (SCr) and urine output criteria. Most recently, the Kidney Disease Improving Global Outcomes (K-DIGO) group has produced a unifying definition of AKI comprising any of the following:

- Increase in SCr by $\geq 26.5\ \mu mol\ L^{-1}$ ($\geq 0.3\ mg\ dL^{-1}$) within 48 h; or
- Increase in SCr to ≥ 1.5 times baseline, which is known or presumed to have occurred within the prior 7 days; or
- Urine volume $< 0.5\ mL\ kg^{-1}\ h^{-1}$ for 6 h

The K-DIGO criteria for the three stages of AKI are listed **Table 50**.

Epidemiology

The frequency of AKI among in-hospital patients is 2% but is as high as 36% on the first day of intensive care unit (ICU) admission and the prevalence is up to 60% during an ICU admission. The mortality associated with AKI is 10% among ward-based patients and 50% for ICU patents with AKI.

Pathophysiology

AKI is divided into three categories according to cause (**Table 51**):

- Pre-renal (volume responsive) AKI results from anything that causes renal hypoperfusion and a reduction in glomerular filtration rate (GFR)
- Renal (intrinsic) AKI occurs when any part of the nephron (glomerulus, tubule, vasculature and interstitium) is injured
- Post renal AKI occurs if there is urinary obstruction distal to the kidney (ureters, bladder or urethra)

In health, glomerular filtration rate is maintained by auto-regulation across a wide range of mean arterial pressure (MAP) and typically is impaired only when the mean arterial pressure reduces below 80 mmHg. In response to a decrease in renal artery pressure, afferent glomerular arteriolar resistance decreases (mediated by prostaglandins) and efferent glomerular arteriolar resistance increases (mediated by angiotensin II). Non-steroidal anti-inflammatory drugs and angiotensin cardioverting enzyme inhibitors block the auto-regulatory responses in the afferent and efferent glomerular arterioles respectively. With a further reduction in renal artery pressure below the auto-regulatory threshold, blood flow to the post-glomerular capillary bed diminishes, which eventually cause tubular ischaemia and injury. Tubular brush-border membrane and cells slough and obstruct the tubules. Increased intra-tubular sodium concentration polymerises Tamm-Horsfall protein, which forms a gel and contributes to cast formation. Oxidant injury results in vasoconstriction, congestion, hypoperfusion and leukocyte infiltration all of which impairs the renal microcirculation. Although the term acute tubular necrosis is

Table 50 Staging of acute kidney injury (AKI) based on the Kidney Disease Improving Global Outcomes (K-DIGO) criteria		
Stage	Serum creatinine (SCr)	Urine output
1	1.5–1.9 times baseline OR ≥ 26.5 µmol L^{-1} (≥ 0.3 mg dL^{-1}) increase	< 0.5 mL kg^{-1} h^{-1} for 6–12 h
2	2.0–2.9 times baseline	< 0.5 mL kg^{-1} h^{-1} for $\geq$ 12 h
3	3.0 times baseline or Increase in SCr to ≥ 353.6 µmol L^{-1} (≥ 4.0 mg dL^{-1}) or Initiation of renal-replacement therapy or In patients < 18 years, a decrease in eGFR to < 35 mL min^{-1} per 1.73 m^2	< 0.3 mL kg^{-1} h^{-1} for $\geq$ 24 h or Anuria for $\geq$ 12 h

Table 51 Causes of acute kidney injury
Pre-renal (85%) • Hypovolaemia (haemorrhage, sepsis, gastrointestinal loss and burns) • Hypotension (hypovolaemia, cardiac failure and vasodilatation) • Functional acute renal failure (hepatorenal syndrome) • Intra-abdominal hypertension/compartment syndrome
Renal (10%) • Drugs (non-steroidal anti-inflammatory drugs, angiotensin converting enzyme inhibitors, angiotensin receptor blockers, gentamicin, amphotericin, β-lactam antibiotics, acyclovir, methotrexate, cisplatin and tacrolimus) • Iodinated radiocontrast agents • Glomerulonephritis • Vasculitis • Interstitial nephritis • Myeloma • Rhabdomyolysis
Post-renal (5%) • Prostatic enlargement • Renal calculi • Pelvic malignancy

often used it is misleading because only some of the tubular cells are necrotic – most are viable.

Investigations

Assessment of renal function

The GFR is the most commonly used measurement of renal function. The GFR is estimated by measuring creatinine clearance although this overestimates GFR by up to 20% because some creatinine, which is a product of muscle metabolism, is secreted into the tubule. Several formulae enable estimation

of GFR (eGFR) but the one used in the United Kingdom is the four-variable modification of diet in renal disease (4-v MDRD) formula:

eGFR (mL min^{-1} per 1.73 m^2)

= 186
× [(serum creatinine (µmol L^{-1})/ 88.4) – 1.154]
× age (years) – 0.203
× 0.742 if female
× 1.21 if African Caribbean

Although increased SCr and plasma urea are classically used as indicators of AKI, they are insensitive indicators of GFR, becoming abnormal only when GFR decreases by more than 50%. These indicators are also modified by nutrition, use of steroids, gastrointestinal blood, muscle mass and injury, age, sex and fluid resuscitation. A high (>6.0 mmol L^{-1}) or rapidly rising serum potassium may provide an indication for renal replacement therapy in the patient with known AKI.

Several novel biomarkers enable earlier detection of AKI (within 2–6 h) and can be used to monitor interventions. They include cystatin C (Cys C), neutrophil gelatinase-associated lipocalin (NGAL), urinary kidney injury molecule-1 (KIM-1) and interleukin-18 (IL-18). Whether these tests are cost effective in routine clinical practice has yet to be determined.

Diagnosis

Determine whether the diagnosis is likely to be pre-renal, renal or post-renal. In an ICU setting, the majority of patients have a pre-renal cause in association with sepsis, major surgery or trauma. If AKI occurs outside of this context, a renal or post-renal cause must be looked for and treated. Assess intravascular volume, check blood pressure, assess for loin tenderness, rash, oedema, signs of autoimmune disease and check for evidence of urinary obstruction (palpable bladder, poor stream, hesitancy and frequency).

Perform a urine dipstick test – findings include:

- Blood only – trauma, malignancy, stones and rhabdomyolysis
- Blood and protein – glomerulonephritis, vasculitis, urinary tract infection (UTI) and malignant hypertension
- Protein – glomerulonephritis, amyloid, severe hypertension and diabetic nephropathy
- No blood or protein – pre- or post renal, interstitial nephritis and drugs
- Leucocytes and nitrites suggest urinary tract infection

If glomerulonephritis or vasculitis is suspected request an autoimmune screen. Measure immunoglobulins and check the urine for Bence Jones protein. If the patient is oliguric, measure the urinary sodium – a value of ≤ 20 mmol L^{-1} implies pre-renal failure or reduced renal perfusion.

Undertake a renal ultrasound to exclude obstruction and to determine kidney size.

Prevention

In many cases, AKI can be prevented:

- Fluid resuscitation to restore intravascular volume. This can be achieved with crystalloids – avoid hydroxyethyl starch in patients with sepsis – it increases AKI and mortality
- Stop nephrotoxic drugs
- Ensure the MAP is adequate, taking into the account the patient's normal blood pressure – this may mean starting a noradrenaline infusion but first ensure normovolaemia. Consider some form of non-invasive cardiac output monitoring if vasoactive drugs are used
- Ensure an adequate haemoglobin concentration (at least 70 g L^{-1})
- Ensure that the cardiac output is adequate. If restoration of normovolaemia and an adequate MAP fail to restore urine output, consider adding low dose dobutamine in an attempt to increase cardiac output and improve renal blood flow
- Do not use low-dose dopamine – it does not provide renal protection
- In theory, loop diuretics such as furosemide reduce oxygen consumption and therefore ischaemia in the loop of Henle but they do not reduce the incidence of AKI
- In patients with severe liver disease, intense renal vasoconstriction combined with splanchnic vasodilatation can cause hepatorenal syndrome and AKI. Many of these patients also have other pre-renal risk factors, such as hypovolaemia and sepsis, which should be treated, but the addition of terlipressin (1–2 mg 6 h) will constrict the splanchnic circulation and may improve renal function

Further reading

Abuelo JG. Normotensive ischemic acute renal failure. N Engl J Med 2007; 357:797–805.

Bellomo R, Kellum JA, Ronco C. Acute kidney injury. Lancet 2012; 380:756–766.

Croft R, Moore J. Renal failure and its treatment. Anaesth Int Care Med 2012;13:336–342.

Kellum JA, Lameire N, for the KDIGO Acute Kidney Injury Guideline Working Group. Diagnosis, evaluation, and management of acute kidney injury: a KDIGO summary (Part 1). Crit Care 2013; 17:204.

Lameire N, Kellum JA, for the KDIGO Acute Kidney Injury Guideline Working Group. Contrast-induced acute kidney injury and renal support for acute kidney injury: a KDIGO summary (Part 2). Crit Care 2013; 17:205.

Related topics of interest

- Fluid therapy (p 165)
- Renal – treatment of established acute kidney injury (p 302)

Renal – treatment of established acute kidney injury

Key points

- Life-threatening hyperkalaemia should be treated while preparing the patients for renal replacement therapy
- In critically ill patients, continuous renal replacement therapy provides more cardiovascular stability than intermittent haemodialysis
- The Kidney Disease Improving Global Outcomes Guidelines provide valuable recommendations on how to conduct RRT in patients with AKI

Preparation for renal-replacement therapy

If the preventative measures described in the Renal – acute kidney injury topic fail to reverse the acute kidney injury, renal-replacement therapy (RRT) will be necessary. While preparations are being made to start RRT (admission to an intensive care unit, insertion of a large-bore double-lumen venous catheter and setting up of the RRT equipment), treat hyperkalaemia according to the 2012 Renal Association Guidelines (**Table 52**).

Indications for renal-replacement therapy

In critically ill patients, RRT is generally started early after the onset of acute renal failure. It simplifies fluid and nutritional management. Observational data suggest improved outcome by starting RRT early in critically ill patients but this has not been confirmed by randomised controlled trials (RCTs) – one small RCT found no difference in outcome. The broad indications for RRT in the critically ill are pulmonary oedema caused by fluid overload, hyperkalaemia, metabolic acidosis and uraemic complications. A list of the conventional criteria for initiating RRT is given in **Table 53**.

Principles of dialysis and filtration

Dialysis describes the diffusion of solute across a semi-permeable membrane and down a concentration gradient. Filtration is the movement of solute by convection across a semi-permeable membrane – it is

Table 52 Treatment of hyperkalaemia (Renal Association Guidelines 2012)	
Step 1	Protect the heart with intravenous calcium. If there are ECG changes consistent with hyperkalaemia give calcium 6.8 mmol (10 mL calcium chloride or 30 mL calcium gluconate).
Step 2	Shift K^+ into cells with an insulin-glucose infusion (indicated if K^+ is ≥ 6.0 mmol L^{-1}).
Step 3	Shift K^+ into cells with salbutamol 10–20 mg by nebuliser (indicated if K^+ is ≥ 6.0 mmol L^{-1}).

Table 53 Indications for renal-replacement therapy

- Anuria (negligible urine output for 6 h)
- Severe oliguria (urine output < 200 mL over 12 h)
- Hyperkalaemia (≥ 6.5 mmol L^{-1})
- Severe metabolic acidosis (pH < 7.2) caused by renal failure
- Volume overload (especially pulmonary oedema or to create space for drugs and nutrition)
- Creatinine > 300–600 mmol L^{-1} and/or rising > 100 mmol L^{-1}day^{-1}
- Urea > 30 mmol L^{-1} and/or rising > 16–20 mmol L^{-1} day^{-1}
- Clearance of dialysable nephrotoxins and other drugs
- Encephalopathy

particularly effective for middle molecular weight molecules. Dialysis is particularly efficient for small molecules such as K^+, Na^+ and urea. Dialysis can be undertaken continuously or intermittently. The size of the molecules removed by filtration will depend on the cut off point (size of the holes) of the artificial membrane. Membranes designed for dialysis or filtration are most commonly made of polyacrylynitrile. This is a biocompatible material and is unlikely to cause significant complement activation.

Renal-replacement-therapy techniques

Methods of renal replacement include:
- Intermittent haemodialysis
- Continuous haemodialysis and/or haemofiltration
- Peritoneal dialysis – very rarely used today

Intermittent haemodialysis

Intermittent haemodialysis (IHD) is undertaken rarely in critical care units within the United Kingdom (UK). Continuous techniques (described below) are more widely available and, in the critically ill patient with multiple organ failure, cause less haemodynamic instability. Critically ill patients do not tolerate the rapid changes in plasma osmolality and intravascular volume that can occur with IHD. Renal units treating patients with 'single-organ' acute renal failure or chronic renal failure typically use IHD. Many American critical care physicians also prefer to use IHD for managing renal failure in the critical care unit. Studies comparing IHD with continuous renal replacement therapy (CRRT) in critically ill patients have shown no difference in mortality but cardiovascular stability is better with CRRT.

Continuous renal replacement therapies

The following techniques are used for continuous RRT in the critical care unit:
- Continuous venovenous haemofiltration (CVVH)
- Continuous venovenous haemodialysis (CVVHD) or haemodiafiltration (CVVHDF)

Venous access is obtained with a single, wide-bore, double-lumen cannula. The Kidney Disease Improving Global Outcomes (KDIGO) Guidelines recommend the following sites in order of preference:
- First choice: right jugular vein
- Second choice: femoral vein
- Third choice: left jugular vein
- Last choice: sub-clavian vein with preference for the dominant side

A pump delivers blood to the filter (**Figure 17**) ideally at flows of 200–250 mL min^{-1}, although achieving such flows depends on the quality of venous access. The excellent urea clearance achieved with CVVHDF is sufficient for even the most catabolic patients. Modern machines enable control of blood, dialysate, effluent (filtrate and/or spent dialysate) and replacement fluid flows, thus providing good control of the patient's fluid balance. The rate of fluid replacement is selected based on the desired fluid balance. In many cases, at least some of the replacement fluid is returned before the filter, which prolongs filter life. Many critical care physicians use the CVVH mode alone; this produces adequate urea and creatinine clearance in most patients. There has been controversy about the potential for CVVH to remove clinically significant quantities of inflammatory mediators in patients with severe sepsis – it probably does not.

The recent KDIGO Guidelines recommend delivering an effluent volume of 20–25 mL kg^{-1} h^{-1} for CRRT in AKI. There are often frequent interruptions in CRRT so this will require prescription of a higher effluent volume (typically 30–35 mL kg^{-1} h^{-1}).

Replacement fluid

Correction of metabolic acidosis can be achieved by including lactate, acetate, citrate or bicarbonate in the replacement fluid. Original replacement solutions most commonly contained lactate but it is not well-metabolised by patients with liver impairment. Use of bicarbonate replacement

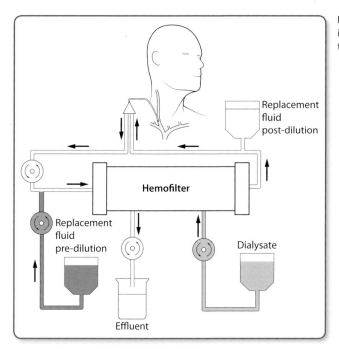

Figure 17 Circuit components in continuous renal replacement therapy.

fluid is now preferred because it results in better correction of acidosis, especially if there is liver impairment. Bicarbonate is unstable in solution and these solutions are therefore prepared immediately before use – the bicarbonate will remain in solution for at least 6 h.

Anticoagulation

Unless the patient has a significant coagulopathy, anticoagulant therapy is necessary to prevent clotting of the filter and extracorporeal circuit. In patients not at risk from bleeding, the most widely used method of anticoagulation is unfractionated heparin: following a bolus of 3000 units, a heparin infusion is started at 10 U kg^{-1} and adjusted to maintain an APTT at 1.5–2 times the control value. Low molecular weight heparin can also be used. In those few patients who develop heparin-induced thrombocytopenia (HIT), KDIGO recommendations are to use direct thrombin inhibitors (e.g. argatroban) or factor Xa inhibitors (e.g. danaparoid or fondaparinux); alternatively regional anticoagulation with citrate can be used. In patients at risk from bleeding some clinicians have used regional anticoagulation with unfractionated heparin infused pre-filter and protamine infused post-filter. But heparin has a much longer half-life than protamine and the patient is exposed to the risks of protamine (anaphylaxis, hypotension and platelet dysfunction) – for these reasons, the technique is not recommended in the KDIGO guidelines. Some clinicians use epoprostenol (2.5–5 ng kg^{-1} min^{-1}) in patients at risk of bleeding but this is not particularly good at preventing filter clotting and does not eliminate bleeding risk.

The use of citrate regional anticoagulation is becoming increasingly popular and is recommended in the KDIGO guidelines as the technique of choice for CRRT. This technique involves infusing citrate pre-filter; this chelates calcium – the target is an ionised calcium of 0.25– 0.35 mmol L^{-1} post-filter. Calcium chloride is infused post-filter to restore normal plasma calcium values. The advantages of citrate anticoagulation are:
- Avoids systemic anticoagulation and therefore reduces the risk of bleeding
- Avoids risk of HIT

- Prolongs filter life

The disadvantages of citrate anticoagulation are:

- It requires careful monitoring to avoid hypocalcaemia
- It can cause a metabolic alkalosis
- Citrate metabolism is reduced in hepatic impairment, and during hypotension, hypovolaemia and hypothermia. It is contraindicated in shock with muscle hypoperfusion
- It is more complex than other techniques

Nutrition

Renal replacement therapy enables critically ill patients to receive protein and calories in quantities required by their catabolic state. Wherever possible, this is given by the enteral route. A significant quantity of non-urea nitrogen is lost across the filter thus it may be appropriate to increase the nitrogen content of feeds given to patients receiving RRT.

Diuretic phase

The oliguric or anuric phase of established AKI lasts typically for about 2 weeks, although there is considerable variation in this period. The return of renal function presents with a diuresis. At this stage urine output is high, but renal function may still be poor. A rising urea and creatinine may indicate the need for a few more days of RRT. Clinicians often prescribe furosemide after stopping CRRT – this will increase urinary volumes and sodium clearance but does not shorten duration or renal failure – the practice is discouraged in the KDIGO guidelines.

Further reading

Tolwani A. Continuous renal replacement therapy for acute kidney injury. N Engl J Med 2012; 367:2505–2514.

Bellomo R, Kellum JA, Ronco C. Acute kidney injury. Lancet 2012; 380:756–766.

Croft R, Moore J. Renal failure and its treatment. Anaesth Int Care Med 2012; 13:336–342.

Alfonzo A, Soar J, MacTier R, et al. Clinical Practice Guidelines. Treatment of Acute Hyperkalemia in Adults. London: UK Renal Association, 2012.

Kellum JA, Lameire N, for the KDIGO Acute Kidney Injury Guideline Working Group. Diagnosis, evaluation, and management of acute kidney injury: a KDIGO summary (Part 1). Crit Care 2013; 17:204.

Lameire N, Kellum JA, for the KDIGO Acute Kidney Injury Guideline Working Group. Contrast-induced acute kidney injury and renal support for acute kidney injury: a KDIGO summary (Part 2). Crit Care 2013; 17:205.

Related topics of interest

Respiratory support – invasive

Key points

- Invasive mechanical ventilation is supportive therapy that is frequently lifesaving but not necessarily primarily therapeutic
- Invasive mechanical ventilation aims to avoid further lung damage whilst allowing time to treat the underlying illness
- Complications arise from the need for sedation, the impact on cardiovascular dynamics, the risk of infection, and ventilator-induced lung injury

Definitions

Mechanical ventilation describes partial or total replacement of spontaneous ventilation. The patient interface determines whether the ventilation is invasive (i.e. via oral tracheal tube or tracheostomy) or non-invasive (using a mask (nasal or full face) or a hood). Improved alveolar ventilation reduces Pa_{CO_2}), and oxygenation is improved with high FI_{O_2} delivery and reduced veno-arterial shunt by recruiting unventilated lung units with the use of positive end expiratory pressure (PEEP) as well as inspiratory positive pressure.

Indications for invasive mechanical ventilation

Despite didactic lists of indications for ventilation and trigger values of Pa_{O_2} and Pa_{CO_2}, in practice, the combination of respiratory failure, patient fatigue, conscious level, inability to clear secretions and inadequate response to non-invasive ventilation dictate the need for invasive mechanical ventilation.

Complications

Ventilation is not primarily therapeutic – the benefit is supportive while the underlying disease (e.g. pneumonia and heart failure) is treated. A major aim when selecting a ventilatory strategy is therefore minimisation of harm.

The complications include:
- Those associated with tracheal intubation, including risk of infection and laryngeal/tracheal trauma
- Those associated with sedation. Sedation and mechanical ventilation lead to atrophy of respiratory muscles. While difficult to detect, this is a major cause of subsequent failure to wean
- Ventilator induced lung injury (VILI). Lung disease is often heterogeneous in distribution with areas of normal compliance (normal ventilation) and areas of very low compliance (low or no ventilation). Excessive volumes and/or pressures will lead to over-distension of the ventilated 'normal' lung with high shear forces between ventilated and non-ventilated lung units. This causes alveolar damage VILI, and alveolar disruption can results in pneumothorax and/or subcutaneous and mediastinal emphysema ('volutraum/barotrauma'). Damaged areas of lung also release inflammatory mediators, causing or worsening the SIRS response ('biotrauma')
- Increased mean intra-thoracic (pleural) pressure reduces right ventricular filling and cardiac output. So tissue oxygen delivery may fall despite an increase in red blood cell oxygen content. Transmission of airway pressure to the pleural space depends on lung and chest wall compliance. The effect is therefore attenuated in disease such as ARDS
- If there is limitation of expiratory flow (e.g. bronchospasm) the lungs may not have emptied before inspiration is triggered. This leads to progressive increase in the end expiratory lung volume, referred to as dynamic hyperinflation, breath-stacking and increased intrinsic-PEEP (PEEPi), and is a potent cause of both barotrauma and cardiovascular collapse. Observation of the expiratory flow waveform will warn whether this is happening (expiratory flow should approach zero before the next breath)

Ventilator settings

Mechanical ventilation has a number of components and different manufacturers use different terms for each, with the potential for confusion. Observation of ventilator settings along with pressure and flow tracings allows an understanding of what the machine is doing. There are four major functions of the ventilator.

- Mandatory breaths. The ventilator will deliver breaths at the set rate by cycling from expiratory pressure to a determined inspiratory pressure (pressure control ventilation, PCV) or by delivering a user determined inspiratory volume (volume control ventilation, VCV). With PCV, lung compliance determines tidal volume and with VCV lung compliance determines inspiratory pressure. While historically VCV utilised a constant inspiratory flow, most ventilators will now permit VCV using constant pressure as for PCV. This results in a high initial inspiratory flow that is exponentially reducing and may improve spatial and temporal distribution of ventilation. Some modes attempt to match machine breaths with spontaneous patient breaths [synchronised intermittent mandatory ventilation (SIMV)]
- Assistance of spontaneous breaths. Patient breaths are detected using a drop in pressure or change in flow within the breathing system. The machine will then support the breath by applying a user defined pressure (pressure support) or volume (volume support). Patient breaths that are not assisted may lead to respiratory fatigue and failure to wean. Spontaneous breathing may reduce respiratory muscle atrophy and is thought to be beneficial. Therefore, some form of inspiratory assist should always be provided
- The pressure during expiration can be altered in an attempt to improve oxygenation by recruiting collapsed/consolidation lung units. On mandatory ventilation this is termed PEEP, if applied during fully spontaneous respiration throughout the respiratory cycle then this represents continuous positive airway pressure (CPAP)
- Inspired oxygenation concentration is set

When setting the ventilator each of these components should be considered, i.e. inspiratory volume or pressure plus rate, level of assist, expiratory pressure and F_{IO_2} (**Table 54**).

These settings are titrated against the patient's Pa_{O_2} and Pa_{CO_2} and comfort. Carbon dioxide elimination can be improved further by increasing the tidal volume (or peak pressure) or by increasing the respiratory rate. Oxygenation can be improved further by increasing F_{IO_2}, increasing PEEP, by prolonging the inspiratory time, or by further recruiting collapsed lung units (e.g. using prone ventilation). Prolonging the inspiratory time will raise mean airway pressure and create $PEEP_i$. Prolonged exposure to an $F_{IO_2} > 0.5–0.6$ may cause pulmonary oxygen toxicity and it may be better to increase PEEP and/or prolong the inspiratory time once this concentration is required. It is not necessary to achieve 'normal' arterial blood gases and when there is actual or potential ARDS,

Table 54 When initiating mechanical ventilation, typical initial settings might be:	
PEEP	5 cmH$_2$O
Tidal volume (VCV mode)	6–8 mL kg^{-1} predicted body weight
Inspiratory pressure (PCV mode)	20 cmH$_2$O (15 above PEEP)
Frequency	10–15 min^{-1}
I:E ratio	1:2
Pressure trigger	–1 to –3 cmH$_2$O
Flow trigger	1–2 L min^{-1}
Pressure support	20 cmH$_2$O (15 above PEEP)

volume and pressure limited ventilation should be used, with acceptance of modest hypoxia (to $Pao_2 > 8$ kPa, $Spo_2 > 88\%$) and hyper-carbia. With normal lungs, ventilation can be titrated to 'normal' levels of oxygenation and CO_2. Use a tidal volume of 6–8 mL kg^{-1} predicted body weight and where possible, inspiratory plateau pressure should be limited to < 35 cmH$_2$O (higher pressures are acceptable if the chest wall compliance is low). This should reduce over distension of relatively compliant areas of lung (**Figure 18**).

Alternative modes and therapies

Reverse I:E ratio

Lengthening inspiratory time improves oxygenation by directly increasing mean airway pressure. If insufficient time is available for expiration there is potential for dynamic hyperinflation, which also increase mean airway pressure but may be dangerous. There is no evidence for outcome benefit.

Nitric oxide

Nitric oxide (NO) causes vasodilatation in ventilated lung areas, secondarily reducing perfusion to poorly ventilated regions.

V/Q matching improves and oxygenation increases in 60–70% of patients. Use of NO does not improve outcome from ARDS and its use in the treatment of adults is now uncommon.

Tracheal gas insufflation

Infusing oxygen by catheter into the airway at the level of the carina both improves oxygenation (partly by simply increasing the mean Fio_2) and CO_2 elimination. There is no evidence for outcome benefit and there is potential for harm.

Prone ventilation

In ARDS, placing the ventilated patient prone improves the distribution of ventilation and therefore V/Q matching. Around 60% of patients will show improvement in oxygenation which may be sustained by changing periodically from front-to-back. Complications include dislodgement of tubes and lines, cardiovascular instability and pressure sores. The recent PROSEVA study suggests a mortality benefit for patients with severe ARDS.

Extracorporeal CO_2 removal

Arterio-venous or pumped veno-venous circuits pass blood over a gas permeable membrane. CO_2 elimination is achieved and

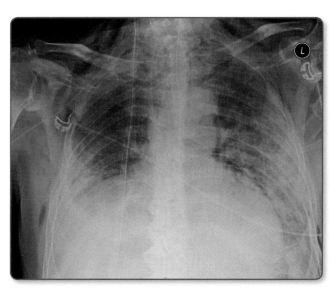

Figure 18 Chest X-ray: Patient with ARDS after right middle and lower lobe resection for carcinoma. Bilateral infiltrates, surgical emphysema, tracheostomy and R PICC.

to a lesser extent, oxygenation. Suggested benefits are avoidance of ventilation and in ventilated patients the potential to significantly reduce tidal volume and/or respiratory rate to 'rest' the lungs and avoid VILI. This remains an experimental technique. Limb ischaemia from access catheters is a potential problem.

Extracorporeal membrane oxygenation

Partial cardiopulmonary bypass using similar systems to those used during cardiac surgery provide near total oxygention and CO_2 removal permitting complete lung 'rest' with similar but larger therapeutic benefit compared with extracorporeal CO_2

removal (ECCOR). Although study results are equivocal, availability and use of the technique is spreading.

High-frequency oscillatory ventilation

A diaphragm oscillating at 3–20 Hz (3–9 Hz in adults) induces CO_2 elimination and a system of CPAP provides oxygenation. In theory, high-frequency oscillatory ventilation (HFOV) is ideal for lung-protective ventilation; peak airway pressures are reduced, mean airway pressure is increased and lung volume is maintained throughout the respiratory cycle. The recent OSCILLATE and OSCAR trials failed to show outcome benefit.

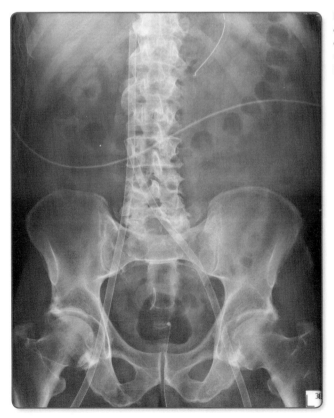

Figure 19 Abdominal X-ray: cannulae for VV ECMO, return cannula positioned in R atrium under TOE control, outflow cannula in IVC.

Further reading

Stewart NI, Jagelman TA, Webster NR. Emerging modes of ventilation in the intensive care unit. Br J Anaesth 2011; 107:74–82.

The Acute Respiratory Distress Syndrome Network. Ventilation with lower tidal volumes as compared with traditional tidal volumes for acute lung injury and the acute respiratory distress syndrome. N Engl J Med 2000; 342:1301–1308.

Peek GJ, Mugford M, Tiruvoipati R, et al. Efficacy and economic assessment of conventional ventilatory support versus extracorporeal membrane oxygenation for severe adult respiratory failure (CESAR): a multicentre randomised controlled trial. Lancet 2009; 374:1351–1363.

Guérin C, Reignier J, Richard JC, et al. Prone positioning in severe acute respiratory distress syndrome. N Engl J Med 2013; 368:2159–2168.

Ferguson ND, Cook DJ, Guyatt GH, et al. High-frequency oscillation in early acute respiratory distress syndrome. N Engl J Med 2013; 368:795–805.

Young D, Lamb SE, Shah S, et al. High-frequency oscillation for acute respiratory distress syndrome. N Engl J Med 2013; 368:806–813.

Related topics of interest

Respiratory support – non-invasive techniques

Key points

- Patient optimisation must be performed prior to non-invasive ventilation
- In conditions such as COPD, NIV has revolutionised care
- CPAP and NIV are the main non-invasive techniques used

Impairment of pulmonary gas exchange causes hypoxaemia with or without hypercarbia. Non-invasive respiratory support techniques aim to produce adequate oxygenation and acceptable carbon dioxide excretion.

Acute hypoxaemic (Type I) respiratory failure

This is the commonest form of respiratory failure and is associated with virtually all acute diseases of the lung, which generally involve fluid filling or collapse of alveoli. Hypoxaemia is due to ventilation/perfusion (V/Q) mismatch, true shunt (areas of zero (V/Q) or, most often, a combination of the two. True shunt occurs when alveoli are completely collapsed, totally consolidated or filled with oedema fluid. V/Q mismatch is caused by regional variations in compliance and perfusion abnormalities.

Ventilatory (Type II) respiratory failure

Inadequate alveolar ventilation (ventilatory failure) with resultant hypercarbia can be due to:

- Central nervous system depression: drugs, head injury, stroke and infection
- Neuromuscular disease: Guillain–Barré syndrome, myasthenia gravis, and spinal trauma
- Chest wall/pleural disease: pneumothorax, flail chest and pleural effusion

- Upper airway obstruction: laryngeal oedema, infection, and foreign body
- Small airway disorders: asthma, chronic obstructive pulmonary disease (COPD)
- Failure to compensate for increased carbon dioxide production
- Failure to compensate for an increase in dead space and re-breathing
- A combination of these factors

In the patient breathing room air, hypoventilation causes hypoxaemia (alveolar gas equation, Arterial blood gases – analysis). This is easily corrected by increasing F_{IO_2}. In the patient breathing air, pulse oximetry is a fair monitor of alveolar ventilation as an increased P_{aCO_2} causes a decreased P_{aO_2} and arterial oxygen saturation. When oxygen is being given, pulse oximetry will not reflect hypoventilation and arterial blood gas analysis is required to assess P_{aCO_2} and pH. An increase in dead space, either physiological dead space or dead space due to inappropriate breathing system design will result in hypercarbia if the patient is unable to increase minute ventilation to compensate. It is important to consider excessive equipment dead space when hypercarbia occurs in a patient receiving any form of respiratory support.

Assessment

Acute respiratory failure causes life-threatening derangements in arterial blood gases and acid-base status whereas the effects of chronic respiratory failure are often less dramatic and not as readily apparent. Shortness of breath (dyspnoea) often accompanies respiratory failure. An increase in respiratory rate (tachypnoea) is a good indicator of critical illness. Once respiratory failure is suspected on clinical grounds, an arterial blood gas analysis will confirm the diagnosis and assist in the distinction between acute and chronic forms.

This helps to assess the severity of respiratory failure and guide management. Visible cyanosis is present when the concentration of deoxygenated haemoglobin in the capillaries or tissues is at least 5 g dL^{-1}. Confusion and somnolence can occur in respiratory failure. Myoclonus and seizures can also occur with severe hypoxaemia. Polycythaemia is a complication of long-standing hypoxaemia.

Simple measures to improve respiratory function

Particular groups of patients at high risk of complications include those with known respiratory disease, depressed level of consciousness, impaired cough, chest trauma, and post-operative upper-abdominal and thoracic surgery. Attention should be directed to:

Treating the underlying condition: In practice, there may be difficulties in identifying the underlying condition. For example, in theory, differentiating infection from heart failure should be easy but in practice it can be very difficult. Empirical treatment in these situations is justifiable.

Airway opening manoeuvres: Airway obstruction may be subtle and must always be corrected.

Posture: Sitting the patient up reduces the weight of the abdominal contents on the diaphragm, increases functional residual capacity (FRC), reduces the central blood volume, improves ventilation and reduces left ventricular diastolic pressure. Early mobilisation including sitting out in a chair, standing and walking will help prevent atelectasis, and help maintain muscle function and strength.

Analgesia: Pain after thoracic or abdominal surgery or trauma inhibits diaphragmatic movement, deep breathing and sighing resulting in a reduced FRC and lung collapse. Inhibition of coughing leads to sputum retention. Use a multimodal approach to treat pain aggressively using paracetamol, opioids, non-steroidal anti-inflammatory drugs and neural blockade as appropriate.

Physiotherapy is an important part of respiratory support. Deep breathing exercises, particularly in conjunction with incentive spirometry improve lung expansion and FRC. Coughing improves sputum clearance.

Humidification with oxygen therapy will preserve mucociliary clearance, reduce viscosity of secretions and reduce collapse and infection.

Infection control should be scrupulous to reduce the chances of cross-infection and nosocomial pneumonia.

Oxygen therapy

Hypoxic patients should be given supplementary oxygen. Titrate the inspired concentration (FIO_2) to normalise the patient's oxygen saturation. In some patients with severe COPD, giving oxygen may reverse hypoxic pulmonary vasoconstriction and increases V/Q mismatch. The subsequent increase in dead space may then cause hypercarbia. This mechanism, and not the removal of 'hypoxic drive', explains why some COPD patients become progressively hypercarbic with high concentration oxygen. The British Thoracic Society recommends targeted oxygen therapy guided by pulse oximetry:

- 94–98% for adults less than 70 years
- 92–98% for adults over 70 years
- 88–92% for those at risk of hyper-capnic respiratory failure

The age cut-off of 70 years is arbitrary. Recent observational data from acute medical admissions suggests a 'normal' oxygen saturation of 96–98% irrespective of age. Whether correcting oxygen saturation to a normal range with oxygen therapy improves outcome is not known.

Variable performance devices

These devices comprise the facemask (e.g. 'MC' mask and 'Hudson' mask) and nasal prongs. They do not deliver a constant FIO_2. Most oxygen delivery systems enable a maximum flow of 15 L min^{-1}. The patient's peak inspiratory flow may reach more than 30 L min^{-1}, even during quiet breathing. Thus, a variable amount of room air is inspired along with the delivered oxygen.

In the acutely dyspnoeic patient, peak inspiratory flow may be many times that of the normal subject and the actual FIO_2 will be lower and even less predictable. Despite this, these devices are safe as long as oxygenation is being monitored. They have the advantage of being simple and inexpensive.

Nasal prongs are well-tolerated and do not interfere with eating and drinking. They are not as effective in mouth breathing patients. High flow nasal delivery systems are available but their benefit is unclear at present.

Fixed-performance devices

A constant F_{IO_2} can be achieved by delivering the air/oxygen mixture at flows that exceed the patient's peak inspiratory flow, or by providing a reservoir bag of gas mixture from which the patient breathes. These devices may not perform as expected in the presence of high peak inspiratory flows or abnormal breathing patterns.

The Venturi mask uses the Bernoulli principle: a moving gas has a lower pressure than stationary gas. Oxygen is forced through a small orifice producing a high-velocity jet which 'sucks' ambient air into the entrainment chamber. The volume of air entrained and thus the F_{IO_2} is a fixed function of the oxygen flow and the characteristics of the Venturi.

The Ventimask has separate Venturis for each F_{IO_2} and the correct oxygen flow must be given. Other systems employ a fixed Venturi but with a variable aperture to regulate air intake. Typically, to achieve an F_{IO_2} of 0.6, the oxygen flow is set at 15 L min^{-1} and the total gas mixture flow is 30 L min^{-1}, which exceeds peak inspiratory flow for the normal patient.

The 'reservoir' mask uses a collapsible bag into which high flow fresh oxygen is delivered and from which the patient inspires. Valves prevent inspiration from ambient air and prevent expiration into the reservoir bag. The system is designed to provide as high a F_{IO_2} as possible. In practice there is inspiratory leakage of ambient air and thus a F_{IO_2} of 1.0 cannot be achieved.

Continuous positive airway pressure

Continuous positive airway pressure (CPAP) is indicated in any patient with hypoxia unresponsive to simple methods of oxygen

delivery. Failure of alveolar ventilation may also be an indication for CPAP if improvement in compliance and reduction in the work of breathing improve alveolar ventilation significantly. Patients with profound hypoventilation require mechanical ventilation. CPAP is usually inappropriate for patients with reduced consciousness.

CPAP has several effects:

- Increase in FRC. A low FRC causes atelectasis and lung collapse, leading to V/Q mismatch and reduced pulmonary compliance with increased airway resistance, which increases the work of breathing. Restoration of a normal FRC will improve oxygenation and reduce the work of breathing
- Reopening closed alveoli (recruitment). This occurs as part of the general improvement in FRC
- Reduction in left ventricular transmural pressure. This is of value in left ventricular failure and may be the main way in which CPAP improves oxygenation in acute cardiogenic pulmonary oedema. CPAP does not necessarily drive pulmonary oedema fluid back into the circulation and total lung water may not change despite clinical improvement
- Reducing threshold work. In patients experiencing auto-PEEP or dynamic hyperinflation, the inspiratory muscles have to work to drop the alveolar pressure from its positive, end-expiratory value to less than the upper airway pressure (normally zero) before inspiratory gas flow occurs. This is termed threshold work and may be significant. By increasing the airway pressure CPAP reduces the work required to initiate inspiratory flow
- Airway splinting. CPAP is a specific treatment for obstructive sleep apnoea and is often of value in patients with temporary airway problems
- Delivery of high F_{IO_2}. Because CPAP systems are closed, with no re-breathing, the chosen inspired oxygen concentration can be delivered reliably, up to and including 100% oxygen

Adverse effects:

- Hypotension. An increase in intra-thoracic pressure reduces right ventricular end diastolic volume and can precipitate hypotension in the presence of hypovolaemia

- Barotrauma. As with any form of pressure therapy, over-inflation and gas trapping are possible, although frank barotrauma is rare
- Discomfort. Patients frequently find the CPAP mask uncomfortable and claustrophobic; patient refusal of mask CPAP is common
- Gastric distension. When CPAP is delivered by facemask, gastric inflation can occur. Although this is an indication for gastric decompression, prophylactic placement of a nasogastric tube is not required in every patient
- Pulmonary aspiration. Vomiting or regurgitation into a tight-fitting CPAP mask may result in massive aspiration
- Pressure necrosis. This may be helped by the use of a hydrocolloid or similar dressing placed over vulnerable areas such as the bridge of the nose. Alternatively helmet or full-face masks can be used

When used in the treatment of obstructive sleep apnoea, a nasal mask is often effective and is better tolerated by the patient. In patients with manifest respiratory failure, a facemask or helmet is usually necessary.

Airway pressure is kept at a specified level (typically 5–15 cmH$_2$O) throughout the respiratory cycle of spontaneously breathing patients. This requires inspiratory gas at flows in excess of the patient's maximal inspiratory flow capacity and a threshold resistor in the expiratory limb of the breathing system. Check the continuity of the positive pressure by examining the expiratory valve; it should stay open throughout the respiratory cycle. An alternative, but less efficient, method for providing CPAP utilises a pressurised reservoir of fresh gas such as a spring-loaded concertina-style reservoir bag.

Non-invasive ventilation

Non-invasive ventilation (NIV) via a facemask, nasal mask or helmet mask can be used instead of conventional ventilation via a tracheal tube. The technique and problems are similar to those described for CPAP. The indications and timing for NIV include:

- Prevent the need for tracheal intubation and invasive ventilation in acute respiratory failure
- Alternative to tracheal intubation and conventional ventilation in established respiratory failure
- Weaning tool in resolving respiratory failure
- Prevention of re-intubation of trachea after weaning from conventional ventilation

Studies show a benefit of NIV in acute exacerbations of COPD in terms of reducing ICU admissions, need for tracheal intubation and overall mortality.

Patients with neutropaenia and respiratory failure are another group who show significant benefit from NIV over invasive ventilation.

There is also increasing evidence that NIV may be useful in patients with other causes of acute respiratory failure, e.g. pulmonary oedema.

Non-invasive ventilation augments tidal volume by sensing inspiratory effort and providing pressure support to the patient. When flow stops, the pressure returns to the preset CPAP level. This results in a decrease in respiratory rate, decreased work of breathing improved alveolar ventilation and possible avoidance of tracheal intubation. However, NIV has limitations and is not successful in every patient. Patient comfort and compliance are critical for success.

Non-invasive ventilation can be provided by conventional ventilators and by simpler, specifically designed, ventilators. The preferred mode is CPAP with pressure support (often referred to as bi-level positive airway pressure). It may be necessary to try several masks to provide effective ventilation that is comfortable for the patient. The level of medical and nursing care required initially to establish and maintain NIV is often much higher than required for conventional ventilation.

The benefits of avoiding the need for tracheal intubation include:

- Lower incidence of ventilator associated pneumonia

- Avoidance of sedative drugs
- Allows patient to talk

In patients with acute respiratory failure in who NIV is not effective, a decision to proceed to intubation should be made within 4 hours in order to improve survival.

Intubation if appropriate is also the treatment of choice in late (> 48 h) NIV failure.

Weaning should initially occur during the day with extended periods off NIV for meals, and other activities (e.g. physiotherapy).

Further reading

Young D, Lamb SE, Shah S, et al. High-frequency oscillation for acute respiratory distress syndrome. N Engl J Med 2013; 368:806–813.

O'Driscoll BR, Howard LS, Davison AG. BTS guideline for emergency oxygen use in adult patients. Thorax 2008; 63:vi1–68.

Royal College of Physicians, British Thoracic Society, Intensive Care Society. Non-invasive ventilation in chronic obstructive pulmonary disease: management of acute type 2 respiratory failure, Concise guidance to good practice, No.11. London: RCP, 2008.

Burns KE, Adhikari NK, Keenan SP, Meade MO. Noninvasive positive pressure ventilation as a weaning strategy for intubated adults with respiratory failure. Cochrane Database Syst Rev 2010:CD004127.

Smith GB, Prytherch DR, Watson D, et al. S(p)O(2) values in acute medical admissions breathing air--implications for the British Thoracic Society guideline for emergency oxygen use in adult patients? Resuscitation 2012; 83:1201–1205.

Related topics of interest

Scoring systems

Key points

- Scoring systems are in common use in the ICU
- They can be used in audit, outcome prediction and for research
- Predictions should be used only for populations and not for individuals

Background

The choice of scoring system depends on the data available and the outcome being evaluated. For example; Child-Pugh scores are useful only in patients with chronic liver disease. Physiological-based systems enable comparisons across disease groups or between critical care units. This is beneficial as it is common to have a disease process affecting several organ systems. **Figure 20** demonstrates the classification of scoring systems.

Scoring systems require collection of data relating to several variables; these are weighted using population data to derive a probability. Mortality is the most common outcome calculated.

Data are collected on the first day of admission to critical care and, depending on the scoring system, also on subsequent days at defined intervals. Multiple regression analyses are used to analyse data from massive multi-centre and multi-national databases and subsequently to generate the scoring systems.

Effective scoring systems must be:

- *Valid* – able to predict mortality accurately for a given population
- *Calibrated* – perform across a range of predicted mortalities
- *Discriminate* – be accurate between predicated and observed mortalities

Acute physiology and chronic health evaluation (APACHE)

This is one of the oldest scoring systems. APACHE II remains the most widely used scoring system in the world. It incorporates both acute physiological derangement and chronic health status.

An acute physiological score is measured from: pulse rate, mean blood pressure, temperature, respiratory rate, $PaO_2:FIO_2$, haematocrit, white cell count, creatinine, urine output, urea, sodium, albumin, bilirubin, glucose, acid base and GCS. Chronic health variables measured are: acquired immunodeficiency syndrome, cirrhosis, hepatic failure, immunosuppression, lymphoma, leukaemia, myeloma or metastatic tumour. Weighted categories also include age, admission diagnosis, admission source, emergency surgery and thrombolytic therapy. The score uses the 'worst values' (those furthest from the normal range) recorded during the first 24 h of admission.

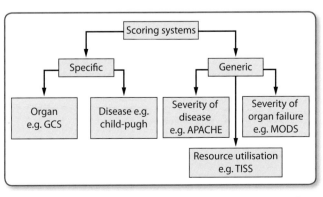

Figure 20 GCS: Glasgow coma scale, MODS: multiple organ dysfunction score, APACHE: acute physiology and chronic health evaluation, TISS: therapeutic intervention scoring system.

APACHE IV uses a database of 110,000 patients from 104 units in North America and was published in 2006. In addition to mortality probabilities, it includes prediction equations for length of stay to enable efficiency comparisons. It shows good discrimination (0.88) and calibration, with a ratio of observed to predicted mortality close to 1.0.

The strongest outcome predictor is acute physiological score, followed by disease group and age.

APACHE II calculators are freely available online (www.globalrph.com/apacheii.htm).

Simplified acute physiology score (SAPS)

Originally this scored only acute physiology variables. Later versions include weightings for chronic health. The outcome data includes length of stay prediction. SAPS III is the current version and, although derived from a smaller database than APACHE, it has great breadth involving over 300 units globally (lack of breadth is a common limitation of other scoring systems). It displays good discrimination (0.84) and calibration. It is scored within the first hour of admission.

Mortality prediction model (MPM)

MPM consists of two parts, measuring 16 variables at admission, and a further 13 variables at 24 h. It can be repeated daily. It is simple to use with a binary scoring system; each variable is either present or absent. Although the original version was based on data from just one unit, it is now in its third incarnation with data from 135 ICUs involving over 120,000 patients. It demonstrates good discrimination (0.81).

Multiple organ dysfunction score (MODS)

The MODS measures a single variable from each organ system to quantify dysfunction. It

weights scores on a scale of 0–4 over six organ systems; scoring – heart rate, PaO_2/FiO_2 ratio, GCS, creatinine, bilirubin and platelets. It is simple to perform and can be repeated to guide patient management.

Sequential organ failure assessment (SOFA)

Initially validated on sepsis data, this score has now broadened to include measures of non-septic organ dysfunction. Variables are scored 1–4 over six organ systems: cardiovascular, respiratory, neurological, renal, hepatic and haematological. It is calculated at 24 h and repeated at 48 h intervals. The average value is used to predict mortality with a rapid change in score suggesting poor prognosis.

Intensive Care National Audit and Research Centre (ICNARC)

Concerns about international differences in databases led a UK group to develop ICNARC. The 'Case Mix Programme' includes data from approximately 240 UK critical care units relating to over 1 million admissions. It has drawn from previous scoring systems and uses acute physiological data, chronic health, age, source and reason for admission and CPR status. It is scored using data for the first 24 h after admission. The acute physiological variables are weighted to give a maximum score of 100. These include: heart rate, systolic blood pressure, temperature, respiratory rate, $PaO_2:FIO_2$, pH, urea, creatinine, sodium, urine output, white blood cell and GCS.

To date, ICNARC has out-performed existing scoring systems; the data is also discriminate, calibrated and validated. It can be used for audit, outcome predictions and as a comparator of critical care units.

Summary

All scoring systems have their limitations. Probabilities reported are for a population and not an individual patient. They are useful only for predicting outcomes in the populations from which the data are generated, i.e. most are not applicable outside of critical care.

Finally, when making comparisons, mortality and length of stay are not the only indicators of quality of care.

Further reading

Zimmerman JE, Kramer AA, McNair DS, Malila FM. Acute Physiology and Chronic Health Evaluation (APACHE) IV: Hospital mortality assessment for today's critically ill patients. Crit Care Med 2006; 34:1297–1310.

Harrison DA, Parry G, Carpenter JR et al. A new risk prediction model for critical care: The Intensive Care National Audit & Research Centre (ICNARC) model. Crit Care Med 2007; 35:1091–1098.

Vincent JL, Moreno R. Clinical review: scoring systems in the critically ill. Crit Care 2010; 14:207.

Related topics of interest

- Quality indicators (p 284)

Sedation

Key points

- The goals of sedation are to reduce anxiety, relieve dyspnoea, enhance analgesia and enable mechanical ventilation and therapeutic procedures
- There is no ideal single sedative drug
- One of the commonest sedation strategies in adult intensive care units is the combination of propofol and an opioid
- A sedation scoring tool should be used to optimise the sedation level

General principles

Sedatives help to relieve anxiety, encourage sleep, help the patient to synchronise with the ventilator and permit therapeutic procedures. The requirements for sedation vary greatly depending on the patient's pathology, psychological state and intensity of the medical and nursing procedures being undertaken. Improving the patient's environment may help to reduce the need for drugs. Effective communication and appropriate reassurance will help to relieve the patient's anxiety. Many patients receiving mechanical ventilation will require sufficient sedation to keep them comfortable yet rousable to voice. Patients with a tracheostomy who are receiving assisted modes of ventilation may not require any sedation. Where indicated, regional analgesia will prevent the need for large doses of systemic analgesia. Deep sedation is required for non-physiological modes of ventilation (e.g. inverse ratio), prone ventilation or control of intracranial hypertension or seizures.

The ideal sedative

The ideal sedative would possess the following properties:

- Anxiolysis
- Analgesia
- Hypnosis
- Amnesia
- Reduce delirium
- Titratability
- Predictable effect
- Rapid elimination
- Lack of cardiovascular and gastrointestinal side effects
- No development of tolerance
- Low cost

No single drug meets all of these ideals and for this reason it is common to use a combination of drugs. However, even this approach rarely achieves all of the objectives.

Drug administration

Sedatives are given usually by bolus or by continuous intravenous infusion (**Table 55**). Inhalational sedation with isoflurane or sevoflurane has been described but is rarely used – these volatile agents are occasionally used to treat severe asthma but in these cases they are being used for their bronchodilator properties and not primarily for sedation. Continuous infusion is a convenient method of drug administration but may produce over sedation if the patient's conscious level is not assessed frequently. Bolus dosing will reduce the incidence of over sedation but is less convenient for nursing staff. In patients who are receiving mechanical ventilation, daily interruption of sedative drug infusions may reduce the duration of mechanical ventilation and the length of stay on the critical care unit; however, if a strict protocolised approach is used, routine interruption of sedation may not be beneficial. Currently, unless there are specific contraindications, it is common practice to stop sedative drug infusions each morning.

Drugs

Sedative drugs

Propofol and benzodiazepines are the commonest sedatives used in critical care. Benzodiazepines produce excellent sedation, anxiolysis and amnesia but can

Table 55 Drugs used for sedation, analgesia and paralysis			
Drug	Bolus	Infusion	Comments
Propofol	0.5–2 mg kg^{-1}	1–3 mg kg^{-1} h^{-1}	Causes hypotension
Midazolam	25–50 µg kg^{-1}	50–100 µg kg^{-1} h^{-1}	Prolonged effects in the critically ill
Clonidine	75–300 µg kg^{-1} 8 h	0.05–0.4 µg kg^{-1} h^{-1}	Can cause hypotension
Dexmedetomidine		0.2–1.5 µg kg^{-1} h^{-1}	Expensive, analgesic properties; can cause bradycardia and hypotension
Morphine	0.1–0.2 mg kg^{-1}	40–80 µg kg^{-1} h^{-1}	Active metabolites accumulate in renal failure
Fentanyl	1–5 µg kg^{-1}	2–7 µg kg^{-1} h^{-1}	Cumulative with prolonged infusion
Alfentanil	15–30 µg kg^{-1}	20–120 µg kg^{-1} h^{-1}	Relatively expensive
Remifentanil	0.5–1 µg kg^{-1}	6–12 µg kg^{-1} h^{-1}	Ultra-short acting, but expensive
Atracurium	0.5 mg kg^{-1}	0.1–0.5 mg kg^{-1} h^{-1}	Metabolised independently of renal/hepatic function

cause delirium. All benzodiazepines are extensively metabolised in the liver. Sepsis will reduce blood flow to the liver and will impair the metabolism of benzodiazepines. The active metabolite of midazolam, α-hydroxymidazolam, is shorter acting than the metabolites of diazepam but accumulates with prolonged infusion and adds to the sedative effects of midazolam.

Propofol is an intravenous anaesthetic. It is eliminated rapidly from the central compartment and full recovery of consciousness is achieved reasonably quickly even after infusions for many days. Hepatic and renal dysfunction has no clinically significant effect on the metabolism of propofol. Propofol reduces systemic vascular resistance and causes hypotension. The propofol infusion syndrome (bradycardia associated with lipaemic plasma, fatty liver enlargement, metabolic acidosis, rhabdomyolysis and myoglobinuria) has been reported in adults and children and is generally associated with prolonged infusions of high doses (more than 5 mg kg^{-1} h^{-1} for more than 48 h). Children are more susceptible to the propofol infusion syndrome, probably because of low glycogen storage and higher dependence on fat metabolism, and for this reason propofol sedation is generally avoided in those under 16 years. When propofol is used in combination with an opioid, typical infusion rates to achieve adequate sedation are 1.5–3 mg kg^{-1}h^{-1}.

Clonidine is an α$_2$-adrenoceptor agonist. It has analgesia, sedative and anxiolytic properties and can be given by bolus dose (75–300 µg 8 h), continuous infusion (up to 4 µg kg^{-1}h^{-1}) or by nasogastric tube (50–600 µg 6–8 h). It is particularly suitable for sedating patients withdrawing from chronic alcohol abuse, during weaning from long-term ventilation or in patients with tetanus. Dexmedetomidine, a highly selective α$_2$-agonist, has recently been approved for use as a sedative in the United Kingdom – it has been available in the United States for several years. Dexmedetomidine provides sedation and anxiolysis via receptors in the locus ceruleus, analgesia via receptors in the spinal cord and attenuation of the stress response with no significant respiratory depression. In comparison with midazolam, it reduces the time patients spend on ventilators and produces less delirium. Bradycardia can be problematic and it is expensive.

Haloperidol, an anti-psychotic drug, can be used to treat delirium on the ICU. It is given in bolus doses of 1–2.5 mg (commencing with 0.5 mg in the elderly and very frail). Recently, a low dose infusion of 0.5 mg h^{-1} for 12 h has been shown to reduce the incidence of delirium in elderly patients after non-cardiac surgery.

Analgesic drugs

Opioids produce effective analgesia and anxiolysis, and reduce respiratory drive. The respiratory depression produced by opioids may help the patient to synchronise with the ventilator. Excessive doses will cause apnoea and prevent the use of patient-triggered modes of ventilation. They also cause gastrointestinal stasis, which impairs absorption of enteral feed and causes constipation requiring aperients. Morphine is cheap and remains a popular choice for analgesia and sedation in critical care. It is metabolised mainly in the liver to morphine-3-glucuronide and morphine-6-glucuronide. The latter is a potent analgesic and is excreted in the urine. Considerable accumulation of this metabolite occurs in patients with renal impairment and for this reason morphine is normally avoided in patients with renal failure.

Fentanyl is a synthetic opioid that is commonly used in anaesthetic practice. In single doses, fentanyl has a short duration of action. However, redistribution rather than the clearance determines duration of action. Thus, after a prolonged infusion, recovery from fentanyl can take a considerable time, i.e. the context-sensitive half-life is prolonged (200 min after a 6 h infusion and 300 min after a 12 h infusion). Alfentanil is shorter acting than fentanyl. The action of alfentanil is terminated by clearance rather than distribution; thus following a prolonged infusion, accumulation is less likely (short context-sensitive half-life). However, in critically ill patients even the clearance of alfentanil can be variable. Remifentanil is an ultra short acting opioid and now it is off patent, and therefore less expensive, it is used increasingly as a sedative in the critical care unit. It has a very short context-sensitive half-life (3–4 min): no residual opioid activity is present within about 10 min of stopping its infusion, regardless of the duration of administration.

Assessment of sedation

It is important to optimise the patient's sedation so that they are calm and pain free and yet sufficiently rousable to co-operate with physiotherapists and nursing staff. A protocolised approach using a sedation scoring system will reduce the risk of over or under sedation. The Richmond Agitation-Sedation Scale (**Table 56**) is generally considered the most valid and reliable sedation assessment tool (aim for score of 0 to –1 in most patients) but the simpler Ramsay Sedation Scale is used more widely:
Awake levels:
1. Patient anxious and agitated or restless, or both.
2. Patient cooperative, orientated and tranquil.
3. Patient responds to commands only.

Table 56 Richmond Agitation-Sedation Scale (RASS)		
Score	Term	Description
+4	Combative	Overtly combative, violent, immediate danger to staff
+3	Very agitated	Pulls or removes tube(s) or catheter(s); aggressive
+2	Agitated	Frequent non-purposeful movement, fights ventilator
+1	Restless	Anxious but movements not aggressive or vigorous
0	Alert and calm	
−1	Drowsy	Not fully alert; has sustained awakening (eye-opening/eye contact) to voice (>10 s)
−2	Light sedation	Briefly awakens with eye contact to voice (<10 s)
−3	Moderate sedation	Movement or eye opening to voice (but no eye contact)
−4	Deep sedation	No response to voice, but movement or eye opening to physical stimulation
−5	Unrousable	No response to voice or physical stimulation

Asleep levels dependent on response to glabellar tap or loud auditory stimulus:

4. Brisk response.
5. Sluggish response.
6. No response.

Levels 2–4 are appropriate for most patients. The level of sedation must be assessed regularly, particularly when the sedatives are given by infusion. Physical methods of measuring sedation have been described. Most are used primarily for assessing depth of anaesthesia and many are based on electroencephalography (e.g. Bispectral Index). None of these systems are in routine clinical use.

Further reading

Barr J, Fraser GL, Puntillo K, et al. Clinical practice guidelines for the management of pain, agitation, and delirium in adult patients in the intensive care unit. Crit Care Med 2013; 41:263–306.

Mehta S, Burry L, Cook D, et al. Daily sedation interruption in mechanically ventilated critically ill patients cared for with a sedation protocol: a randomized controlled trial. J Am Med Assoc 2012; 308:1985–1992.

Kress JP. Pohlman AS, O'Connor MF, Hall JB. Daily interruption of sedative infusions in critically ill patients undergoing mechanical ventilation. N Engl J Med 2000; 342:1471–1477.

Jakob SM, Ruokonen E, Grounds RM, et al. Dexmedetomidine vs midazolam vs propofol for sedation during prolonged mechanical ventilation. Two randomized controlled trials. J Am Med Assoc 2012; 307:1151–1160.

Jamadarkhana S, Gopal S. Clinidine in adults as a sedative agent in the intensive care unit. J Anaesthesiol Clin Pharmacol 2010; 26:439–445.

Related topics of interest

Seizures – status epilepticus

Key points

- Emergency treatment of patients with status epilepticus involves closely monitoring airway, respiratory and cardiovascular function
- First line treatment for patients with convulsive status epilepticus is a benzodiazepine (lorazepam or diazepam) followed by phenytoin
- If first line treatment fails, you should transfer the patient to an intensive care unit and give an anaesthetic agent

Epidemiology

Status epilepticus (SE) describes prolonged or repetitive convulsive or non-convulsive seizures that continue without a period of recovery (return of consciousness) between attacks. Traditionally defined as lasting longer than 30 min, more recent suggestion is seizure activity for more than 5 min as self-termination of seizure after this time point is uncommon. SE may arise in known epileptics (epilepsy has a prevalence of 1:200) or in non-epileptic individuals. SE is most common (around 80 cases per 100,000) in those >60 years old. During SE the brain is at risk of secondary injury from hypoxia, hypotension, cerebral oedema and direct neuronal injury. The risk of permanent brain damage and death is proportional to the duration of seizures. Mortality rates of 4–40% are described.

Pathophysiology

- Idiopathic epilepsy (particularly associated with medication non-compliance and changes in medication). This group has a good prognosis
- Infection (meningitis, abscess, encephalitis, malaria, HIV associated toxoplasmosis and lymphoma)
- Head injury
- Intracranial tumour (primary and secondary)
- Cerebrovascular disease (haemorrhage, thrombosis, embolism, eclampsia and cerebral vasculitis)
- Drug-induced/overdose (local anaesthetics, tricyclic antidepressants, theophylline, amphetamines, cocaine, LSD and insulin)
- Drug withdrawal (benzodiazepines and alcohol)
- Metabolic (hypoglycaemia, hyponatraemia, hypocalcaemia, hyperpyrexia, uraemia, hepatic failure, pyridoxine deficiency and porphyria)
- Non-epileptic status (known previously as pseudoepilepsy)

Clinical features

Status epilepticus may present as:
- Generalised tonic-clonic seizures without full neurological recovery between attacks
- Focal epileptic seizures without impaired consciousness
- Non-convulsive seizures with impaired consciousness

Airway compromise: During seizures the airway is compromised and there is risk of aspiration.

Hypoxia is common because of inadequate ventilation combined with high oxygen requirements of continuous muscle activity. Hypercarbia occurs due to increased CO_2 production and reduced ventilation.

Metabolic changes: Hyperthermia, dehydration, acidosis, rhabdomyolysis, hyperkalaemia and, occasionally, renal impairment are caused by excessive muscle activity. Hypo- or hyperglycaemia can occur, both of which may result in secondary brain injury.

Cerebral consequences: Brain oedema may occur due to increased cerebral blood flow, hypercapnia, impaired venous drainage (position and raised venous pressure). Hypertension is common and may further add to cerebral oedema. Hypotension will usually signify hypovolaemia.

Investigations and diagnosis

- Blood biochemistry (glucose, sodium, calcium, magnesium, phosphate and liver function)
- Arterial blood gas
- Drug screen for suspected drugs
- Urinalysis
- Anticonvulsant drug levels
- Brain CT or MRI to identify structural brain lesions
- Lumbar puncture (contraindicated if raised ICP or space-occupying lesion suspected)
- ECG and echocardiography to exclude cardiac embolism
- EEG is required in all patients presenting with epilepsy. It will differentiate secondary generalised (focal seizures) from primary generalised seizures. It will occasionally detect sub-clinical epileptic activity in the absence of external signs of convulsions

Treatment

Management of SE should follow ABC priorities. Specific therapy should be directed to the underlying problem. Tracheal intubation may be required to enable airway protection in those who remain deeply comatose for a prolonged period. Ensure adequate ventilation, avoid excessive hyperventilation and maintain adequate circulating volume. Avoid hypotonic solutions, which will increase cerebral oedema. Correct hypoglycaemia and if alcoholism or impaired nutrition is suspected, give thiamine i.v.

Choice of anticonvulsant

1. **Status epilepticus (grand mal)**
- Initial (early) SE: Give lorazepam 4 mg i.v. over 2 min; this can be repeated after 15 min if seizures persist. Lorazepam is more effective than diazepam as therapeutic levels persist in the brain for a longer period (up to 24 h). Clonazepam 1 mg IV and repeated if needed is an alternative. When intravenous access is unavailable buccal midazolam 5–10 mg is an option or rectal administration of diazepam will provide peak serum concentrations within 10–30 min.
- Established SE: If seizures persist despite lorazepam, give phenytoin 15–18 mg kg^{-1} i.v. at 50 mg min^{-1}. Alternatively, give fosphenytoin 15–20 mg phenytoin equivalent (PE) kg^{-1}. Fosphenytoin is a pro-drug of phenytoin and is less likely to cause hypotension, arrhythmias and phlebitis. Phenobarbital may also be used in addition or as an alternative: bolus of 10–15 mg kg^{-1} at a rate of 100 mg min^{-1}
- Refractory SE. If seizures persist 20 min after giving phenytoin, induce general anaesthesia with propofol or thiopental
2. **Tonic-clonic (grand mal):** Drug options include sodium valproate, carbamazepine, phenytoin or thiopental.
3. **Partial (focal)**
- Psychomotor: Carbamazepine and phenytoin
- Absence (petit mal): Sodium valproate and ethosuxamide
- Myoclonic: Clonazepam and sodium valproate

Gabapentin, lamotrigine or vigabatrin may be added when control is difficult.

There is little data on the newer agents, e.g. leviteracetam. Check and correct anticonvulsant levels in known epileptics. Manage cerebral oedema with measures including optimal head and neck positioning, adequate oxygenation, avoidance of hypotension, sedation, strict temperature control, controlled hyperventilation and osmotic diuretics. Consider steroids for those with a known tumour, arteritis or parasitic infections. Consider surgery for space-occupying lesions (e.g. haemorrhage, abscess or tumour). Correct any hyperthermia. Maintain a brisk diuresis if there is any evidence of rhabdomyolysis. There is no role for long-acting muscle relaxants purely to control seizures. Continuing seizure activity implies inadequate anti-convulsant levels. Occasionally, paralysis may be required to facilitate ventilation if there is associated severe lung injury or for the control of ICP. If neuromuscular blockade is used, continuous EEG monitoring is mandatory to assess seizure activity.

Non-convulsive status

Outcome from SE is directly related to the duration of seizures, the incidence of secondary brain injury and the underlying pathology. SE will eventually burn itself out with resultant irreversible brain damage. Overt seizure activity may be markedly reduced or clinically absent but EEG will demonstrate continued seizure activity. The prognosis in this situation is extremely poor; anticonvulsant therapy must be used aggressively to avoid reaching this situation. Regardless of the initiating stimulus, status appears to enter a stage where seizures are perpetuated by excess excitatory amino acids, primarily glutamate. Ketamine, which has excitatory amino acid blocking activity, has been suggested as potentially useful in this situation but clear evidence to support its use is lacking. The importance of continuous EEG to enable continuous monitoring of SE is clear.

Non-epileptic status

Non-epileptic status (pseudoepilepsy) is a diagnosis of exclusion. Simulated seizures may be differentiated from true epilepsy by features such as atypical movements (e.g. asynchronous limb and rolling movements), the presence of eye lash reflexes, resistance to eye opening, normal pupil responses during convulsion, retained awareness or vocalisation and normal tendon reflexes and plantar responses immediately after convulsion. They may be brought on by approaching the patient, are often recurrent and are seen in individuals who have some knowledge of what epilepsy looks like (health care workers or relatives of epileptics). Non-epileptic status is more common in females with a history of psychological disturbance. Occasionally, the diagnosis will become clear only on EEG monitoring.

Further reading

Neligan A, Shorvon SD. Frequency and prognosis of convulsive status epilepticus of different causes: a systematic review. Arch Neurol 2010; 67:931–940.

Costello D, Cole A. Treatment of acute seizures and status epilepticus. J Intensive Care Med 2007; 22:319–347.

Walker M. Status epilepticus: An evidence-based guide. Br Med J 2005; 331:673–677.

National Institute for Health and Clinical Excellence (NICE). The epilepsies: the diagnosis and management of the epilepsies in adults and children in primary and secondary care, Clinical Guideline 137. London: NICE, 2012.

Related topics of interest

- Coma (p 116)
- Meningitis and encephalitis (p 217)

Selective oropharyngeal and digestive tract decontamination

Key points

- Selective oropharyngeal decontamination (SOD) and selective digestive tract decontamination (SDD) are strategies to reduce secondary infection in critically ill patients
- SOD/SDD comprises four key components: oral and local application of non-absorbable antibiotics, systemic antibiotics, optimal hygiene practice and surveillance of efficacy
- Evidence for the impact of SOD/SDD on patient outcome is conflicting and uptake is minimal because of concern about generating resistant pathogens

Introduction

Selective oropharyngeal decontamination (SOD) and selective digestive tract decontamination (SDD) are used to prevent potential infection in mechanically ventilated patients. Treatment includes non-absorbable antimicrobial agents in the oropharynx and gastrointestinal tract and short-term intravenous antibiotics. SOD uses topical therapy alone whereas SDD includes intravenous drugs.

Rationale

The normal flora of any healthy individual includes six potential pathogens: *Streptococcus pneumoniae, Haemophilus influenzae, Moraxella catarrhalis* in the throat; *Escherichia coli* in the gut; and *Staphylococcus aureus* and *Candida albicans* in both the throat and gut.

There are nine 'abnormal' bacteria that are carried by individuals with underlying disease. Of these, eight are aerobic Gram-negative bacilli (AGNB): *Klebsiella, Enterobacter, Citrobacter, Proteus, Morganella, Serratia, Acinetobacter* and *Pseudomonas*; and one is methicillin-resistant *Staphylococcus aureus* (MRSA).

In critical illness, a patient's normal flora is replaced partly by abnormal flora. Organism growth is also more rapid than normal leading to high grade carriage of both normal and abnormal flora. The increased numbers of colonising organisms predispose the patient to infection.

- Primary endogenous infection: these infections occur within the first week of the intensive care unit (ICU) stay, and are the result of colonisation and overgrowth of normal or abnormal pathogens that were part of the patient's flora on admission to the ICU
- Secondary endogenous infection: these infections are caused by pathogens that were not part of the patient's flora on admission to ICU but instead are acquired during their stay in hospital or on the ICU. Colonisation and overgrowth of the pathogen occurs in the oropharynx and gut leading to the infection. These infections usually occur after the first week on ICU
- Exogenous infection occurs when pathogens acquired on the ICU or elsewhere are directly introduced into a previously sterile organ. These infections can develop at any time during the ICU stay
- Hospital acquired infections can be due to both endogenous and exogenous sources of pathogens

Critical illness affects native flora promoting overgrowth and an increase in more abnormal organisms. Gut overgrowth is the putative mechanism preceding primary and secondary endogenous infection, and is a risk factor for the development of resistance. Clinically significant gut overgrowth is defined as $\geq 10^5$ potential pathogens (including normal bacteria, yeasts and abnormal AGNB) per mL of gastrointestinal secretion. Reducing or eliminating these organisms may prevent endotoxin translocation and infection. Thus, the aim is to prevent secondary colonisation by any potentially pathogenic commensals (whether part of the patient's flora or acquired) and maintain normal intestinal flora.

This is achieved by use of high-concentration topical and systemic anti-microbials effective against normal and abnormal pathogens. Primary endogenous infections are treated with intravenous antibiotics, secondary endogenous infections are treated with the local application of enteral antibiotics, and exogenous infections are controlled with hygiene measures.

Method

There are four components to SOD/SDD therapy:

1. Selective eradication of the oropharynx and gut, which aims to reduce secondary endogenous and exogenous infection:
   - Application of non-absorbable antibiotics (polymyxin E, tobramycin and amphotericin B) in the form of a gel, paste or lozenge to the mouth
   - Gut decontamination with the same antibiotics administered as a suspension via a nasogastric tube
     The oral paste is used to prevent gut overgrowth of abnormal AGNB. If methicillin-resistant staphylococcal cover is required, enteral vancomycin is added. Amphotericin B or nystatin address fungal overgrowth. In practice, it is difficult to get antibiotics made up specifically and the paste is difficult to administer and smear adequately.
2. Systemic prophylactic antibiotics which aim to control primary endogenous infection:
   - High-dose parenteral cefotaxime for four days from time of admission
     Cefotaxime is used as its spectrum covers both normal and most abnormal bacteria.
3. High standards of hygiene to prevent cross-contamination, secondary endogenous and exogenous infection including hand-washing, apron use at the bedside, strict asepsis technique with any procedures and surgery, high nurse-patient ratio and use of cubicles.
4. Regular surveillance cultures of throat and rectal swabs to monitor efficacy of SOD/

SDD therapy. Surveillance sampling of the throat and gut is the only method of detecting overgrowth.

SOD uses oropharyngeal topical application of the mouth paste only. SDD involves oropharyngeal and gut decontamination with the topical antibiotic mixture as well as systemic cefotaxime.

Evidence

The use of SOD/SDD is very controversial.

A current review of all randomised controlled trials and meta-analyses demonstrated that SOD/SDD reduces the incidence of lower airways infection (by 72%), blood stream infection (by 37%) and mortality (by 29%) with minimal emergence of resistance or increased detection of *Clostridium difficile* toxin.

However, there is conflicting evidence about resistance. Some studies show that SDD is associated with less resistance compared with conventional systemic antibiotics. Others suggest SDD causes a gradual increase of resistant AGNB in the respiratory tract and a significant increase in the gastrointestinal tract after SDD discontinuation. Effect on mortality rates was not clinically significant.

It is speculated that SDD may promote gut overgrowth of intrinsically resistant bacteria such as MRSA, vancomycin-resistant *Enterococcus* and exert selection pressure on plasmid-mediated extended-spectrum β-lactamases.

Colistin is one of the antibiotics that can be used in SOD/SDD. With the rise in carbapenem-resistant Gram-negative bacilli, the effects of topical colistin use on resistance must be determined before it is implemented routinely.

One study concluded that SOD is as effective as SDD for improving patient outcome, thus questioning the role of intestinal decontamination and systemic cefotaxime.

A formal cost-benefit analysis has not been carried out; however, SOD/SDD appears to be cost-effective, and when analysed per survivor, there is a reduction in costs with

SDD because of the shorter length of ICU stay and reduced use of systemic antibiotics.

The 2012 Surviving Sepsis Campaign guidelines recommend investigation of SOD/SDD as a strategy to reduce the incidence of ventilator-associated pneumonia (VAP).

For critically ill patients with severe sepsis, oropharyngeal decontamination with oral chlorhexidine is recommended to reduce VAP risk; however, antibiotic-based SOD/SDD is not currently recommended.

Further reading

Silvestri L, de la Cal MA, van Saene HK. Selective decontamination of the digestive tract: the mechanism of action is control of gut overgrowth. Intens Care Med 2012; 38:1738–1750.

Oostdjik E, de Smet A, Blok HE, et al. Ecological effects of selective decontamination on resistant Gram-negative bacterial colonization. Am J Respir Crit Care Med 2010; 181:452–457.

de Smet AM, Kluytmans JA, Cooper BS, et al. Decontamination of the digestive tract and oropharynx in ICU patients. N Engl J Med 2009; 360:20–31.

Daneman N, Sarwar S, Fowler RA, Cuthbertson BH. Effect of selective decontamination on antimicrobial resistance in intensive care units: a systematic review and meta-analysis. Lancet Infect Dis 2013; 13:328–341.

Related topics of interest

Sepsis – management

Key points

- Mortality rates associated with septic shock are in the range of 40–70%
- Resuscitation follows the standard airway, breathing and circulation approach
- The 2012 Surviving Sepsis Guidelines detail treatment recommendations

Patients with sepsis and septic shock who require admission to the critical care unit have an extremely high mortality, which may exceed 50%. Timely diagnosis and management is essential. The key steps in the management of sepsis are undertaken simultaneously where possible and comprise:

1. Resuscitation
2. Diagnosis
3. Appropriate antibiotics after culture specimens have been taken
4. Source control
5. General supportive measures to preserve life and limit organ dysfunction

Resuscitation

The standard airway, breathing and circulation approach to resuscitation is undertaken. Bundles of care are defined by the Surviving Sepsis Campaign (**Table 57**).

Airway and breathing

Immediate intubation and ventilation may be necessary where there is airway obstruction, respiratory failure or impaired consciousness. Extreme care is required when intubating a septic patient because induction of anaesthesia may induce profound hypotension and even cardiac arrest. After intubation, a lung-protective ventilation strategy is used.

Circulation

Management of the circulation is often the immediate priority at presentation. Check the heart rate and blood pressure. Perfusion can be impaired in the absence of hypotension and is assessed as follows:

a. Clinical signs, such as capillary refill time or mental confusion.
b. Urine output – measured hourly.
c. Lactate – can be measured by many blood gas analysers from an arterial, venous or capillary blood sample. An elevated lactate may reflect anaerobic metabolism due to inadequate oxygen delivery to the tissues (exacerbated if there is reduced lactate clearance by the liver).
d. Central venous oxygen saturation ($ScvO_2$). A sample is taken from a central venous

---

Table 57 Surviving sepsis campaign bundles

The Surviving Sepsis Campaign* (SSC) proposes two care bundles:

To be completed within 3 h
1. Measure plasma lactate level.
2. Obtain blood cultures prior to administration of antibiotics.
3. Administer broad spectrum antibiotics.
4. Administer 30 mL kg^{-1} crystalloid for hypotension or lactate $\geq$ 4 mmol L^{-1}.

To be completed within 6 h
1. Infuse vasopressors (for hypotension that does not respond to initial fluid resuscitation) to maintain a mean arterial pressure $\geq$ 65 mmHg.
2. In the event of persistent arterial hypotension despite volume resuscitation (septic shock) or initial lactate $\geq$ 4 mmol L^{-1}:
   – Measure central venous pressure (target $\geq$ 8 mmHg).
   – Measure central venous oxygen saturation (target $\geq$ 70%).
3. Re-measure lactate if initial lactate was elevated (target – normalization of lactate).

* SCC: International body that publishes evidence-based recommendations intended to provide guidance for the clinician caring for the patient with severe sepsis and septic shock.

catheter (CVC) and evaluated in a blood gas analyser. Some types of CVC can measure oxygen saturations *in vivo* utilising spectrophotometry. A low $ScvO_2$ (<70%) reflects inadequate oxygen delivery to the tissues, i.e. oxygen extraction from the capillary blood is higher than normal. Occasionally an extremely high $ScvO_2$ (>90%) is seen in sepsis because of mitochondrial dysfunction resulting in failure of oxygen utilisation at the cellular level (cytopathic hypoxia).

e. Specific devices may be used to assess the adequacy of intravascular volume replacement and cardiac output. There are many modalities available including trans-thoracic echocardiography, pulse contour cardiac output monitoring derived from an arterial catheter, pulmonary arterial catheterisation and the oesophageal Doppler.

In order to effectively manage the circulation as described, early urinary, arterial and often central venous catheterisation is undertaken.

Fluid therapy

The initial management of severe sepsis and septic shock usually requires the administration of a fluid bolus of at least 30 mL kg⁻¹. Further fluid boluses are guided by objective measures of the adequacy of the circulation.

The choice of intravenous fluid used for resuscitation is contentious. Crystalloids (e.g. normal saline or Ringer's lactate solution), artificial colloids (gelatins and hydroxyethyl starches), and human albumin solution have been used to a variable extent in different centres and in different countries. Recent trials have cast doubts on the safety of starch solutions in sepsis, particularly with respect to worsening of renal function and, in one high-quality study, increased 90-day mortality. As a result of these studies, hydroxyethyl starch products were withdrawn in the United Kingdom (UK) in June 2013. There is some evidence that gelatin solutions may also cause renal injury and, in the absence of clear benefit, many clinicians avoid them in patients with sepsis. Some recent analyses suggest improved mortality

with albumin compared with other fluids in sepsis. The 2012 Surviving Sepsis Guidelines recommend that crystalloids be used as the initial fluid of choice in the resuscitation of severe sepsis and septic shock (strong recommendation). These guidelines also suggest 'the use of albumin in the fluid resuscitation of severe sepsis and septic shock when patients require substantial amounts of crystalloids' (weak recommendation); however, 'substantial amounts' of crystalloid are not defined. Recent clinical guidelines published by the National Institute for Health and Care Excellence also advocate crystalloid fluid resuscitation in septic patients, supplemented, if necessary, with albumin.

In the absence of impaired tissue perfusion, maintain a haemoglobin concentration of 7–9 g dL⁻¹. Blood transfusion to a haemoglobin value of 10 g dL⁻¹ has been advocated by one group, which showed improved outcome in a cohort of patients with septic shock treated with an early goal-directed therapy protocol; however, blood transfusion was only one of several therapies given to the treatment group in this trial and further larger studies are ongoing.

Vasoactive drugs

Once the circulating volume has been restored, if inadequate perfusion persists, a vasoactive drug infusion will be necessary. In the presence of an adequate cardiac output and vasodilation, a vasopressor such as noradrenaline is indicated with adrenaline used occasionally as a second line therapy. Where myocardial contractility is impaired, intense vasoconstriction may further reduce cardiac output and oxygen delivery. In this case, use a positive inotrope such as dobutamine or levosimendan. Plasma vasopressin concentration is reduced in sepsis and replacement results in vasoconstriction and reduces noradrenaline requirements. The exact place and dosing regimen of vasopressin in the management of sepsis has yet to be established.

When a patient presents *in extremis* with profound hypotension, it may be necessary to give a vasoactive drug before an adequate circulating volume has been restored. Maintenance of blood pressure with vasopressors, thereby compensating for significant hypovolaemia will cause further organ dysfunction and should be continued only very briefly.

Diagnosis

Undertake a thorough history and examination, looking for symptoms (e.g. rigors or productive cough) and signs (e.g. pyrexia or rash) that may suggest the presence of sepsis and the likely primary site of infection. Target investigations such as laboratory tests and radiological imaging to give further information on the site of infection. Inflammatory markers such as white cell count and C-reactive protein (CRP), whilst fairly widely available, cannot be relied upon to distinguish sepsis from the systemic inflammatory response (SIRS) with a non-infective aetiology. As well as aiding the initial diagnosis of sepsis, CRP may have a role in assessing resolution of infection or failure of therapy by following trends in levels. Procalcitonin and various other biomarkers currently under investigation are purported to be more specific for sepsis than SIRS; however, the place of these is still debated and the gold standard investigation has yet to be found.

Samples for microbiological culture are taken from all potential sites of infection before antibiotic administration when possible, including sputum, urine, CSF and pus depending on the clinical presentation. Blood cultures are taken with strict attention to aseptic technique as contaminants can erroneously influence management.

Antibiotics

Delays between presentation and administration of antibiotics in sepsis will increase mortality. Give antibiotics immediately after cultures have been taken, within one hour of presentation. The general principle is to initiate therapy with broad-spectrum agents chosen depending on the likely site of infection, local antibiotic sensitivity patterns, tissue penetration and patient factors such as renal dysfunction. The likely organisms may differ between immunocompetent patients and immunocompromised individuals where opportunistic and fungal infections should be borne in mind. The results of cultures will enable narrowing of the spectrum of antibiotic therapy, thereby reducing the selection of drug-resistant species such as MRSA and *Clostridium difficile*. Discuss all cases of sepsis regularly with a microbiologist.

Source control

Where the source of infection is known or suspected, control it as soon as possible, for instance removal of an infected central venous catheter, drainage of an empyema or in the case of intra-abdominal sepsis, laparotomy to enable washout of infected material and prevent further contamination.

General supportive measures

Having performed initial resuscitation, routine ICU management is continued to preserve organ function and limit further damage such as a lung protective ventilatory strategy and enteral nutrition.

The role of corticosteroids

Addisonian crises are not a common feature of the multiple organ dysfunction syndrome associated with sepsis; however, relative adrenal insufficiency may develop and is associated with a worse outcome. For many years, corticosteroids have been used to treat this insufficiency and to reduce the excessive inflammatory response associated with sepsis. High-dose steroids, commonly used in the 1970s and 1980s (e.g. methyl prednisolone 30 mg kg^{-1}) worsen outcome overall in sepsis, despite earlier resolution of shock, and are not used. Several more recent trials have resulted in a resurgence of the use of steroids in lower doses (around 200 mg day^{-1} of intravenous hydrocortisone). There is reasonable evidence of a reduction in the use of vasopressors but mortality is unchanged. Steroids in these doses are given to patients in many critical care units with septic shock where arterial pressure does not improve despite adequate fluids and moderate to high dose vasopressors (e.g. noradrenaline ≥ 0.25 mcg kg^{-1} min^{-1}). Do not use an ACTH stimulation (Synacthen) test to assess adrenocortical response because it is difficult to interpret in this setting. Steroid therapy is usually tapered rapidly once vasopressor therapy has been stopped.

Other therapies

Sepsis is thought to result from an imbalance in the pro-inflammatory, anti-inflammatory and coagulation systems; attempts have been made to influence these and many other parts of the inflammatory response. Agents have been trialled to neutralise endotoxin, reduce inflammatory mediator concentrations and antagonise their effects. The naturally occurring anticoagulants, activated protein C and antithrombin, showed initial promise as therapies. Attempts have been made to reduce production and effects of the vasodilator nitric oxide (e.g. nitric oxide synthase inhibitors). Anti-oxidants and non-steroidal anti-inflammatory drugs have been studied. None of these treatments have shown benefit in large trials and some have shown harm; the search for the magic bullet for sepsis continues.

Further reading

Russell JA. Management of sepsis. N Engl J Med 2006; 355:1699–1713.

Mackenzie I, Lever A. Management of sepsis. Br Med J 2007; 335:929–932.

Angus DC, van der Poll T. Severe sepsis and septic shock. N Engl J Med 2013; 369:840–851.

Dellinger RP, Levy MM, Rhodes A, et al. Surviving Sepsis Campaign: International Guidelines for Management of Severe Sepsis and Septic Shock. Crit Care Med 2013; 41:580–637.

The surviving sepsis campaign. http://www.survivingsepsis.org/Pages/default.aspx.

Related topics of interest

Sepsis – pathophysiology

Key points

- Sepsis is the systemic inflammatory response syndrome caused by infection
- The infective trigger is recognised by the innate immune system, which then results in the production of inflammatory mediators
- The compensatory anti-inflammatory response syndrome exists to minimise the systemic effects of local inflammation
- There is considerable inter-individual variation in response to infection and outcome from sepsis – genetic polymorphisms are partly responsible for this variation

Introduction

Sepsis exists when there is a systemic inflammatory response to infection. The clinical presentation can vary considerably depending on the site of infection, the infecting organism and the host response to the invading micro-organism. The symptoms and signs can be precisely mimicked by non-infective causes [the systemic inflammatory response syndrome (SIRS)], such as sterile acute pancreatitis, and the pathophysiology may be identical with the exception that the trigger is not microbial.

The inflammatory cascade combat infections of the host by:

1. Recognising a trigger, i.e. some component of the invading organism.
2. Signalling to attract various parts of the body's immune system, such as neutrophils, to kill the invading organisms and remove damaged or non-host material.
3. The process is then shut down to confine the response to the area of injury and prevent widespread damage to the host.

When this response becomes excessive, causing a generalised rather than localised response, there may be cellular hypoxia, damage to distant host tissues and organ dysfunction, and occasionally death.

Trigger

Inflammation requires a trigger, which may be infective or non-infective (in the case of SIRS rather than sepsis). Infective triggers include endotoxin (lipopolysaccharide) from Gram-negative bacterial cell membranes, components of Gram-positive cell walls (e.g. peptidoglycans and lipoteichoic acid), toxins such as toxic shock toxin-1, viral DNA, or fungal antigens.

Recognition

Recognition of the trigger by the host usually involves innate immunity. Numerous types of cell surface receptor such as the family of Toll-like receptors or the CD14 receptor on monocytes/macrophages recognise broad patterns of antigens such as those listed above. Prior exposure is not necessary to trigger a response (i.e. this defence mechanism against infection exists at birth) and no long-lasting immunity is conferred on the host. This contrasts with the adaptive immune system where prior exposure to the antigen is required and a highly specific memory is developed with the aim of preventing re-infection.

Mediator release

Having recognised the trigger, various inflammatory mediators are released from leucocytes, including cytokines [small polypeptides, e.g. tumour necrosis factor (TNF) and interleukins (IL) such as IL-1 and IL-8], platelet activating factor, leukotrienes, thromboxane and prostaglandins. The complement system is activated.

These inflammatory mediators cause polymorphonuclear leucocyte (neutrophil) proliferation (with further mediator release) as well as systemic effects such as increased capillary permeability (causing a protein-rich oedema), fever, raised metabolic rate and catabolism. Inducible nitric oxide synthase causes increased nitric oxide production from the endothelium resulting in vasodilatation.

Neutrophils, under the influence of adhesion molecules, roll along the endothelium, adhere and then migrate into the tissues releasing various toxic substances including reactive oxygen species (e.g. superoxide).

Coagulation is activated and fibrinolysis impaired causing microvascular thrombosis, clotting factor consumption and possibly bleeding.

The compensatory anti-inflammatory response syndrome

Various anti-inflammatory substances are released, designed to counteract the excess pro-inflammatory mediators. These include anti-inflammatory cytokines (e.g. IL-4 and IL-10), soluble TNF receptors, IL-1 receptor antagonist and naturally occurring anti-coagulants (e.g. protein C). In localised infection, this process prevents the systemic effects of inflammation. An inadequate compensatory anti-inflammatory response syndrome (CARS) may explain the excessive systemic inflammation of sepsis.

Both an excessive anti-inflammatory response as well as increased lymphocyte apoptosis (programmed cell death) may result in a degree of sepsis-induced immunosuppression possibly contributing to a second peak in infection rates during a critical illness; for example, ventilator associated pneumonia or catheter-related sepsis.

Cellular hypoxia

There are several mechanisms by which cells become hypoxic as a result of the systemic inflammatory response:

1. **Vasodilation** due to increased nitric oxide production results in relative hypovolaemia and distributive shock. Vasopressin secretion may also be reduced.
2. **Oedema** results from increased capillary permeability and altered capillary hydrostatic pressure leading to a barrier to oxygen diffusion from erythrocyte to the cells and may also cause extrinsic compression of capillaries. This fluid loss from the intravascular compartment, which may account for many litres, may then cause hypovolaemic shock.
3. **Myocardial dysfunction** resulting in a low cardiac output (and in extreme cases cardiogenic shock) may be present in sepsis. Rather than the classical description of these patients all having a high cardiac output, many have impaired contractility including patients with and without prior cardiovascular disease. Circulating myocardial depressant substances are thought to be responsible.
4. **Microvascular thrombosis** due to activation of coagulation and impairment of fibrinolysis may reduce oxygen delivery to the tissues.
5. **Derangements in vasomotor auto-regulation** may cause shunting of blood away from tissue capillary beds.
6. **Mitochondrial dysfunction** may occur such that oxygen utilisation is impaired despite adequate or even supra-normal oxygen delivery, so-called cytopathic hypoxia or 'cryptic shock'.

The end result is anaerobic metabolism, lactic acidosis and cellular dysfunction/death. Reperfusion of previously hypoxic tissues can cause further release of damaging reactive oxygen species.

Organ dysfunction

The combination of tissue hypoxia and cellular damage by substances such as reactive oxygen species may precipitate organ dysfunction. The clinical presentation will depend on the organ system involved and the severity of the dysfunction. All organ systems can be affected by the inflammatory response, including:

1. **Cardiovascular:** lactic acidosis and hypotension with either a high or a low cardiac output.
2. **Respiratory:** increased pulmonary capillary permeability results in interstitial and alveolar oedema and acute lung injury or the acute respiratory distress syndrome.
3. **Renal:** acute (usually oliguric) kidney injury.

4. **Hepatic:** deranged liver function tests, cholestasis and impaired clearance of bacteria and endotoxin by the reticulo-endothelial system.
5. **Gastrointestinal:** stress ulceration, failure of enteral nutrition and possibly translocation of endotoxin or intestinal bacteria into the systemic circulation driving the inflammatory response and causing new infections.
6. **Nervous system:** an altered conscious level or delirium is common (the so-called septic encephalopathy which may be contributed to by an impaired blood-brain barrier). A polyneuropathy of peripheral nerves is one of the causes of weakness in critically ill septic patients.
7. **Coagulation:** disseminated intravascular coagulation and thrombocytopenia may result in thrombosis, bleeding or both.

There is considerable inter-individual variation in response to infection and outcome from sepsis. Genetic polymorphisms cause variability in the production of cytokines between individuals. For example, individuals who are homozygous for high production of tumour necrosis factor (TNF), a pro-inflammatory cytokine, have a higher mortality from sepsis than heterozygotes who produce less TNF. There is also considerable differences in the severity of illness caused by different species of the same family of micro-organism, e.g. infection with staphylococci or streptococci producing the 'superantigen' toxic shock syndrome toxin cause more severe illness than those which do not.

PIRO (predisposing factors, infection, response to the infection and organ dysfunction) is a system for classifying septic patients. It gives a more precise description of the patient and how they are affected by their illness.

The management of sepsis in the intensive care unit revolves around limiting the derangements in homeostasis caused by failing organ systems as well as preventing further damage whilst specific treatments such as antibiotics or surgery eradicate infection.

Further reading

Singh S, Evans TW. Organ dysfunction during sepsis. Intensive Care Med 2006; 32:349–360.

Abraham E, Singer M. Mechanisms of sepsis-induced organ dysfunction. Crit Care Med 2007; 35:2408–2416.

Gentile LF, Cuenca AG, Efron PA, et al. Persistent inflammation and immunosuppression: a common syndrome and new horizon for surgical intensive care. J Trauma Acute Care Surg 2012; 72:1491–1501.

Angus DC, van der Poll T. Severe sepsis and septic shock. N Engl J Med 2013; 369:840–851.

Related topics of interest

- Sepsis and SIRS (p 336)
- Sepsis – management (p 329)

Sepsis and SIRS

Key points

- Sespis causes 20,000 deaths each day worldwide
- Precise definitions, relating to both infection-related and non-infective causes of systemic inflammation, have been agreed internationally
- Causes of the systemic inflammatory response syndrome include infection, trauma, burns, pancreatitis, anaphylaxis, tissue ischaemia, transfusion reactions, drug reactions, cardiopulmonary bypass, fat embolism and the post-cardiac-arrest syndrome

Introduction

The four clinical signs of inflammation as described by Celsus in the 1st century AD comprised: dolor (pain), rubor (redness), calor (heat) and tumor (swelling). Functio Laesa (loss of function) was added later. This localised inflammatory process is a short-term response to a localised insult resulting in eradication of infection (where the cause is infective) and healing of injured tissue, e.g. a boil on the skin or a small cut. Where the inflammatory response is confined to the area of tissue injury it is usually beneficial and the patient is unlikely to require admission to the intensive care unit (ICU). When the inflammatory response is excessive and 'spills over' into the systemic circulation it may become harmful.

Incidence and outcome

Most critically ill patients will exhibit evidence of systemic inflammation sufficient to be classified as having SIRS at some point during their illness. Outcome will vary enormously depending on the cause of inflammation.

Sepsis occurs in 750,000–900,000 patients annually in the United States resulting in 200,000 deaths. In the European Union, the incidence of sepsis is 90 cases per 100,000 population. Globally, sepsis causes 20,000 deaths per day. The Sepsis Occurrence in Acutely Ill Patients study of over 3000 European intensive care admissions documented an incidence of sepsis of 25% at admission and over 35% at some stage during the ICU stay. Mortality in this study was 27% for patients with sepsis and >50% for patients with septic shock.

Definitions

Precise definitions, relating to both infection-related and non-infective causes of systemic inflammation, have been agreed internationally.

1. Infection describes the inflammatory response to the presence of micro-organisms or the invasion of normally sterile host tissue by those organisms.
2. Bacteraemia is the presence of viable bacteria in the blood.
3. The systemic inflammatory response syndrome (SIRS) is diagnosed when the patient has two of the following four abnormalities:
- Temperature > 38 °C or < 36 °C
- Heart rate > 90 beats min^{-1}
- Respiratory rate > 20 breaths min^{-1} or Pa_{CO_2} < 4.3 kPa
- White blood cell count > 12,000 cells mL^{-1} or < 4000 cells mL^{-1} or > 10% immature cells (band forms)
4. Sepsis is SIRS resulting from infection.
5. Severe sepsis is sepsis associated with organ dysfunction, hypoperfusion or hypotension. Perfusion abnormalities may include, but are not limited to, lactic acidosis, oliguria or an acute alteration in mental status.
6. Septic shock is sepsis with hypotension (systolic blood pressure < 90 mmHg or a reduction of > 40 mmHg from baseline) and perfusion abnormalities (see severe sepsis above) or the requirement for vasoactive drugs despite adequate fluid resuscitation in the absence of other causes for hypotension.

7. The multiple organ dysfunction syndrome (MODS) exists when there is altered organ function in an acutely ill patient such that homeostasis cannot be maintained without intervention. While there are no universally agreed definitions of organ dysfunction, there are several organ failure assessment scores (e.g. the Sequential Organ Failure Assessment score or the MODS), which define the severity of organ dysfunction in (cardiovascular, respiratory, renal, hepatic, neurological and coagulation systems).

Causes of SIRS

The causes of SIRS other than infection are numerous and include trauma, burns, pancreatitis, anaphylaxis, tissue ischaemia, transfusion reactions, drug reactions, cardio-pulmonary bypass, fat embolism, the post-cardiac-arrest syndrome and many others. The pathophysiology, clinical features and management will vary depending on the cause but are broadly similar to those of sepsis with the exception of the use of antimicrobial agents.

Further reading

Levy MM, Fink MP, Marshall JC, et al. 2001 SCCM/ ESICM/ ACCP/ ATS/ SIS International sepsis definitions conference. Crit Care Med 2003; 31:1250–1256.

Vincent JL, Sakr Y, Sprung CL, et al. Sepsis in European intensive care units: results of the SOAP study. Crit Care Med 2006; 34:344–353.

Abraham E, Singer M. Mechanisms of sepsis-induced organ dysfunction. Crit Care Med 2007; 35:2408–2416.

Related topics of interest

Sickle cell disease

Key points

- Sickle cell disease is an autosomal recessive inherited haemoglobinopathy characterised by a mutation on chromosome 11 resulting in the production of haemoglobin S
- Sickle cell anaemia is characterised by vaso-occlusive, aplastic and sequestration crises, hyposplenism and haemolytic anaemia
- Treatment is mainly supportive with prevention of sickling and the use of top-up or exchange transfusions if necessary

Epidemiology

Sickle cell disease represents a group of inherited haemoglobinopathies endemic in Africa, Mediterranean countries, the Middle East and India. It is thought that over 10,000 people have sickle cell disease in the United Kingdom.

Pathophysiology

Sickle cell disease is due to a mutation on chromosome 11, resulting in a substitution of valine for glutamic acid in position 6 of the β haemoglobin (Hb) chain forming HbS. It is inherited with an autosomal recessive pattern and distribution between the sexes is equal. Patients may present with a homozygous state (HbSS, sickle cell anaemia), heterozygous state (HbSA, sickle cell trait), or a combination state with another haemoglobinopathy such as thalassaemia (HbS/β-thal) or Haemoglobin C (HbSC disease). Desaturation causes polymerisation of the insoluble HbS chains forming aggregates called tactoids inside the red blood cell, distorting its contour into a rigid sickle shape. These abnormal cells result in erythrostasis, microvascular occlusion, thrombosis and tissue infarction in one or more organ systems – classical sickle crises. Sickling is initially reversible, however once potassium and water are lost from the cell it becomes irreversible. Homozygous (HbSS) cells sickle at an oxygen saturation of about 85% (Pao_2 5.2–6.5 kPa) whereas heterozygous cells (HbSA) tend to sickle at saturations lower than that of venous blood, i.e. below 40% (Pao_2 3.2–4.0 kPa).

Clinical features

The clinical features depend on the type of sickle cell disease and the degree and distribution of sickling.

Sickle cell trait is associated with some protection against falciparum malaria, patients generally have a normal life expectancy, have mild or no anaemia, and rarely sickle under normal conditions, although care is needed with flying and under anaesthesia. There is however an increased risk of pulmonary infarcts.

Sickle cell anaemia becomes apparent after 3–4 months of age when there is a change from fetal (HbF) to adult haemoglobin (HbA). Patients are universally anaemic. The most common manifestations of sickle cell anaemia are vaso-occlusive crises which may present as an acute abdomen (visceral sequestration), acute chest syndrome (pneumonia-like with dyspnoea, cough, haemoptysis and pleuritic pain secondary to recurrent pulmonary infarctions), stroke, priapism, dactylitis or long bone ischaemia and aseptic necrosis. Acute chest syndrome is the most common cause for sickle cell anaemia patients to be admitted to critical care.

'Sequestration crises' occur mainly in children, with sudden pooling of erythrocytes within the spleen resulting in worsening of anaemia and hypotension. This may be fatal without transfusion. By adulthood, most patients have small atrophied spleens ('auto-splenectomy') from recurrent splenic sequestration crises and they therefore require prophylactic antibiotics and immunisation in the same way as any other asplenic patient.

Aplastic crises are characterised by a shutdown of erythropoiesis in the bone marrow caused by infection with parvovirus 19 or folate deficiency.

There may be skeletal and soft tissue

deformities from marrow hyperplasia and hypertrophy of extra-splenic lymphoid tissue. Frontal bossing and a prominent maxilla may make intubation challenging and enlarged adenoids and tonsils predispose to obstructive sleep apnoea.

Investigations

A 'Sickledex' test is simply a screening tool using de-oxygenation of blood with metabisulphite to look for HbS sickling. It will be positive in both sickle cell anaemia and sickle cell trait. In sickle cell trait however, the haemoglobin level and blood film will be normal.

In sickle cell anaemia, the haemoglobin is usually 60–90 gL^{-1} with increased reticulocytes. A blood film will show sickling, target cells and Howell-Jolly bodies (with splenic atrophy). There may be a reactive leucocytosis and thrombocytosis.

The gold standard investigation is Hb electrophoresis which will not only differentiate between HbA, HbS, HbC and thalassaemia, but also give the relative proportions of each haemoglobin. This is particularly relevant in crises where treatment aims at keeping the HbS level <30%.

Investigations during a crisis should be directed at the organ system in question, but routinely include chest X-ray, ECG with or without an echocardiogram, blood cultures, urine dipstick and MSU. The focus should be on discovering any sources of sepsis (a common precipitant for crises) and on detecting complications, e.g. lung infarction or myocardial ischaemia. Abdominal ultrasound or computed tomography (CT) scan may be of value in the patient presenting with abdominal pain in order to exclude other pathologies.

Diagnosis

Prenatal diagnosis is offered to susceptible families and in the United Kingdom, there is routine neonatal screening. Screening in the emergency situation can be with the Sickledex test; however, Hb electrophoresis is the diagnostic tool of choice.

Treatment

Patients with sickle cell disease are often well known to their local haematology department and there should be close liaison between hospital teams to optimise management. Patients are managed by a multidisciplinary team and receive lifestyle advice as well as routine prophylactic antibiotics, vaccinations and folic acid supplements. Hydroxycarbamide (hydroxyurea) may be used to increase levels of HbF and reduce the frequency of crises; however, it is associated with myelosuppression and may need to be discontinued with acute illness.

At the present time, there is no cure for sickle cell disease except bone marrow transplantation which carries a significant mortality. Therefore, the management consists of prophylaxis, support and treatment of complications.

Avoidance of sickling is the main aim when a patient with sickle cell anaemia or sickle cell trait presents for surgery. This is achieved by keeping patients hydrated, well-oxygenated, normothermic and pain free prior, during and after the surgery. Consideration should be given to transfusing the patient to an Hb of approximately 100 gL^{-1} to optimise their haematocrit and minimise their HbS levels prior to surgery. This may also be achievable by hydroxycarbamide if time permits. Tourniquets should be used with caution and the limb meticulously exsanguinated. Critical care admission for post-operative care is advisable in all sickle cell anaemia patients undergoing moderate or major surgical procedures. Non-invasive ventilation has been used successfully to aid oxygenation and reduce the risk of acute chest crises.

Vaso-occlusive crises are treated with rest, intravenous (IV) hydration, analgesia, oxygen and broad-spectrum antibiotics for any infection. Morphine is frequently required to manage the associated severe pain.

Aplastic or sequestration crises require transfusion, aiming to raise the haemoglobin by 20–30 gL^{-1} to alleviate symptoms. Exchange transfusion may be required for patients with stroke, acute hepatic sequestration, acute chest syndrome or multi-organ failure.

Complications

Cholelithiasis is common as with other causes of haemolytic anaemia, and is often a reason for surgery. Chronic anaemia and microinfarcts may lead to an ischaemic cardiomyopathy. Long-standing and recurrent pulmonary infarctions cause pulmonary hypertension which has an extremely high mortality. Micro-infarction of the renal vasculature results in a loss of concentrating ability, proteinuria and end-stage renal failure in some patients. Sickle cell disease patients are prothrombotic and should receive appropriate thromboprophylaxis while in hospital.

Further reading

Wilson M, Forsyth P, Whiteside J. Haemoglobinopathy and sickle cell disease. Contin Educ Anaesth Crit Care Pain. 2010; 10:24–28.

Hoffbrand AV, Moss PAH. Essential Haematology, 6th edn. Chichester: Wiley-Blackwell, 2011:99–104.

Kumar P, Clark M. Clinical Medicine, 8th edn. London: Saunders Elsevier 2012:392–395

Related topics of interest

- Analgesia in critical care – advanced (p 28)
- Blood and blood products (p 51)
- Hypothermia (p 186)

Skin and soft tissue infections

Key points

- Necrotising fasciitis is a lethal, progressive soft tissue infection that spreads rapidly
- Pain disproportionate to other symptoms and signs is the clinical feature that can differentiate necrotising fasciitis from cellulitis
- Early effective surgical debridement of necrotising fasciitis reduces mortality

Epidemiology

Skin and soft tissue infections are common but fulminant infections requiring admission to critical care are relatively rare. The incidence of necrotising fasciitis in the United Kingdom is approximately 500 cases per year.

Pathophysiology

The skin is colonised by bacteria and acts as a barrier to infection. Factors that predispose to infection include trauma and disruption of anatomical integrity, ischaemia, immunocompromise or the presence of virulent colonising bacteria. Pre-existing conditions that increase the risk include diabetes mellitus, hepatic cirrhosis, malnutrition, renal failure, steroid use, vascular disease, malignancy and advanced age.

Impetigo is a superficial infection caused by group A streptococci or *Staphylococcus aureus*.

Erysipelas is a superficial dermal infection, typically caused by beta-haemolytic Streptococci.

Cellulitis is an infection extending below the superficial fascia; it is most commonly caused by beta-haemolytic streptococci (groups A, B, C, G and F) but can be caused by other Gram-positive and negative organisms. Cellulitis presenting with necrosis includes anaerobic infections with *Clostridium* or non-clostridial anaerobes and may be mixed with Gram-negative species.

Necrotising fasciitis is a deeper infection differentiated from cellulitis by the origin of the infection. In cellulitis, infection begins at the junction of superficial fascia and dermis whereas in necrotising fasciitis it starts at the level of the deep fascia and subcutaneous fat. Infection spreads rapidly through fascial planes causing extensive tissue damage. Rapid spread is helped by the release of enzymes, endotoxins and exotoxins. Interruption of the microcirculation and thrombosis of blood vessels causes local necrosis, overlying skin ischaemia and loss of sensation.

Type I infections are polymicrobial caused by one or more anaerobic species (e.g. *Bacteroides*, *Clostridium* or *Peptostreptococcus*) combined with one or more facultative anaerobic Streptococci and Enterobacteriaceae (e.g. *E coli*, *Enterobacter* or *Proteus*). Type I infections are most common and typically affect the perineum (known as Fournier's gangrene), head and neck or trunk areas of immunocompromised individuals.

Type II infections are caused by group A streptococci sometimes with coexisting *Staphylococcus aureus* infection. Type II infections typically affect the extremities and often occur in healthy individuals.

Type III Gram-negative (typically Vibrio species) and type IV fungal infections are rare.

Clinical features

A systemic inflammatory response may be present with even superficial infections. Erysipelas causes lymphatic blockade and a painful well-demarcated erythematous area. In cellulitis, the borders are less easily defined. Cellulitis tends to feature most commonly on the lower extremities and face. If organisms are gas-producing crepitus may be present, blistering and bullae are rare. Erysipelas has an acute onset of symptoms, cellulitis presents more gradually.

Necrotising fasciitis can occur spontaneously, may follow local trauma and can even arise as a complication of Varicella infection. Severe pain is a key symptom often out of keeping with other features, pain may precede skin changes by up to 48 h. Lymphangitis does not occur in true necrotising fasciitis but may be present in other more superficial necrotising soft tissue infections. Haemorrhagic bullae, crepitus, ulceration and superficial necrosis develop as deeper structures are affected but these are a late feature and may not occur until day 5 or later. Necrotising fasciitis is associated with streptococcal toxic shock syndrome in up to 50% of cases when caused by exotoxin producing streptococci.

Investigations

Radiological imaging can determine the depth and extent of infection. Magnetic resonance imaging is probably the most useful and can identify necrotic, inflamed or oedematous tissue. Ultrasound and computed tomography have been used to demonstrate fasciial thickening and the presence of fluid collections or gas. Imaging may detect infections earlier in their course but should not delay surgical intervention.

Creatine kinase levels can be raised in necrotising fasciitis and hypocalcaemia occurs as a consequence of calcium deposition in necrotic tissue. Other laboratory tests reflect the associated degree of organ dysfunction.

Blood cultures should be taken and are positive in approximately 60% of patients with group A *Streptococcus* related necrotising fasciitis but only 20% of type I necrotising fasciitis. Blood cultures are positive in less than 5% of cases of cellulitis and erisypelas. Samples from debrided tissue and aspirates should be gram-stained and cultured. Histology confirms fasciial involvement but diagnostic changes are usually visible macroscopically.

Scoring systems have been developed to help differentiate between cellulitis and necrotising fasciitis. For example, The Laboratory Risk Indicator for Necrotising Fasciitis score, is a score based on 6 domains: CRP, WBC, haemoglobin, plasma sodium, creatinine and glucose. The greater the degree of abnormality the higher the likelihood of necrotising fasciitis.

Diagnosis

Diagnosis relies on the clinical presentation and findings at surgical exploration. Treatment is indicated before culture results are available. Necrotising fasciitis is notoriously difficult to diagnose and patients are at risk of being diagnosed with cellulitis and managed less aggressively. Close observation of patients with soft tissue infections is key to identify patients whose disease is progressing or not responding as expected.

Findings at surgery that support a diagnosis of necrotising fasciitis include fascial necrosis, myonecrosis, and loss of fascial integrity or adherence to surrounding tissues. There is often a lack of bleeding during dissection and presence of foul 'dishwater' pus.

Treatment

Broad-spectrum empirical antibiotic therapy and for necrotising fasciitis surgical exploration and debridement form the mainstay of treatment. Debridement of infected and necrotic tissue removes the source of infection and toxins and should leave only healthy tissue that can be penetrated by antibiotics. Early surgery improves mortality in necrotising fasciitis and delay or inadequate initial debridement increases mortality. Antibiotic therapy is tailored to culture results but clindamycin is often included to reduce toxin production. Multi-organ failure is a feature of necrotising fasciitis and goal-directed resuscitation needs to occur in parallel to surgical intervention. Intravenous immunoglobulin to bind exotoxins is indicated in critically ill patients with Streptococcal or Staphylococcal necrotising fasciitis. Re-look surgical examination is indicated at regular intervals to debride further necrosis until the process stops.

Complications

Mortality from soft tissue infections depends on the extent and site of tissue involvement, the infecting bacteria and the physiological reserve and co-morbidities of the patient. The rate of progression of necrotising fasciitis can vary from over a few days to rapid deterioration and death within hours of presentation. Necrotising fasciitis has a high mortality reported between 20% and 40%. Reconstructive surgery and rehabilitation should be considered only when infection is fully eradicated. The hospital length of stay averages 33 days for survivors.

Further reading

Sarani B1, Strong M, Pascual J, et al. Necrotizing fasciitis: current concepts and review of the literature. J Am Coll Surg 2009; 208:279–288.

Wong CH1, Khin LW, Heng KS, et al. The LRINEC (Laboratory Risk Indicator for Necrotising Fasciitis) score: a tool for distinguishing fasciitis from other soft tissue infections. Crit Care Med 2004; 32:1535–1541.

Davoudian P, Flint NJ. Necrotizing fasciitis. Contin Educ Anaesth Crit Care Pain 2012; 12:245–250.

Anaya DA, Dellinger EP. Necrotizing soft-tissue infection: diagnosis and management. Clin Infect Dis 2007; 44:705.

Related topics of interest

- Antibiotics, antivirals and antifungals (p 34)
- Sepsis – management (p 329)
- Sepsis – pathophysiology (p 333)

Sodium

Key points

- Hyponatraemia is very common
- Neurological deterioration associated with acute hyponatraemia is a medical emergency and requires partial correction with sodium replacement
- Mortality associated with hypernatraemia can be in excess of 60%

Sodium is the principal extracellular cation. Normal plasma values are in the range 133–145 mmol L^{-1} with a requirement of 1–2 mmol kg^{-1} day^{-1}.

Hyponatraemia

Hyponatraemia is the most common electrolyte abnormality seen in hospitalised patients. It is associated most commonly with increased total body water and sodium, and is compounded by giving hypotonic intravenous (i.v.) fluids.

Pathophysiology

Hyponatraemia may occur in the presence of low, normal or high total body sodium; normal, reduced or increased circulation volume; and may be associated with a low, normal or high serum osmolality. Basic mechanisms involve:

- Shift of water out of cells secondary to osmotic shifts: hyperglycaemia, mannitol and alcohol
- Shift of sodium into cells to maintain electrical neutrality: hypokalaemia
- Excessive water retention:
  - Renal failure
  - Oedematous states: congestive heart failure, nephrotic syndrome, cirrhosis, hypoalbuminaemia – syndrome of inappropriate anti-diuretic hormone (SIADH)
- Excessive water administration: glucose infusions and absorption of irrigation solutions
- Excessive sodium loss: renal and bowel loss
- Translocational hyponatraemia
- Hyperglycaemia: accounts for up to 15% of cases of hyponatraemia; every 5.6 mmol L^{-1} increase in serum glucose causes the serum Na^+ to decrease by 1.6 mmol L^{-1}

Causes of hyponatraemia associated with volume depletion are:

- Renal loss: diuretics, osmotic diuresis (glucose and mannitol), renal tubular acidosis, salt-losing nephropathy and mineralocorticoid deficiency/antagonist
- Non-renal loss: vomiting, diarrhoea, pancreatitis, peritonitis and burns

Causes of hyponatraemia associated with normal or increased circulating volume include:

- Water intoxication: postoperative 5% glucose administration, TURP (transurethral resection of the prostate) syndrome, SIADH and renal failure
- Oedematous states: congestive heart failure, cirrhosis and nephrotic syndrome
- Glucocorticoid deficiency and hypothyroidism

Clinical features of hyponatraemia

The rate of change of serum sodium is more important than the absolute concentration. Symptoms are rare with a serum sodium concentration > 125 mmol L^{-1}.

- Mild: confusion, nausea, cramps and weakness
- Severe (Na^+ value usually < 120 mmol L^{-1}): headache, ataxia, muscle twitching, convulsions, cerebral oedema, coma and respiratory depression

Diagnosis

Assess the patient's urine volume and level of hydration (circulating volume), the nature of any i.v. fluid replacement and recent administration of diuretics. Exclude hyperglycaemia and measure simultaneous urine and plasma osmolalities. The urine osmolality is inappropriately high with SIADH and advanced renal failure. In SIADH, the serum osmolality is <280 mosmol kg^{-1} and the urine osmolality is inappropriately raised (>100 mosmol kg^{-1}, and urine Na^+ >30 mmol L^{-1}). There should also be an absence of renal, thyroid and adrenal disease and no recent diuretic administration. The urine sodium will be increased despite a normal salt and water intake. The signs of SIADH improve with fluid restriction.

Treatment

Follow the ABC priorities and treat the underlying disorder. The rate of correction of the hyponatraemia depends on the underlying condition and the clinical features.

In chronic causes with mild or no symptoms, hyponatraemia should be corrected slowly over a period of days; rapid correction may precipitate osmotic demyelination (previously known as central pontine myelinolysis). There is increased risk of de-myelination in the presence of malnutrition, alcoholism, hypokalaemia and severe burns and in elderly females taking thiazides. Correct chronic hyponatraemia by:

- Stopping all hypotonic fluids
- Fluid restriction
- Giving demeclocycline or lithium (ADH antagonists)
- Giving furosemide

The rate of correction of acute and symptomatic hyponatraemia is more difficult to dictate. The morbidity from acute cerebral oedema is worse in children, females (particularly during menstruation and elderly females on thiazides) and psychiatric patients. Acute hyponatraemia developing over less than 48 h carries a high risk of permanent neurological damage and rapid partial correction of the hyponatraemia is indicated. Depending on the underlying cause, rapid partial correction of hyponatraemia may be accomplished by:

- Stopping all hypotonic fluids
- Hypertonic saline (e.g. 3% sodium chloride solution at 1 mL kg h^{-1})
- Use of diuretics (furosemide is best given by low-dose infusion)
- Frequent measurement of electrolytes with adjustment of therapy

For acute symptomatic hyponatraemia with severe neurological signs, the aim is to increase the serum sodium by 1–2 mmol L^{-1} h until symptoms resolve, but not to exceed an increase of 12 mmol L^{-1} in 24 h. A 4–6 mmol L^{-1} increase in serum sodium over 6 h is sufficient for immediate rescue from severe complications. For chronic symptomatic hyponatraemia or acute hyponatraemia with no neurological signs or when neurological signs have resolved, aim for a correction rate of < 0.4 mmol L^{-1} h^{-1} for the first 24 h and < 0.3 mmol L^{-1} h^{-1} thereafter.

The main causes of morbidity associated with hyponatraemia are cerebral oedema, respiratory failure and hypoxia. The relation and risk of osmotic demyelination associated with rapid correction is unclear. The risks of rapid correction must be weighed against the risk of continued symptomatic hyponatraemia.

Hypernatraemia

Hypernatraemia results from inadequate urine concentration, losses of hypotonic fluids by various routes or from excessive administration of sodium. Patients who are unable to drink have lost their major defence against hypernatraemia. High-risk groups include infants and the elderly and patients on hypertonic infusions and osmotic diuretics.

Pathophysiology

Hypernatraemia may be seen in the context of low, normal or high total body sodium (See **Table 58** for causes of hypernatraemia).

Low total body sodium and hypernatraemia results from loss of both sodium and water, but the water loss is proportionately greater. It is caused by hypotonic fluid loss from the kidney or gut and is accompanied by signs of hypovolaemia.

Increased total body sodium and hypernatraemia usually follows administration of hypertonic sodium-containing solutions.

Normal total body sodium and hypernatraemia is caused by loss of water in greater proportion than sodium. This usually results from renal losses due to central or nephrogenic diabetes insipidus (DI). Initially, euvolaemia is maintained, but uncorrected water loss will lead eventually to severe dehydration and hypovolaemia.

Table 58 Causes of hypernatraemia
Hypotonic fluid loss: • Loop diuretics   • Osmotic diuresis: urea, mannitol, hyperglycaemia   • Renal disease   • Post-obstructive diuresis   • Post-acute tubular necrosis (ATN) diuresis   • GI losses: vomit, diarrhoea, NG losses,
Sodium gain: • Fluids: Hypertonic saline, sodium bicarbonate   • Feed   • Primary hyperaldosteronism   • Cushings disease
Pure water loss: • Insensible losses: skin, respiratory   • Decreased oral intake   • Diabetes insipidus: Cranial and nephrogenic

Diabetes insipidus

DI is caused by impaired reabsorption of water by the kidney. Water reabsorption is regulated by ADH, which is secreted by the posterior pituitary. Cranial DI is caused by lack of ADH production or release, while nephrogenic DI results from renal insensitivity to the effects of circulating ADH.

Causes of cranial DI

- Head injury
- Neurosurgery
- Pituitary tumour (primary: pituitary, craniopharyngioma, pinealoma; secondary: breast)
- Pituitary infiltration (sarcoid, histiocytosis and tuberculosis)
- Meningitis/encephalitis
- Guillain–Barré syndrome
- Raised intracranial pressure
- Drugs (ethanol and phenytoin)
- Idiopathic

Causes of nephrogenic DI

- Drugs (lithium, demeclocycline and amphotericin B)
- Congenital nephrogenic DI
- Chronic renal failure
- Sickle cell disease
- Hypokalaemia
- Hypocalcaemia

Diagnosis

Polyuria (may be >400 mL h^{-1}) in the presence of a raised serum osmolality (>300 mosmol kg^{-1}) is suggestive of DI. The diagnosis is confirmed by measuring urine and plasma osmolalities simultaneously. In DI, the urine osmolality is inappropriately low (<300 mosmol kg^{-1} and often <150 mosmol kg^{-1}) in the presence of an abnormally high serum osmolality. The effects of osmotic and loop diuretics must be excluded.

Psychogenic polydipsia (compulsive water drinking) is differentiated by the presence of a low serum osmolality (<280 mosmol kg^{-1}) with a low urine osmolality and often associated with hyponatraemia.

Clinical features

Signs and symptoms of hypernatraemia are often non-specific and include lethargy, irritability, confusion, nausea and vomiting, muscle twitching, hyper-reflexia and spasticity, seizures and coma.

Treatment

Treatment of DI follows the ABC priorities. Treat the underlying pathology and replace water (usually as 5% i.v. glucose). Vasopressin may be given (caution in coronary artery disease and peripheral vascular disease). Desmopressin has a longer half-life and less vasoconstrictor effect.

In nephrogenic DI, stop the causative drug. Thiazides (e.g. chlortalidone) have a paradoxical antidiuretic effect. Chlorpropamide and carbamazepine may be beneficial.

Morbidity and mortality tend to be higher in acute severe hypernatraemia than in chronic hypernatraemia. Mortality associated with chronic severe hypernatraemia (serum sodium >160 mmol L^{-1}) can be as high as 60%, while acute severe hypernatraemia is associated with mortality rates of up to 75%. Neurological damage is common in those surviving severe hypernatraemia. Correction should be slow (<2 mmol L^{-1} h^{-1} and no more than 10 mmol L^{-1} day^{-1}) to avoid the risk of cerebral oedema.

Further reading

Overgaard-Steensen C. Initial approach to the hyponatremic patient. Acta Anaesthesiol Scand 2011; 55:139–148.
Sterns RH, Hix JK, Silver S. Treatment of hyponatremia. Curr Opin Nephrol Hypertens 2010; 19:493–498.
Kumar S, Berl T. Sodium. Lancet 1998; 352: 220–228.
Reynolds RM, Padfield PL, Seckl JR. Disorders of sodium balance. Br Med J 2006; 332:702–705.

Related topics of interest

Spinal injuries

Key points

- Suspect spinal injury in all trauma victims
- Missed or delayed diagnosis of spinal column injury may lead to a 7.5-fold increase in neurological injury
- Treatment is aimed at minimising secondary damage

Epidemiology

The incidence of spinal cord injuries is 15–40 per million population per year (16 per million in the United Kingdom). Men aged 15-35 years are most commonly affected and 25% of this cohort has alcohol as a contributing factor. Common mechanisms of trauma are motor vehicle crashes (45%), falls (20%), sports injuries (15%) and physical violence (15%) although this varies with country. There is an emerging bimodal age distribution with a second peak in adults over 65 due to falls.

Injury to the cord can be expected in 1–3% of major trauma victims; the risk is approximately 8% if the victim is ejected from a vehicle. Fifty percent of patients with damage to the spinal cord have other injuries. Spinal injury must be suspected in all severely injured patients. The risk of cervical spine injury is 10–15% if the patient is unconscious and injury is due to a fall or motor vehicle crash. Five to ten percent of patients with significant head and facial trauma have associated cervical spine injury.

The majority of spinal injuries (55%) involve the cervical region. In adults, the commonest sites are C_5/C_6 and T_{12}/L_1.

Pathophysiology

Primary neural damage results directly from the initial insult - transection, compression, contusion, shear injury and vascular injury.

Secondary neural injury may be caused by mechanical disruption after failure to immobilise, hypoxia (ventilatory impairment from cord damage or chest trauma), hypotension (hypovolaemia, sympathetic blockade, myocardial dysfunction), oedema, haemorrhage into the cord and hyper/hypoglycaemia.

Clinical features of acute injury

Complete cord injury

In complete cord injury all motor function, sensation and reflexes are lost below the level of the lesion.

The initial injury causes immediate massive sympathetic activity with a sudden rise in systemic vascular resistance and blood pressure. Acute myocardial infarction, cerebrovascular accident or fatal arrhythmias may ensue. All voluntary and reflex activity ceases below the level of the lesion (spinal shock).

Airway

There is increased risk of aspiration due to impaired upper airway reflexes and gastric stasis. Premonitory signs of vomiting may be absent. There may be associated facial trauma, retropharyngeal haemorrhage and oedema.

Breathing

Cord injury above C_3 leads to loss of diaphragmatic function, apnoea and death if artificial ventilation is not commenced. Nerves from T_2-T_{12} innervate the intercostal muscles and patients with cord injury above this level are reliant on diaphragmatic breathing with limited expansion, decreased tidal volumes and impaired cough. Residual volume is increased and the functional residual capacity reduced.

Circulation

Loss of sympathetic vasoconstrictor tone (above T_6) causes neurogenic shock. Cord damage above T_2 disrupts the sympathetic innervation of the heart, causing loss of reflex tachycardia, impaired left ventricular function and the risk of severe bradycardia or asystole following unopposed vagal stimulation.

Neurology

Spinal shock refers to the muscle flaccidity and areflexia that occurs after spinal injury. It may last for 48 h to 9 weeks.

Temperature

Hypothermia may be precipitated by heat loss due to peripheral vasodilatation.

Gastrointestinal tract

Paralytic ileus may last for several days.

Genitourinary

Bladder atony necessitates catheterisation.

Biochemical and endocrine

Increased ADH secretion leads to water retention with a dilutional hyponatraemia. Glucose intolerance may occur. Nasogastric losses may cause a hypokalemic, hypochloraemic metabolic alkalosis. Hypoventilation causes respiratory acidosis.

Thromboembolism

Cord injury is associated with a high incidence of DVT and PE.

Incomplete cord injury

Incomplete cord lesions classically present as four main clinical syndromes:

- Anterior cord syndrome. This is caused by ischaemic damage to the cord following aortic trauma or cross-clamping where blood supply from the anterior spinal artery is disrupted. There is damage to the corticospinal and spinothalamic tracts with paralysis and abnormal touch, pain and temperature sensation. The posterior columns are unaffected; joint position and vibration sense are preserved
- Central cord syndrome. In this syndrome, the central grey matter is damaged. Paralysis with variable sensory loss is greater in the upper limbs than the lower limbs because nerves to the upper limbs are located nearer to the centre of the cord. Bladder dysfunction presents as urinary retention
- Brown-Séquard syndrome. This refers to hemisection of the cord, due usually to penetrating trauma. There is ipsilateral paralysis and loss of vibration and joint position sense with contralateral loss of pain and temperature sensation
- Cauda equina syndrome. This presents with loss of bowel and bladder function with lower motor neurone signs in the legs following a lumbar fracture. Sensory changes are unpredictable

Investigations

Clearing the spine in trauma patients.

All life-threatening haemodynamic and pulmonary problems should be addressed before a prolonged cervical spine evaluation is undertaken.

1. There are validated clinical decision rules regarding imaging of patients not at high risk. These include the National Emergency X-Radiography Utilization Study (NEXUS) Low-risk Criteria (NLC) the Canadian C spine rule.
   NLC state that an X-ray is not needed if the patient meets all five of the following:
   i. Alert
   ii. Not intoxicated
   iii. No posterior midline tenderness
   iv. No distracting pain
   v. No neurological deficits
2. Plain X-ray will suffice if there is no severe mechanism of injury and no neurological deficit. C spine views must be adequate including lateral pictures from occiput to the upper T1 vertebral body, AP view showing the spinous processes of C2 – T1 and an open mouth odontoid view showing the lateral masses of C1 and the entire odontoid process.
3. CT scans of the entire spine should be obtained if
   i. X-ray views are inadequate.
   ii. A fracture has been demonstrated at one level on X-ray.
   iii. There is history of high energy trauma and the patient is not clinically assessable.
   iv. Any neurological signs.
   v. Major trauma having CT imaging to assess head, chest and abdomen.
   vi. Criteria for high risk of cervical spine trauma.

- High speed motor vehicle accident (MVA) >35 mph
- Death at the scene
- Fall >3 m
- Closed head injury
- Neurological signs
- Multiple limb fractures

4. MRI is less sensitive than CT for fractures but will demonstrate soft-tissue and ligamentous injury and give a better indication of the severity of the cord injury. It may also demonstrate vascular injury and spinal cord injury without radiographic abnormality (SCIWORA).

Before removing spinal immobilisation, all imaging should be reviewed by a clinician with expertise in interpreting these studies If the cervical spine X-rays are normal but the patient complains of significant neck pain, flexion and extension views have been advocated but now largely superseded by MRI.

There should be a protocol for clearing the cervical-spine in obtunded patients who are unable to complain of pain or neurologic deficit since prolonged unnecessary immobilization is detrimental, e.g. raised ICP and pressure areas from cervical collars, increased risk of pneumonia from supine position, and increased risk of thromboembolism. Evidence supports that if a helical CT with 1 mm cuts and 3D reconstruction is normal cervical collars may be removed.

Thoracic and lumbar injuries are similarly excluded by examination, X-rays (AP and lateral) and targeted CT and/or MRI.

Diagnosis

Diagnosis is on the basis of clinical examination and imaging. A careful neurological examination with meticulous documentation is essential. It is important to determine the presence of any motor or sensory function below the level of a lesion, since this has important prognostic implications. The patient should be log-rolled to assess for local tenderness and palpable 'step-off' deformity.

Patients may demonstrate diaphragmatic breathing, hypotension without tachycardia if the lesion is above level of cardioaccelerator sympathetic outflow (T_2), areflexia or priapism. A routine PR is no longer advocated.

Treatment

Secondary damage to the cord is reduced by immobilisation, minimising spinal hypoxia and hypoperfusion, and by ensuring the patient is fully resuscitated before transfer to a specialist centre.

Airway with cervical spine control

Manual in-line stabilisation of the neck is maintained until a correctly sized hard collar and lateral support and tape are fitted. Early intubation should be undertaken if consciousness is depressed. Manual in-line stabilisation must be maintained throughout a rapid sequence induction of anaesthesia. Tracheostomy is done for long-term ventilation after any surgery to the cervical spine is completed.

Breathing

The patient is given sufficient oxygen to maintain $Spo_2 > 95\%$ and assisted ventilation instituted as required. Close monitoring of ventilation is essential, as deterioration may occur insidiously over several days. Muscle power is reduced, sputum clearance is poor, and pneumonia is common. Early intubation must be considered since respiratory complications account for the majority of deaths after spinal injury. Suxamethonium must be avoided after the first 24 h for a year following injury since it may precipitate severe hyperkalaemia. Other respiratory problems include neurogenic pulmonary oedema, ARDS and pulmonary emboli. As spinal shock resolves, increasing muscle tone improves ventilation. Vital capacity may increase by 65–80%, enabling the patient to be weaned from mechanical ventilation.

Circulation

An adequate blood pressure must be maintained to perfuse the damaged cord and decrease secondary injury. Most patients will stabilise with fluid loading alone but some may require vasopressors and inotropic support. Hypotension must not be attributed to spinal injury without excluding hypovoaemia due to haemorrhage. Invasive blood pressure and central venous pressure monitoring are usually appropriate. Prolonged postural hypotension may require long-term oral therapies.

Neurology

Initial treatment serves to minimise secondary injury. Methylprednisolone given within 8 h was previously recommended but any small outcome benefit appears to be outweighed by harm (e.g. infection, poor wound healing or acute myopathy) and most centres have abandoned its use.

Patients should be transferred to a specialist centre within 24 h of injury. Limited evidence supports early decompression leading to shorter intensive care and hospital stays.

Only 1% of patients who have no cord function after 24 h will achieve functional recovery. Recovery to a chronic state with abnormal reflex activity occurs over several months. Following the phase of spinal shock, 50–80% of patients with lesions above T_7 will demonstrate episodes of autonomic dysreflexia. Stimulation below the level of the lesion causes a mass spinal sympathetic reflex that would normally be inhibited from above. Patients develop a sudden, marked rise in blood pressure and compensatory severe bradycardia, with flushing and sweating above the level of the lesion. This may be so extreme as to cause seizures, cerebrovascular accidents or cardiac arrest. Triggering factors include distended bladder or bowel, cutaneous irritation from pressure sores and medical procedures. Management is preventive and regional or general anaesthesia may be required to avoid crises precipitated by surgery despite the absence of sensation.

Gastrointestinal tract

Patients require stress ulcer prophylaxis and benefit from early enteral feeding. Percutaneous gastrostomy may be used for long-term feeding if swallowing is inadequate. Bowel management with laxatives is needed.

Genitourinary

Indwelling catheters are required at least initially.

Musculoskeletal

The patient may develop contractures and muscle spasms after resolution of spinal shock. There is chronic loss of bone mass and osteoporosis.

Skin

Meticulous nursing and 2 h turning is needed to prevent pressure sores.

Thromboembolism

Prophylaxis with TED stockings, calf compression devices and s.c. low molecular weight heparin is required for a minimum of 8 weeks.

Psychological

Reactive depression is common and multidisciplinary team support and guidance is essential. Clear advice and honesty are paramount. Support groups will help the family.

Spinal injuries in children

The low incidence of bony spinal injury (0.2% of all paediatric fractures and dislocations) is due to the mobility of the spine in children that can dissipate forces over a larger area. Treatment is similar to adults. Infants and children under 8 years old may require padding placed under the back to achieve the neutral position in which to immobilise the cervical spine.

SCIWORA

There is no obvious injury to the spine in up to 55% of children with complete cord injuries. The upper cervical cord is usually affected where there is greatest mobility. It occurs most commonly in children under 8 years old but detection rates in adults have increased with increased use of MRI.

Further reading

Como JJ, Diaz JJ, Dunham CM, et al. Practice management guidelines for identification of cervical spine injuries following trauma: update from the eastern association for the surgery of trauma practice management guidelines committee. J Trauma 2009; 67:651–659.

Consortium for Spinal Cord Medicine. Early acute management in adults with spinal cord injury: a clinical practice guideline for health-care professionals. J Spinal Cord Med 2008; 31:403–479.

Harrison P, Cairns C. Clearing the cervical spine in the unconscious patient. Contin Educ Anaesth Crit Care Pain 2008; 8:117–120.

Related topics of interest

Stress ulceration prophylaxis

Key points

- Stress ulcers are multiple, superficial, well demarcated and commonly located in the stomach fundus/body. Stress ulcers were once a common cause of death in the critically ill
- Multi-modal prevention has significantly reduced mortality
- Nosocomial pneumonia is a complication of stress ulceration prophylaxis

Epidemiology

The incidence of mucosal injury, identified by endoscopy, is in the range 75–100% within the first 24 h of admission to the intensive care unit (ICU). However, the incidence of overt bleeding without gastric prophylaxis is 2–25%. Mortality of patients with clinically important bleeding is five times higher compared with critically ill patients without bleeding.

Pathophysiology

Stress ulceration or stress-related mucosal damage is distinct from peptic ulceration. Ulcers are superficial, well-demarcated, often multiple, lack surrounding oedema, and are commonly located in the fundus/body of the stomach or the first part of the duodenum.

Prevention of ulcer formation in the healthy stomach relies on a delicate balance between acid production and mucosal defence. Stress ulceration was originally thought to be caused by excessive acid production, which might occur following head injury (Cushing's ulcer) or burns (Curling's ulcer). The exact pathophysiology of stress ulceration formation is not entirely clear but reduced mucosal defence, secondary to local hypoperfusion from sepsis and shock, is thought to be more important in critically ill patients. Reperfusion injury following resuscitation may exacerbate this process.

Clinical features

- Haematemesis
- Melaena
- Decrease in haemoglobin
- Cardiovascular instability ($\uparrow$ pulse rate $\downarrow$ blood pressure)

Investigations

Endoscopy remains the gold standard for identifying upper GI pathology. The finding of occult blood on testing of either gastric aspirate or faecal material produces an unacceptably high incidence of false positive results.

Risk factors

Two main major risks factors for clinically significant bleeding from stress ulceration are:

- Mechanical ventilation for > 48 h
- Coagulopathy (platelets <50, INR >1.5, APTT >2 times upper limit of normal)

Other risk factors have also been described:

- Anticoagulation therapy
- Shock
- Sepsis
- Multi-organ failure, especially renal and hepatic failure
- Multiple trauma
- Burns > third of total body surface area
- Head injury
- Previous history of peptic ulceration/ upper GI bleeding
- Organ transplant recipient

Treatment

- Treat the critical illness
- Nutrition
- Pharmacological prophylaxis

Data on gastric ulceration were collected predominantly in the 1980s to 1990s when it was common practise for critically ill patients to be kept nil by mouth. The decrease in clinically significant bleeds to less than 4% has been put down to better overall ICU care, prophylaxis and enteral feeding.

Nutrition

Animal models have shown that enteral feeding reduces stress-induced mucosal damage. A recent meta-analysis of a subgroup of data in three RCTs suggested that in patients fully enterally fed, pharmacological prophylaxis did not reduce the risk of bleeding any further. Instead mortality was purported to be higher as a consequence of the complications of pharmacological prophylaxis (see below).

Antacids

Antacids decrease the incidence of both microscopic and macroscopic bleeding from the upper GI tract. Aim to keep the pH of the gastric content higher than 4.0. This requires regular measurement of pH by either aspiration of gastric content from a gastric tube or using a pH probe. Antacids must be given frequently (every 2–4 h). They may produce hypermagnesaemia, hyperaluminaemia, alkalosis, hypernatraemia, constipation or diarrhoea. Frequent administration of antacids may represent a large volume load to a non-functioning gut. For these reasons antacids are impractical in the ICU.

H_2-receptor antagonists

These include cimetidine, ranitidine, famotidine and nizatidine. They are as effective as antacids in reducing clinically significant bleeding compared with placebo but are associated with several complications. The most important clinical side effect is the risk of nosocomial pneumonia because of loss of the bacteriocidal effect of gastric acid. This promotes bacterial colonisation of the stomach and subsequently the nasopharynx, and is then followed by aspiration into the trachea. Strategies to reduce the incidence of nosocomial pneumonia include nursing the patient with the head of the bed elevated and the use of sub-glottic suction devices in intubated patients.

Sucralfate

This is the basic aluminium salt of sucrose octasulphate. It is given via a nasogastric tube. It does not raise intra-gastric pH, but polymerises and adheres to damaged ulcerated mucosa. It also binds bile salts and increases mucosal production of mucus and bicarbonate. Sucralfate is less effective than H_2-receptor antagonists in preventing stress ulceration. It may be associated with a lower incidence of nosocomial pneumonia but data are conflicting on this point.

Proton pump inhibitors

Omeprazole is a hydrogen-potassium ATPase receptor antagonist. It binds irreversibly to the gastric parietal cell proton pump, markedly reducing the secretion of hydrogen ions. It may be less effective in fasting patients, but in critically ill patients it maintains the gastric pH above 4.0.

Omeprazole is probably the drug of choice for secondary prevention following a GI bleed. Proton pump inhibitors (PPIs), of which omeprazole is one, reduce the efficacy of platelet inhibition by clopidogrel, potentially increasing the risk of cardiovascular events. PPIs compare favourably with H_2-receptor antagonists in prophylaxis efficacy but have not been tested against placebo.

Misoprostol

It is an analogue of prostaglandin E. Misoprostol inhibits basal and stimulated gastric acid secretions and also increases gastric mucus and bicarbonate production. The role of misoprostol in the prevention of stress ulceration has yet to be established.

Complications

These are similar to those of peptic ulceration and include bleeding, perforation and obstruction. The latter two are rare from stress ulceration.

Complications of management

- Nosocomial pneumonia
- *C. difficile*

In theory, an increase in gastric pH may facilitate proliferation of *C. difficile*, but this is unproven.

Further reading

Marik PE, Vasu T, Hirani A, Pachinburavan M. Stress ulcer prophylaxis in the new millennium: a systematic review and meta-analysis. Crit Care Med 2010; 38:2222–2228.

National Institute for Health and Clinical Excellence (NICE). Acute upper gastrointestinal bleeding: Management, Clinical Guidance CG141. London: NICE, 2012.

Related topics of interest

Stroke

Key points

- Prompt treatment may significantly reduce mortality and morbidity
- Ongoing research and guidelines based on expert opinion have increased the number and type of patients who are considered for thrombolysis after ischaemic stroke
- Decompressive craniectomy is considered under specific circumstances

Epidemiology

Stroke accounts for approximately 11% of all deaths in the United Kingdom and represents an age-adjusted annual death rate of 200 per 100,000 population. The mortality rate following a stroke is 20–25%. Almost a million people in England live with effects of a stroke.

Pathophysiology

Approximately 80–85% of strokes are ischaemic; the remainder are haemorrhagic. Ischaemic causes include:

- Large artery atherosclerosis
- Cardiac embolism
- Small vessel occlusion
- Stroke of other determined aetiology, e.g. arterial dissection, blood disorders, vasculitis
- Stroke of undetermined aetiology

Risk factors for the development of an acute ischaemic stroke (AIS) include hypertension, smoking, alcohol, hyper-cholesterolaemia, obesity, diabetes, sleep apnoea, polycythaemia and atrial fibrillation. Prevention or treatment of these risk factors will reduce the likelihood of an AIS.

Clinical features

The clinical presentation depends on the site of ischaemia or infarction. The most common presentation follows an infarction in the internal capsule caused by an occlusion of a branch of the middle cerebral artery (MCA). This causes weakness on the contralateral side to the infarct, which may progress to hemiparesis or hemiplegia and facial weakness. Aphasia may occur if the dominant hemisphere is affected. Seizures and headaches are uncommon. Initially, affected limbs will be flaccid and areflexic; this is followed by return of reflexes. A gradual improvement in power may occur over days, months or years.

Investigations

Recognition, rapid assessment and distinguishing between ischaemic and haemorrhagic stroke are fundamental to stroke management. Most strokes occur in the community and a reliable screening tool that can be used by the public and paramedics will improve the speed of detection. Initial imaging comprises typically non-contrast brain computed tomography (CT). This rapidly excludes haemorrhage but may not demonstrate infarction. Magnetic resonance imaging (MRI) or diffusion weighted MRI (DWMRI) may be available in some centres and can show an infarct more reliably. Imaging is performed immediately or at most within one hour, if the patient meets any of the following criteria:

- Thrombolysis or early anticoagulation treatment may be indicated
- Taking anticoagulation therapy
- Known bleeding tendency
- Glasgow Coma Score < 13
- Progressive or fluctuating symptoms
- Papilloedema, neck stiffness or fever
- Severe headache with onset of symptoms

Further investigations are undertaken simultaneously with imaging and treatment. These include blood tests (full blood count, coagulation and thrombophilia screens, ESR, vasculitis screen and other auto-antibodies, infection screen and lipid profile), chest X-ray and ECG. Later investigations include carotid Doppler, echocardiogram and MR angiography.

Diagnosis

The diagnosis is made by clinical assessment and diagnostic imaging.

Treatment

The primary treatment objectives are to restore cerebral blood flow and maintain normal physiology and homeostasis.

- Maintain in the normal range blood glucose (4–11 mmol L^{-1}), blood pressure, arterial blood oxygenation (SpO$_2$ > 94%), and core temperature
- Treat hypertension only if there is a hypertensive emergency or if a patient is a candidate for thrombolysis and the BP is 185/110 mmHg or higher
- Admission to a critical care area for airway protection and neuroprotective strategies may be necessary
- Thrombolysis is increasingly used for the treatment of AIS: intravenous alteplase (recombinant tissue plasminogen activator) 0.9 mg kg^{-1} (maximal dose 90 mg). Thrombolysis can only be given once an intracerebral bleed has been excluded in a centre with trained staff, immediate access to imaging and a specialist acute stroke service. The BP should ideally be 185/110 mmHg or less
- Any patient without an intracerebral bleed or other contraindication should be considered for thrombolysis if it can be started <3 h from onset of symptoms. Patients aged < 80 years who fulfil criteria and are within 3–4.5 h of symptom onset are also considered. Patients within 3–6 h after symptom onset are considered on an individual basis
- All patients with non-haemorrhagic AIS are prescribed antiplatelet treatment; those with dyspepsia are given an anti-reflux drug
- Patients already on statin treatment should continue it but do not start statin treatment immediately following an AIS and do not anticoagulate routinely

Consider decompressive craniectomy in patients who have sustained a MCA infarct and meet the following criteria:

- 60 years of age or younger
- Clinical, neurological deficits in keeping with MCA infarct
- National Institute of Health Stroke Scale (NIHSS) of > 15
- CT demonstrating evidence of an infarct of at least 50% of the MCA territory or an infarct volume of > 145 cm^3 as demonstrated by DWMRI

Refer within 24 h; the procedure should be performed within 48 h of symptom onset. Local stroke services will have established protocols for the management of stroke patients.

Complications

The main complication in the treatment of AIS with thrombolysis is intracranial haemorrhage. In a recent multi-centre trial (IST-3), fatal and non-fatal symptomatic intracranial haemorrhage within 7 days occurred in 7% of patients in the treatment group compared with 1% in the control group. There were also more deaths within 7 days in the treatment group (11%) compared with the control group (7%). Between 7 days and 6 months there were less deaths in the treatment group; by 6 months, the number of deaths in each group was the same. Functional outcome was improved in the treatment group.

Other complications relate to the residual functional impairments caused by the infarct: difficulty with mobilising, dysphasia, dysphagia, nutritional problems, risk of pressure sores and impaired capacity to understand and/or communicate.

Further reading

Intercollegiate Stroke Working Party. National clinical guideline for stroke, 4th edn. London: Royal College of Physicians, 2012.

Sandercock P, Wardlaw JM, Lindley RI, et al. The benefits and harms of intravenous thrombolysis with recombinant tissue plasminogen activator within 6 hours of acute ischaemic stroke (the third international stroke trial [IST-3]): a randomised controlled trial. Lancet 2012; 379:2352–2363.

National Institute for Health and Clinical Excellence (NICE). Diagnosis and initial management of acute stroke and transient ischaemic attack (TIA), Clinical Guideline CG68. London: NICE, 2008.

Related topics of interest

- Hypertension (p 179)
- Subarachnoid haemorrhage (p 359)
- Traumatic brain injury (p 396)

Subarachnoid haemorrhage

Key points

- Prognosis correlates closely with the clinical state on admission
- Aetiology is best determined by digital subtraction angiography
- Nimodipine improves neurological outcome

Epidemiology

Blood can be found in the subarachnoid space following intracranial haemorrhage of any cause. The term subarachnoid haemorrhage (SAH) is generally applied to a spontaneous haemorrhage, usually from a ruptured intracranial aneurysm (85%). Non-aneurysmal (10%) and rarer causes [e.g. arteriovenous malformation (AVM), cocaine abuse and mycotic aneurysm] make up the remainder.

Aneurysmal sub-arachnoid haemorrhage

The prevalence of intracranial aneurysms in the general population is high (0.4–6%). The incidence of rupture is 6–8 per 100,000 population per year. Most aneurysms occur sporadically. Risk factors include hypertension, cigarette smoking, alcohol abuse and positive family history (2–5 times risk in first degree relatives). Disease associations include Ehlers–Danlos syndrome, Marfan's syndrome, neurofibromatosis and polycystic kidney disease. Approximately 80% of aneurysms occur on the anterior cerebral circulation and 20% on the posterior circulation.

Idiopathic sub-arachnoid haemorrhage

Approximately 10% of patients presenting with spontaneous SAH have a normal angiogram. If perimesencephalic distribution on CT and negative angiogram patients have a good prognosis.

Ruptured cerebral arteriovenous malformation

Ruptured AVM presents more commonly with intra-parenchymal or intra-ventricular haemorrhage than SAH. Arteriovenous malformation rupture generally occurs at a younger age (mid-20s) than aneurysm rupture (mid-50s and rising). Up to 20% of patients with an AVM will also have one or multiple associated intracranial aneurysms.

Pathophysiology

The exact pathophysiology of aneursymal SAH is not clear. The risk factors suggest a degenerative process is involved with inflammation within arterial walls leading to aneurysm formation. Some important pro-inflammatory mediators (e.g. NF-kappaB, TNF-a, reactive oxygen species and toll-like receptor 4) have been identified.

Clinical features

Most aneurysms are clinically silent until they rupture. SAH classically presents with a sudden-onset severe headache often associated with nausea and vomiting. This is followed by decreased level of conscious (50%) and/or meningeal irritation (35%). Neurological abnormalities such as cranial nerve palsy, seizures or lateralising signs depend on the site and severity of the bleed. A warning headache prior to SAH is reported in up to 43% and generally occurs 1–3 weeks prior to major SAH.

The prognosis following SAH correlates closely with the clinical state on admission. Clinical grading scores – e.g. Hunt and Hess Scale and World Federation of Neurological Surgeons (WFNS) Scale – are commonly used to quantify this (**Table 59**). Abnormal S-T segments or T waves exist on the electrocardiograph of 25% of patients, and can be misdiagnosed as myocardial infarction.

Investigations and diagnosis

Detection of sub-arachnoid blood

A non-contrast CT scan of the brain is the investigation of choice. The volume of blood on CT scan is prognostic, and correlates

Table 59 Clinical grading scales for aneurysmal subarachnoid haemorrhage (SAH)		
Grade	Hunt and Hess Scale	WFNS[a] Scale
I	Asymptomatic or mild headache	GCS[b] 15 without motor deficit
II	Moderate to severe headache, nuchal rigidity, cranial nerve palsy	GCS 13–14 without motor deficit
III	Lethargy, confusion, mild focal deficit	GCS 13–14 with motor deficit
IV	Stupor, moderate to severe hemiparesis, early decerebrate rigidity	GCS 7–12 with or without motor deficit
V	Deep coma, decerebrate rigidity, moribund	GCS 3–6 with or without motor deficit

[a]WFNS, World Federation of Neurological Surgeons.
[b]GCS, Glasgow Coma Scale.

with the incidence of vasospasm (see below **Table 60**). CT sensitivity for SAH is nearly 100% in the first 3 days. It is best within 12 h and decreases rapidly after 5 days to only 50% at 1 week. Lumbar puncture should be performed if SAH suspected and CT scan is normal. Xanthochromia in cerebrospinal fluid (CSF) is diagnostic but can take >6 h to form.

Location of aneurysm

CT angiography (CTA) is non-invasive and can guide the type of aneurysm repair. If CTA is inconclusive, four-vessel (bilateral carotid and vertebral) digital subtraction angiography (DSA) is performed. This is more sensitive than CTA and MRI particularly with aneurysms less than 3 mm. DSA has a complication rate of 2%, with neurological morbidity (0.3%) and mortality (0.1%).

Treatment

Initial resuscitation and stabilisation according to ABC are essential. Subsequent care should

Table 60 Fisher Scale for grading subarachnoid haemorrhage (SAH) using computed tomography (CT)	
Grade	CT appearance
1	No SAH on CT
2	Thin SAH (< 1 mm)
3	Thick SAH (> 1 mm)
4	Intra-cerebral or intra-ventricular haemorrhage, with no or thin SAH (< 1 mm)

ideally occur in a neurosurgical centre and concentrates on the following areas.

Prevention of re-bleeding

Re-bleeding from a ruptured aneurysm carries an immediate mortality up to 50%. The risk is 4% in the first 24 h and 1–2% per day for the next 12 days. The cumulative risk is 20% over the first 2 weeks. Worse grade on admission, site of aneurysm, delay to definitive treatment and older age all contribute to the chance of re-bleeding.

Surgical or endovascular repair should occur as soon as possible. Prior to procedure maintain systolic blood pressure under 160 mmHg. Surgery aims to place a clip across the aneurysm neck. Endovascular repair involves radiologically guided placement of soft metallic coils into the aneurysm lumen, which thrombose and obliterate the aneurysm. If possible, coiling is preferred over clipping with an absolute risk reduction of 7% for dependency or death. In experienced hands, the mortality of endovascular repair is approximately 1% and the procedural complication rate is 3–9% (up to 19% in clipping).

Treatment of hydrocephalus

Hydrocephalus is present in approximately 20% of patients with SAH. It usually presents as an acute neurological deterioration and requires urgent surgical CSF drainage. In a small percentage permanent CSF shunt is required.

Prevention and treatment of cerebral artery vasospasm

Angiography demonstrates vasospasm in around 70% of patients following aneurysmal SAH. Approximately half of these develop delayed ischaemic neurological deficits (DIND) ranging from confusion to hemiparesis and coma. The risk of vasospasm increases with higher grades of SAH (**Table 60**). It typically presents around 3–4 days post-SAH and peaks at day 7–10. It may be diagnosed angiographically or using transcranial Doppler sonography. Clinical exam is useful, but less sensitive in higher grades.

Oral nimodipine for 21 days (60 mg given 4 h) improves neurological outcome (number needed to treat 19) following aneurysmal SAH. It should be given to all patients. Intravenous nimodipine can be given if oral route not tolerated. Other medical therapy (statins, magnesium and endothelin-1 antagonists) for DIND show promise and further phase 3 trials are currently underway.

'HHH' (triple H) therapy has previously been used post aneurysm repair and refers to the induction of hypertension, hypervolemia and haemodilution. Maintenance of euvolaemia is now preferred, but avoid hypovolaemia. Induce hypertension if evidence of DIND. If no response medical therapy balloon angioplasty and/or intra-arterial vasodilators (calcium channel blockers and more recently milrinone) can be used.

Seizures

The incidence of seizures in SAH is up to 20% and should be treated if present. Prophylactic treatment prior to aneurysm treatment is not routine.

Complications

Medical complications

Medical complications contribute to significant morbidity and may account for up to 23% of deaths after SAH. The main complications are arrhythmias (35%), pulmonary oedema (23%), hepatic dysfunction (24%), renal dysfunction (7%) and thrombocytopenia (4%). Water and sodium imbalance occurs in 30% of patients after SAH. Causes include inappropriate anti-diuretic hormone secretion, 'cerebral salt wasting' and diabetes insipidus.

Outcome after aneurysmal subarachnoid haemorrhage

Outcome after aneurysmal SAH continues to improve. Mortality in the 1950s was approximately 46%. Mortality today averages 33%, with some specialist centres attaining 20% or lower. Up to 40% of survivors will remain dependent or suffer a significant restriction in lifestyle.

Further reading

Connolly ES Jr, Rabinstein AA, Carhuapoma JR, et al. Guidelines for the management of aneurysmal subarachnoid haemorrhage: a guideline for healthcare professionals from the American Heart Association/American Stroke Association. Stroke 2012; 43:1711–1137.

Molyneux A, Kerr R, Stratton I, Sandercock P, et al. International Subarachnoid Aneurysm Trial (ISAT) of neurosurgical clipping versus endovascular coiling in 2143 patients with ruptured intracranial aneurysms: a randomised trial. Lancet 2002; 360:1267–1274.

Dorhout Mees SM, Rinkel GJ, Feigin VL. Calcium antagonists for subarachnoid haemorrhage Cochrane Database Syst Rev 2007:CD000277.

Related topics of interest

Tetanus

Key points

- Tetanus is a clinical diagnosis and may be confused with other syndromes
- Autonomic instability is common
- Mortality rates of up to 50% are seen in developing countries

Epidemiology

Geographical variation in the incidence of tetanus reflects the implementation of tetanus toxoid vaccination programmes. The incidence in developed countries, where most of the population is immunised, is approximately 0.2/million population with a higher incidence in individuals greater than 65 years old.

Pathophysiology

The clinical syndrome of tetanus results from the production of tetanus toxoid within a host that has been infected with *Clostridium tetani*. This Gram-positive rod-shaped anaerobic bacteria is widely found in the environment existing as a spore in soil and in the gastrointestinal tract of animals. The bacterium becomes inoculated into damaged tissue and subsequently undergoes transformation into a vegetative cell growth state. During this phase, a zinc dependant metalloproteinase called tetanospasmin ('tetanus toxoid') is produced. This 150 kDa polypeptide is released during cell lysis into the systemic circulation. It then binds to peripheral motor nerve axons and via retrograde axonal transport enters the central nervous system. The toxin binds irreversibly to neuronal membrane proteins preventing inhibitory neurotransmitter release and subsequent continued motor neurone stimulation.

Clinical features

The symptoms of tetanus typically develop over days to weeks following an initial inoculation injury. The incubation period ranges from 3–21 days but on average presents by day 8 with most cases occurring within 14 days. Shorter incubation periods are associated with more severe disease and worse outcomes.

There are four main clinical patterns in which tetanus may present:

1. Generalised tetanus is the most common and severest form of the disease. Clinical features include trismus (in up to 98% of cases), dysphagia (83%), risus sardonicus (a sardonic smile resulting from trismus), opisthotonus (involvement of the erector spinae muscles), a board-like rigid abdomen, laryngeal spasm, periods of apnoea and upper airway obstruction and features of autonomic instability. There is no impairment of consciousness and therefore the tetanic muscle spasms are extremely painful.
2. Local tetanus involves hypertonicity and muscle spasms in one limb or body region. It may progress to generalised tetanus.
3. Cephalic tetanus is a form of local tetanus when spasms occur in the region of the head or neck following an inoculating injury. Various clinical manifestations may occur including focal cranial neuropathies (most commonly in cranial nerve VII), trismus and dysphagia followed by progression to generalised tetanus.
4. Neonatal tetanus occurs between days 3 and 28 of life. The typical features include spasms, inability to suck or cry, muscle rigidity, trismus and seizures. The disease usually results from lack of aseptic technique in cutting and covering the umbilical stump.

Investigations

The diagnosis of tetanus is clinical, based on features within the history, clinical examination and disease progression. *Clostridium tetani* may be cultured from the primary wound although this rarely occurs given the delay in presenting symptoms from initial inoculum. However, investigations will often be sought to confirm or exclude other diagnoses that may mimic tetanus. Differential diagnoses to consider include trismus secondary to local oropharyngeal infection, drug induced dystonias, neuroleptic malignant syndrome, hypocalcaemic tetany, epilepsy, meningoencephalitis, rabies, strychnine poisoning and stiff person syndrome. These diagnoses can again be confirmed or excluded predominantly from the clinical history, exposure to any associated agent and from particular clinical signs. The management of strychnine poisoning is identical to that of tetanus although the substance may be confirmed by toxicology testing of urine, blood or gastric contents. Stiff person syndrome is associated with a rapid response to diazepam and the presence of autoantibodies against glutamic acid decarboxylase.

Diagnosis

As previously stated, the diagnosis of tetanus is clinical. The severity of infection can be determined using the Tetanus Severity Score that uses features from the history and clinical features. Different scores are applied to a number of variables including age, time from injury to first symptom, breathing difficulties on admission, co-existing medical conditions, injury entry site, highest systolic blood pressure and heart rate, lowest recorded heart rate and evidence of hyperpyrexia.

Treatment

Toxin that has not already bound to neurones can be neutralised by administering human tetanus immunoglobulin. There is some evidence that intrathecal administration may result in a shorter duration of mechanical ventilation and hospital stay although this has only been confirmed in one clinical trial. Active immunisation with tetanus toxoid is also required as infection with *Clostridium tetani* does not result in immunity.

The production of further tetanus toxoid is prevented by adequate wound toilet, including surgical debridement and the administration of intravenous antibiotics; penicillin, metronidazole, erythromycin, tetracycline, chloramphenicol and clindamycin are effective agents.

Muscle spasms can be effectively controlled using a combination of sedative agents including benzodiazepines, propofol and opioids such as morphine and remifentanil, as well as muscle relaxants. This strategy requires intubation and mechanical ventilation.

Autonomic instability is a common feature of generalised tetanus. It may be managed using a number of agents including magnesium sulphate, beta-blockade and clonidine.

Complications

The key complications of tetanus are those of severe painful muscular spasms, airway compromise, respiratory failure and autonomic instability. Invasive ventilatory support, intravascular access, tracheostomy and prolonged ICU stay all carry additional risks. Most patients survive if modern medical support is available. In developed nations the case fatality rate is approximately 13% increasing to 30% in patients over 65 years. However, the mortality rate is up to 50% in developing countries and accounts for 1 million deaths per year caused by *Clostridium tetani.*

Further reading

Attygalle D, Rodrigo N. New trends in the management of tetanus. Expert Rev Anti Infect Ther 2004; 2:73–84.

Thwaites CL, Yen LM, Glover C, et al. Predicting the clinical outcome of tetanus: the tetanus severity score. Trop Med Int Health 2006; 11:279–287.

Taylor AM. Tetanus. Contin Educ Anaesth Crit Care Pain 2006; 6:101–1104.

Kabura L, Ilibagiza D, Menten J, Van den Ende J. Intrathecal vs. intramuscular administration of human antitetanus immunoglobulin or equine tetanus antitoxin in the treatment of tetanus: a meta-analysis. Trop Med Int Health 2006; 11:1075–1081.

Related topics of interest

Thyroid gland disorders

Key points

- Endocrine emergencies typically involve multiple organ systems and have profound autonomic and metabolic perturbations
- Thyroid hormones partially control thermoregulation and metabolism. They are also involved in growth and nervous system development
- Thyroid gland emergencies are extremes of thyroid hormone excess or deficiency: thyroid crisis and mxyoedema coma
- Most critically ill patients have deranged thyroid hormone concentrations; this is known as the euthyroid sick syndrome

The thyroid gland concentrates iodide and produces tetraiodothyronine (T4) and triiodothyronine (T3). Triiodothyronine has more metabolic activity than T4. Thyroid gland function is regulated by thyroid-stimulating hormone (TSH), which is secreted by the anterior pituitary gland. The secretion of TSH is controlled partly by higher centres such as the hypothalamus via thyrotrophin-releasing hormone (TRH)

Thyroid crisis

A life-threatening clinical syndrome resulting from excessive thyroid hormone (hyperthyroidism).

Epidemiology

Hyperthyroidism has a prevalence of 1%. It affects middle aged women most commonly (10:1 female:male). Thyroid crisis occurs in less than 10% of patients hospitalised for hyperthyroidism.

Pathophysiology

Excessive thyroid hormone results most often from overproduction, release of hormone secondary to damaged thyroid gland and excessive iodine intake including drugs. Thyroid crisis is often precipitated by an inter-current illness, especially infection, trauma, surgery, poorly controlled diabetes or labour.

Clinical features

Signs and symptoms reflect increased sensitivity to circulating catecholamines and a hyper-catabolic state

- Tachycardia and tachyarrhythmias, particularly atrial fibrillation
- Flushing and sweating
- CNS derangement (anxiety, confusion, psychosis and coma)
- Hyperpyrexia
- Abdominal pain, diarrhoea and vomiting
- Dehydration
- High output cardiac failure

It is often difficult to distinguish from other clinical presentations, particularly malignant hyperthermia, neuroleptic malignant syndrome, sepsis and phaeochromocytoma.

Investigation

Thyroid crisis is predominantly a clinical diagnosis. Laboratory investigation confirms high T4 and T3 values. TSH is decreased secondary to negative feedback. However, T4 and T3 values may not correlate with the clinical syndrome if there is inter-current illness and a depression of thyroid hormones as seen in critically ill patients.

Treatment

Treatment is both supportive and specific. Supportive measures include supplemental oxygen (the basal metabolic rate is high), antipyretics (avoid salicylate because it displaces thyroxine from thyroid-binding globulin), cooling, arrhythmia control and treatment of the underlying precipitating cause. Assisted ventilation and sedation may be required. Dantrolene has been used in a few cases where muscle activity is extreme. Specific therapy reduces the synthesis, release and peripheral effects of thyroid hormones.

1. **Beta-blockade:** Intravenous propranolol is used most often, providing there are no contraindications to non-selective beta-blockade. The sympathetic response is obtunded, which reduces symptoms, e.g. tachycardia, fever, tremor and agitation. It also reduces peripheral conversion of T4 to T3.

2. **Thiourea derivatives:** Propylthiouracil is given enterally. It blocks iodination of tyrosine and the conversion of T4 to T3 peripherally. Carbimazole is metabolised to methimazole. It has a slower onset but is longer acting. It is often associated with a temporary reduction in white cell count.
3. **Steroids:** Dexamethasone reduces peripheral conversion of T4 to T3.
4. **Iodide:** Inhibits the synthesis and release of thyroid hormones.

Refractory cases may require plasmapheresis, plasma exchange and haemodialysis to remove thyroid hormone.

Complications

Hypothyroidism.

Myxoedema coma

A potentially fatal clinical syndrome resulting from thyroid hormone deficiency.

Epidemiology

Mortality is high (30–50%). It is encountered typically in elderly females during the winter.

Pathophysiology

It usually occurs in an undiagnosed or inadequately treated hypothyroid patient, or as a consequence of a precipitant in an already diagnosed hypothyroid patient, e.g. inter-current illness, trauma, surgery, drugs, sedatives, hypothermia, treated hyperthyroidism.

Clinical features

- CNS [seizures (25%), stupor, obtunded, coma]
- Hypothermia
- Hypoventilation (hypoxia and hypoventilation)
- Constipation
- Bradycardia, long QT, flat/inverted T waves
- Hypoglycaemia
- Hyponatraemia, with increased total body water but low circulating volume
- Hypophosphataemia
- Hypercholesterolaemia
- Pericardial effusion
- Underlying chronic hypothyroid disease, e.g. cool, dry skin, periorbital oedema, ptosis, macroglossia and generalised skin and soft tissue swelling

Treatment

This is both supportive and specific. Supportive measures include control of the airway, assisted ventilation, active slow warming (quick warming can result in cardiovascular collapse secondary to vasodilatation), inotropes for hypotension and correction of electrolyte imbalance and hypoglycaemia.

Small incremental doses of thyroid replacement are given. There is no clear evidence whether levothyroxine or liothyronine produces the best morbidity/mortality benefit. However, intravenous liothyronine probably works more quickly.

The thyroid gland in critical illness

Serum thyroid hormone concentrations decrease during severe illness. In mild illness, this involves only a decrease in serum T3 values. However, as the severity of the illness increases, there is a decrease in both serum T3 and T4 values. This decrease in serum thyroid hormone concentration has been reported in starvation, sepsis, after surgery, myocardial infarction, following coronary pulmonary bypass and in bone marrow transplant recipients. Although these patients have abnormally low concentrations of circulating thyroid hormones, they are not hypothyroid and usually have low or normal TSH values. The condition has been called the euthyroid sick syndrome or non-thyroidal illness syndrome.

Proposed mechanisms include impaired responsiveness of the thyroid gland to TSH, reduced serum binding of thyroid hormones, or reduced peripheral conversion of T4 to T3. It has been postulated that endogenous cortisol has an inhibitory effect on TSH concentrations in patients with euthyroid sick syndrome. In low T4 and T3 syndromes, those with the lowest plasma T4 values have the highest mortality, but giving T3 or T4 to these patients does not improve outcome. Current recommendations are therefore to not attempt to correct low serum thyroid hormone concentrations in critical illness.

Further reading

Bello G, Ceaichisciuc I, Silva S, Antonelli M. The role of thyroid dysfunction in the critically ill: a review of the literature. Minerva Anestediol 2010; 76:919–928.

Thomas Z, Bandall F, McCowen K, Malhotra A. Drug-induced endocrine disorders in the intensive care unit. Crit Care Med 2010; 38:S219–230.

Klubo-Gwiezdzinska J, Wartofsky L. Thyroid emergencies. Med Clin North Am 2012; 96:385–403.

Related topics of interest

Tracheostomy

Key points

- The main indications for tracheostomy are prolonged ventilation, weaning from ventilatory support, bronchial toilet and upper airway obstruction
- The anticipated benefits of early tracheostomy have not been realised in two randomised controlled trials. The authors of these trials recommended delaying tracheostomy until about 2 weeks after intubation
- Percutaneous dilatational tracheostomy is the preferred insertion technique and has many advantages over surgical tracheostomy

Tracheostomy is one of the most common procedures undertaken on the intensive care unit (ICU) and is required in up to 25% of patients receiving mechanical ventilation. Percutaneous dilatational tracheostomy (PDT) is now the standard technique; surgical tracheostomy is reserved for anatomically complex cases or where there are other contraindications to PDT.

Indications

The main indications for tracheostomy are prolonged ventilation, weaning from ventilatory support, bronchial toilet and upper airway obstruction. Translaryngeal tracheal tubes cause laryngeal damage (particularly to the arytenoids and vocal cords) in two ways: (a) abrasion of the laryngeal mucosa from tube movement during coughing and movement ; and (b) pressure necrosis from the round tracheal tube as it passes through the pentagonal shaped larynx. The advantages of tracheostomy over prolonged translaryngeal tracheal intubation include:

- Less sedation required
- Better oral hygiene
- Enables patient to eat and speak
- Airway fixed more securely enabling greater patient mobility
- Less dead space and work of breathing
- Improved efficiency of airway suctioning

- Faster weaning from mechanical ventilation
- Reduced length of stay in the critical care unit

Timing of tracheostomy

Whether early conversion of tracheal tube to tracheostomy reduces the incidence of laryngotracheal damage is controversial. In the past, a tracheostomy was undertaken only when it was estimated that the patient would be ventilator-dependent for at least 2–3 weeks. Percutaneous techniques reduced considerably the threshold for performing tracheostomies but randomised controlled trials (RCTs) comparing early versus late tracheostomy.

The UK TracMan study assessed the impact of early (day 1–4 of ICU admission; $n = 455$) versus late (day 10 or later; $n = 454$) tracheostomy. There was no difference in 30-day mortality (31% in both groups), no significant difference in ICU or hospital length of stay and no significant difference in antibiotic use. The early group received 2.4 fewer days of sedation. An Italian RCT compared early tracheostomy after 6–8 days of intubation ($n = 145$) with late tracheostomy after 13–15 days of intubation ($n = 119$). The incidence of ventilated associated pneumonia (the primary endpoint) was not significantly different (14%, 95% CI 10–19% versus 21%, 95% CI 15–26%) but the number of ventilator-free days and the incidences of successful weaning and ICU discharge were significantly greater in the early tracheostomy group compared with late tracheostomy group. The 28-day mortality was no different between the early and late groups. The authors of these studies recommend delaying tracheostomy until about 2 weeks after intubation. Studies of early tracheostomy in patients with severe head injury suggest no mortality difference between patients receiving early tracheostomy (3–7 days), versus late tracheostomy or prolonged tracheal intubation, but early tracheostomy reduces total days of mechanical ventilation and ICU length of stay. Therefore, consider early tracheostomy for patients with a severe head injury.

Percutaneous dilatational tracheostomy

Percutaneous dilatational tracheostomy (PDT) was popularised by Ciaglia who described his technique of serial dilatation over a wire in 1985. The Ciaglia technique has evolved into a single dilator system, which is more convenient and faster. Other existing techniques for percutaneous tracheostomy include a single forceps dilatation (Griggs), a single dilator with a screw thread (Frova), a balloon dilatation and translaryngeal tracheostomy (Fantoni). In comparison with surgical tracheostomy, PDT has many advantages and relatively few disadvantages (**Table 61**).

The list of absolute contraindications to PDT has become shorter with increasing experience of the technique. The addition of fibreoptic guidance improves safety and should be used routinely during PDT. This can be achieved either with a flexible bronchoscope or with a semi-rigid scope (e.g. Bonfils). Pre-operative ultrasound scanning of the neck will identify any aberrant or large blood vessels and may reduce the risk of significant bleeding.

Contraindications to PDT

- Absolute
  - The need for immediate airway access (where intubation is impossible in an emergency, cricothyroidotomy remains the technique of choice)
  - Children – this may change as more data become available
- Relative
  - Ill-defined anatomy (inability to feel cricoid, obesity and thyroid enlargement)
  - Coagulopathy (INR >1.5, platelet count < 50,000)
  - Haemodynamic instability
  - Neck extension contraindicated
  - High oxygen ($F_{IO_2} > 0.5$), PEEP (> 10 cmH$_2$O) and ventilatory requirement

Complications of PDT

Comparative studies have shown that the incidence of early complications with PDT is lower than those with surgical tracheostomy. The minimal tissue damage makes infection (0–4% versus 10–30%) and secondary haemorrhage less likely. The limited data available on long-term complications also suggest that PDT is less likely to cause tracheal stenosis than conventional, surgical tracheostomy.

- Immediate complications
  - Hypoxia due to failure of ventilation during procedure (accidental extubation or puncture of the tracheal tube cuff)
  - Misplacement: too high, paratracheal, through posterior wall of trachea into oesophagus
  - Bleeding: minor – common, major – rare

Table 61 Advantages and disadvantages of percutaneous dilatational tracheostomy (PDT) versus open surgical tracheostomy
Advantages of PDT
• No need for the patient to go to the operating theatre
• Short operating time
• Less cost
• Low incidence of wound infection
• Small, cosmetically more acceptable scar
• Low incidence of tracheal stenosis
• Less bleeding
Disadvantages to PDT
• More difficult to replace in an emergency
• Loss of airway during procedure
• Deskills surgeons

- Intermediate complications
  - Early displacement of the tracheostomy tube – very small tracheal stoma makes replacement very difficult without dilators (see below)
  - Obstruction from blood or secretions
  - Infection
  - Secondary haemorrhage
- Late complications
  - Tracheal stenosis (26% when defined by a tracheal stenosis of > 10%)
  - Subglottic stenosis – rare

The technique of PDT

The single-dilator modification of the Ciaglia technique is described. Increase the infusion rates of sedative drugs and give a neuromuscular blocker. Extend the patient's head and neck by placing a pillow under the shoulders. Increase the inspired oxygen concentration to 100% and withdraw the tracheal tube until the top of the cuff is across the cords. Alternatively, the tracheal tube can be replaced with a ProSeal laryngeal mask airway (PLMA).

1. Clean the anterior neck with antiseptic solution and drape the area. Infiltrate the skin and subcutaneous tissues with 1% lignocaine and adrenaline over the space between the second and third tracheal rings.
2. A second operator inserts a bronchoscope through the tracheal tube, or through the PLMA and glottis, so that upper trachea can be seen. Use of videobronchoscopy is ideal because it enables both operators to see the procedure.
3. Load the tracheostomy tube (an 8.0 mm ID tracheostomy tube will be adequate for most patients) on to its dilator.
4. Puncture of the trachea while infiltrating with local anaesthetic will enable bronchoscopic confirmation of the correct position in the midline of the appropriate level.
5. Remove the local anaesthetic needle and insert the cannula from the PDT kit at right angles to the trachea between the second and third rings (ideally). Advance until air is aspirated freely; confirm the correct location through the bronchoscope. Slide the cannula off into the trachea and confirm free aspiration of air.
6. Insert the J wire through the cannula and feed 5–8 cm into the trachea before carefully removing the cannula. There should be no resistance to wire insertion and its advancement towards the carina is confirmed through the bronchoscope.
7. Advance the short introducing dilator over the wire and into the access site. Remove the dilator, leaving the wire in position.
8. Make a small vertical incision (2 mm) through the skin and subcutaneous tissues either side of the wire.
9. Dip the horn-shaped dilator in water to lubricate the hydrophilic coating. Place the dilator over the guiding catheter and advance both over the wire and into the trachea, aligning the proximal end of the guiding catheter with the solder mark on the wire.
10. Advance the dilator, guiding catheter and wire as a single unit into the trachea, as far as the skin level mark on the dilator.
11. Remove the dilator, leaving the guiding catheter and wire in position.
12. Advance the preloaded tracheostomy tube over the guiding catheter and wire into the trachea.
13. With a twisting motion, remove the dilator, guiding catheter, and wire, inflate the tracheostomy cuff and connect the catheter mount and ventilator. Confirm adequate ventilation (including waveform capnography) and secure the tracheostomy tube.

Displaced tracheostomy

In the UK 4th National Audit Project (NAP4), tracheostomy-related events accounted for 18 (50%) of the 36 ICU cases: inadvertent tracheostomy dislodgement occurred in 14 patients, 11 of whom died or sustained hypoxic brain injury. Half all these patients were obese – a factor known to be associated with increased tracheostomy complications. A tracheostomy can be displaced at any time and an individual with advanced airway skills may not be present on the ICU. A recently inserted tracheostomy, particularly a PDT, will be virtually impossible to reinsert without creating a false passage. For this reason, an algorithm enabling ICU staff to manage the airway and establish primary emergency oxygenation pending arrival of expert help is essential. An individual with advanced airway skills can then re-establish a definite airway by oral intubation and/or intubation of the stoma.

Further reading

Young D1, Harrison DA, Cuthbertson BH, Rowan K. Effect of early versus late tracheostomy placement on survival in patients receiving mechanical ventilation: the TracMan randomized trial. J Am Med Assoc 2013; 309:2121–2129.

Mallick A, Bodenham AR. Percutaneous tracheostomy and cricothyrotomy techniques. Anaesth Intensive Care Med 2011; 12:293–298.

Engels PT, Bagshaw SM, Meier M, Brindley PG. Tracheostomy: from insertion to decannulation. Can J Surg 2009; 52:427–433.

Terragni PP, Antonelli M, Fumagalli R, et al. Early vs late tracheotomy for prevention of pneumonia in mechanically ventilated adult ICU patients. A randomized controlled trial. J Am Med Assoc 2010; 303:1483–1489.

Delaney A, Bagshaw SM, Nalos M. Percutaneous dilatational tracheostomy versus surgical tracheostomy in critically ill patients: a systematic review and meta-analysis. Critical Care 2006; 10:R55.

Cook TM, Woodall N, Harper J, Benger J. Major complications of airway management in the UK: results of the Fourth National Audit Project of the Royal College of Anaesthetists and the Difficult Airway Society. Part 2: intensive care and emergency departments. Br J Anaesth 2011; 106:632–642.

Holevar M, Dunham JCM, Brautigan R, et al. Practice management guidelines for timing of tracheostomy: the EAST Practice Management Guidelines Work Group. J Trauma 2009; 67:870–874.

Related topics of interest

- Airway complications on the intensive care unit (p 18)
- Airway management in an emergency (p 21)
- Airway obstruction – upper and lower (p 24)
- Respiratory support – invasive (p 306)
- Weaning from ventilation (p 413)

Transplant medicine

Key points

- Ethical and moral dilemmas often pervade
- There is a need to increase the number of suitable organs for transplantation
- Increasing success is due to advances in drug therapies and surgical techniques

Introduction

Organ transplantation outcomes have improved dramatically over recent years due to advances in surgical techniques, organ preservation, immunosuppressive therapy and clinical management both peri- and post-operatively. Approximately 90% of transplant recipients are alive and well after a year.

NHS blood and transplant is responsible for policies involving patient selection and allocation of donated organs within the United Kingdom (UK). Currently, cardiothoracic, liver, kidney, pancreas, intestinal, tissue, corneal and stem cell transplants are performed in the UK. Risk is associated with the transplant procedure itself, graft dysfunction, potential transmissible infection, rejection and immunosuppression.

The implementation of organ donation recommendations has increased referral rates and donation, especially donation after cardiac death and living donation. Despite this, there remains an acute shortage of suitable organs. Within the UK, at the end of 2012, there were over 7500 patients on the active transplant waiting list. More than 500 patients died while awaiting transplantation and approximately 10% were removed from the transplant list due to deteriorating health. Nearly 4000 organs were transplanted in 2011 to 2012, of which over a quarter of organs were from living donors (UK Transplant Registry).

Patients considered for listing are those who have at least a 50% chance of a 5-year survival rate following transplantation. Ethical and moral dilemmas are often faced; patients may encounter challenging decisions about risking death while waiting for suitable organs known to have better transplant outcomes or accepting organs likely to result in poorer outcomes. There are few absolute contraindications to transplantation: life-limiting co-existing conditions, systemic infection, continued alcohol or substance abuse, uncontrolled psychiatric disorder and inability to comply with treatment regimens.

Screening of transplant donors is limited but includes extensive viral serological testing. Hepatitis C (HCV) positive organs are reserved for HCV-infected recipients. Infections in recipients should be actively treated and may not preclude transplantation.

Transplants may include autograft (autologous transplant of own individual's tissue to another site), isograft (transplant of tissue between genetically identical members of same species), allograft (transplant of tissue between genetically non-identical members of same species) and xenograft (transplant of tissue between members of different species). Graft survival is defined as time from transplant to graft failure. Patient survival is defined as time from transplant to patient death.

Hepatic transplantation

Liver disease is increasing as conditions such as non-alcoholic steatohepatitis and hepatocellular carcinoma emerge in an ageing population. Indications for consideration of liver transplant include:

- Acute liver disease: Paracetamol toxicity, hepatotoxic drugs, acute viral hepatitis, unknown aetiology
- Chronic liver disease:
  - Cholestatic: Primary biliary cirrhosis, Primary sclerosing cholangitis and biliary atresia
  - Parenchymal: Alcoholic liver disease (with demonstrable abstinence for more than six months), autoimmune hepatitis, chronic viral disease, cryptogenic liver disease and malignancy (hepatocellular carcinoma, cholangiocarcinoma)
- Metabolic liver disease: Wilson's disease, haemachromatosis, alpha-1 antitrypsin deficiency

- Others: Budd–Chiari syndrome and trauma

Portopulmonary hypertension and hepatopulmonary syndrome (hypoxaemia and dyspnoea in the presence of acute liver disease) are now regarded as indications rather than contraindications. Liver transplantation is the only treatment proven to be of benefit for acute liver failure; survival is better in those who receive a transplant for acute liver disease compared to those with chronic disease. Contraindications include clinical conditions associated with poor post-transplant outcomes and psychosocial factors. Patients with relative contraindications such as cardiovascular disease are discussed on an individual basis at transplant centres.

The Model for End-stage Liver Disease (MELD) is a commonly used scoring system to select and prioritise patients for transplant.

In the UK, approximately 800 patients received a liver transplant in 2012, mostly with organs donated after brainstem death (DBD). Whole organ cadaveric orthotopic liver transplantation is most common with recipient hepatectomy, revascularisation of the donor graft and biliary reconstruction. Techniques include portal bypass or 'piggyback technique', which preserves the vena cava and provides better haemodynamic stability during the anhepatic phase. Split-liver grafts allow for more than one recipient but are associated with higher risk of complications such as biliary leak. Auxiliary transplantation (liver implantation without recipient hepatectomy) allows immunosuppression to be weaned when native organ function improves but is technically more difficult. Intestinal transplants are often performed concomitantly with liver, renal and pancreas transplantation.

Post-operative care involves managing the complications of post-reperfusion syndrome, significant blood product transfusion and any complications that arise relating to the surgery, pre-existing co-morbidities or immunosuppression. Pulmonary, renal and biliary complications including ventilator associated pneumonia and acute kidney injury are common.

Graft function is monitored by perfusion (using Doppler ultrasound of vessels), bile production, coagulation and biochemistry. Cold and warm ischaemia times greater than 30 min are associated with poorer graft function.

Warm ischaemia time describes the ischaemia of cells and tissues during normothermic conditions. It is the period from point of cross-clamping (or from asystole in non-heart beating donors) until cold perfusion with organ preservation solution is commenced. Warm ischaemia also occurs during implantation when the organ is removed from ice until reperfusion occurs with completed surgical anastomosis. Cold ischaemia is the time when the organ is perfused with cold preservation solution to when it reaches physiological temperature during the implantation procedure.

Immediate failure of the graft/liver transplant may necessitate urgent re-transplantation and is often a result of ischaemic injury or hepatic artery thrombosis.

Outcomes after non-heart beating liver transplantation (donation after cardiac death, DCD) are approaching those donated after brainstem death and have significantly improved. Living donor-related transplantation is performed but carries a risk of death to the donor of 1 in 100.

Cardiothoracic transplantation

Cardiac and lung transplantation forms part of standard management for end-stage cardiorespiratory conditions such as heart failure, intractable angina unsuitable for revascularisation, intractable ventricular arrhythmias, dilated cardiomyopathy, congenital heart disease with pulmonary hypertension and specific lung diseases such as cystic fibrosis.

Stricter age limits apply; other exclusion criteria may include ventilator dependency, irreversible pulmonary hypertension, steroid therapy, active malignancy, active infection including fungal disease, previous thoracic surgery or radiotherapy and psychosocial factors.

In 2006, the International Society for Heart and Lung Transplantation published a consensus statement for the listing and management policies for potential cardiac transplantation candidates.

The physiology of the denervated heart differs to the native heart. Due to surgical technique, the recipient sinoatrial node is retained but does not activate the donor heart. The donor sinoatrial node is not innervated but intrinsically controls the graft heart rate. Only direct-acting drugs affect the donor heart. The denervated heart retains intrinsic control mechanisms of volume response, adrenergic response and conductivity. Denervation alters response to hypovolaemia, hypotension and pain. Arrhythmias are common but may herald rejection. Post-operative management is similar to standard post-cardiopulmonary bypass surgery management with the addition of immunosuppression. Major complications include tracheal dehiscence, bleeding, graft atherosclerosis and vasculopathy.

Donor lungs remain denervated; spontaneous breathing is preserved as this is initiated via chest wall afferents. Bronchomotor tone is retained but cough response is lost below the anastomosis. Complications include tracheal dehiscence, bronchiolitis obliterans, which may suggest graft rejection and acute lung injury following reperfusion.

There is an 80% 1-year survival rate following lung transplantation (similar between DBD and DCD), with slightly higher survival rates for heart-lung transplant.

Renal transplantation

Studies support survival benefit of transplantation relative to dialysis; patients transplanted earlier in their disease course have better outcomes. The majority of transplants are following DBD; however, there are increasing rates of living donation. Altruistic living kidney donation is associated with a donor mortality risk of 1 in 3000.

Various features affect organ acceptance: donor age, presence of hypo- or hypertension, renal impairment, DCD and prolonged ischaemia in transport (this increases the risk of acute tubular necrosis and need for post-transplant dialysis). There is increased graft survival from living donors and machine-perfused kidneys; graft failure

is often due to vascular thrombosis, donor or recipient disease and rejection.

Pancreas transplantation

Pancreas transplantation is often performed for diabetics with life-threatening hypoglycaemic unawareness or concomitantly with liver or intestinal transplantation. Graft thrombosis is a complication, particularly after DCD. Islet cell transplantation is less invasive. There is a lack of long-term survival data as it is only a recently performed procedure.

Stem cell transplantation

A high proportion of haematological malignancies receive haemopoeitic cell transplantation (HCT). Failure of allogenic HCT may result in graft rejection or graft-versus-host disease (GvHD). GvHD presents with rash, gastrointestinal upset and liver dysfunction and is due to donor-derived T-cells reacting with recipient tissue antigens. It is treated with high dose steroids; chronic GvHD requires long-term steroids with or without immunosuppression.

Tissue transplantation

Tissue transplantation is available including eyes (corneal and stem cell transplants), heart valves, skin, bone and tendons. Tissue is more tolerant of ischaemic times. Trained professionals perform retrieval in mortuaries within 12–24 h to minimise microbial load. The 1-year graft survival rate for corneal transplants is approximately 90%.

Graft rejection

Rejection is categorised into hyper-acute (occurring in theatre within minutes), acute (days to weeks), late acute (after 3 months) and chronic (months to years later). Clinical presentation is non-specific and may include rapid graft dysfunction. The gold standard for diagnosis is biopsy. Treatments include plasmapheresis, high dose steroids, intravenous immunoglobulin and anti-proliferative agents.

Rejection occurs due to the recipient mounting an immune response against alloantigens of the donor graft as a result of major histocompatability complex and human leucocyte antigens (HLA). It is mainly T-cell lymphocyte mediated. Ischaemia and reperfusion up-regulate graft HLA-antigen expression.

Factors considered in order to decrease the incidence of graft rejection include:

- Organ matching by weight to within 80–120%
- ABO blood group compatibility
- Negative lymphocyte cross-match (identifies preformed circulating cytotoxic antibodies in the recipient)
- Depletion of donor-specific anti-HLA antibodies (desensitisation therapy)

Immunosuppression

Immunosuppressive agents significantly reduce incidence of rejection but increase susceptibility to opportunistic infections and cancer. High levels are required immediately after transplant and are subsequently reduced according to drug levels. Initial therapy is enhanced by combination with specific monoclonal or polyclonal antibody agents that target lymphocyte subsets, e.g. basiliximab (targets only activated T cells via IL-2 receptor – which are involved in allorecognition and initiation of immune response). It reduces incidence of graft rejection but as yet, is unclear regarding long-term survival rates.

Side effects of immunosuppression include cell lysis, cytokine release and haemodynamic instability, infection [in particular *Pneumocystis (carinii) jiroveci* pneumonia, cytomegalovirus, aspergillus] and malignancy (including virally induced). Immunosuppression is discontinued if the graft fails.

Other drugs used include calcineurin inhibitors which stop T-cell activation, e.g. cyclosporin, tacrolimus. These can cause neurotoxicity, nephrotoxicity and diabetes. Sirolimus is a novel immunosuppressant with antifungal and antiproliferative properties. Other cytotoxics include mycophenolic acid, the active component of MMF (mycophenolate mofetil), which blocks DNA synthesis. It is more potent than azathioprine (which also targets B-lymphocytes), has fewer side effects and is associated with lower rates of acute rejection.

Transplant recipients are at risk of bacterial infections; sepsis is a major cause of ICU re-admission. It is more difficult to recognise infection in transplant recipients, so it is essential to treat early with microbiologically guided therapy and invasive sampling for accurate diagnosis.

Infection risk should be continually assessed and balanced against the need for immunosuppression. Prophylaxis is based on time since transplantation and exposures. It decreases incidence and severity of post-transplant infections using three preventative strategies: vaccination, universal prophylaxis (antibiotics and antivirals for first 3–6 months) and pre-emptive therapy.

Surgical prophylaxis depends on the organ being transplanted and colonisation. Antifungal prophylaxis should be considered for lung, pancreas or liver transplantation. Invasive fungal infection is common after liver transplantation, re-transplantation, massive transfusion, respiratory failure, broad spectrum antibiotic therapy and viral infection (CMV, HCV). The risk of CMV pneumonitis is highest after stem cell transplant followed by lung, pancreas, liver, heart and renal transplantation. The risk is negligible if both donor and recipient are seronegative. The risk of disease is higher if the donor is seropositive and recipient seronegative. Antiviral therapy reduces seroconversion rates and infection risk diminishes after 6 months.

Conclusion

Despite increasing age and obesity of donors, outcomes are improving. However, there is still a need for suitable organs for transplantation, particularly in certain ethnic groups. Advances in immunosuppression have reduced infection, acute rejection rates and side effects, while novel techniques in organ preservation are improving outcomes.

Further reading

Watson CJE, Dark JH. Organ transplantation: historical perspective and current practice. Br J Anaes 2012; 108:i29–42.

Nankivell B, Alexander SI. Rejection of the kidney allograft. N Engl J Med 2010; 363:1451–1462.

NHS Blood and Transplant UK transplant website: www.organdonation.nhs.uk/.

International Society of Heart and Lung Transplantation website: http://www.ishlt.org/publications/guidelines.asp.

Related topics of interest

Transport of the critically ill

Key points

- Critically ill patients may require transfer to access treatment unavailable locally; ultimately this should improve outcome, but transfers carry some risk
- Resuscitation of unstable patients prior to transfer minimises the risk of adverse events during transport
- Organization, preparation and transport team training make patient transfer safer

Introduction

Critically ill patients are frequently transferred to enable them to receive treatment that is likely to improve their outcome and is not available at the original location. Patients can be transferred from the site of injury or illness to the hospital (primary transport), between hospitals (secondary inter-hospital transport) or between locations within the same hospital (secondary intra-hospital transport). Inter-hospital transport can be by road or air (fixed wing or rotary wing crafts).

Reasons for intra-hospital transport
- Diagnostic
- Therapeutic

Reasons for inter-hospital transport
- Investigations
- Specialist care or intervention
- Specialist facilities
- Repatriation
- Non-clinical (bed availability, insurance cover and family proximity)

The same general principles apply to all categories of transport.

Impact of transport

Adverse events

Transport is associated with movement, acceleration and deceleration, posture changes, equipment changes, noise, temperature variation and procedures that have an effect on haemodynamic, respiratory, neurological and psychological patient variables.

Transport of critically ill patients is associated with morbidity and mortality: adverse events occur in up to 70% of transports; serious adverse events requiring intervention during transport occur in 4–9%. Cardiac arrest during transport has an incidence of up to 1.6%. Mechanically ventilated patients have the highest risk of complications during transport. There is an increased risk of ventilator associated pneumonia (VAP) and long-lasting respiratory function deterioration after transport.

Frequent adverse events
- Cardiovascular: hypotension, hypertension, tachycardia, arrhythmias and cardiac arrest
- Respiratory: hypoxia, bronchospasm, pneumothorax, tracheal tube displacement, extubation, hyperventilation, hypoventilation and ventilator dysynchrony. Deterioration in oxygenation lasting hours after transportation. Higher incidence of VAP in mechanically ventilated patients after transport
- Neurological: agitation and intracranial hypertension
- Others: Hypothermia, electrical failure, oxygen failure and tubing and cable disconnection

Benefits

Changes in management after transport for a diagnostic procedure are frequent and range from 25–70% depending on the diagnostic procedure performed and the patient population studied. Surgical, trauma patients and patients requiring coronary intervention benefit the most from diagnostic and therapeutic procedures that require transport (computed tomography imaging, angiography and surgery).

Complete an early risk-benefit analysis whenever transport of critically ill patient is being considered. Consider alternative bedside diagnostic techniques and therapeutic procedures.

Prevention of adverse events

Adverse events during transfer are caused by patient, equipment, team- or organisation-related factors. Adequate resuscitation and physiologic stabilisation before transport reduces the risk of adverse events. Some conditions may only be stabilised with definitive treatment at the destination (e.g. ruptured aortic aneurysms and penetrating unstable trauma).

At least one-third of adverse events are equipment related. Ensure transport drugs and equipment are readily available and regularly checked. Staff involved in transport must be familiar with the equipment used.

The risk of complications is greater when the accompanying personnel are untrained and inexperienced. At least two escorts, including a qualified nurse and an orderly should accompany patients being transported. Unstable patients, those at risk of destabilising during transport, and mechanically ventilated patients must be escorted by a physician appropriately trained in airway management, ventilation, resuscitation and unanticipated emergency procedures. Dedicated specialist transport teams offer consistent high standard of care and are ideal for inter-hospital transport.

Standard operation procedures, protocols and checklists should be available. Quality improvement measures including staff training, regular evaluation and refinement should be implemented.

Transport

Resuscitate and stabilise any unstable patient before transport. Establish effective communication between the transferring, transport and receiving teams and provide a detailed clinical patient handover. Conference calling is useful to assist this.

Assess airway and breathing and secure the airway if there is risk of compromise during transfer. In mechanically ventilated patients, trial the ventilator mode that will be used during transport for 5–10 min to ensure effectiveness and tolerance; ensure suction equipment is available and functional throughout transfer. Check that there is sufficient oxygen for the estimated transport time plus a safety margin.

Obtain and secure adequate venous access and take enough drugs, including pre-prepared vasopressor, inotrope and sedative infusions, for the duration of transport.

Ensure battery operated equipment is fully charged and supported with backup batteries. Minimise the number of infusion pumps and, when feasible, use loaded syringes for bolus administration.

Assess and document immediate pre-transport patient status and transport all relevant documentation with the patient.

During transfer

Patients are transported with, at a minimum, the same level of monitoring they had in the original location (ICU or ED).

Minimum monitoring:
- Constant clinical assessment
- ECG
- Blood pressure (ideally continuous intra-arterial)
- Oxygen saturation
- Respiratory rate
- Heart rate
- Temperature
- Capnography in ventilated patients

Minimum equipment:
- ECG monitor/defibrillator
- Pulse oximeter
- Non invasive blood pressure monitor
- Airway management devices and oxygen source
- Resuscitation drugs, venous access material and intravenous fluids

Other drugs (sedatives, analgesics, muscle relaxants and hypertonic solutions) are included as needed.

More invasive equipment, such as that required for continuous invasive blood pressure, cardiac output, haemodynamic pressures, capnography and intra-cerebral pressure are continued if already in use.

Transport mechanical ventilators enable reliable administration of minute volume, oxygen concentration and PEEP. Trial the ventilator mode to be used during transport before departing the original location.

Cover the patient adequately to prevent hypothermia during transport.

On arrival at the destination, prioritise connection of the ventilator, monitor and infusion pumps to wall oxygen and electricity source so that supplies are preserved for possible return transport.

Inter-hospital transfer

Inter-hospital transport is usually associated with fewer adverse events probably because of greater pre-transfer patient stability, dedicated specialised team involvement and improved organization.

The choice of transport mode is made by the transferring physician, in agreement with the receiving physician and transport team, and will depend on the nature of the illness, urgency, availability, geographical factors, traffic and weather conditions, mobilisation times and cost.

Aeromedical transfer

Aeromedical transport has the advantage of speed, accessibility and specialised staff. Staff involved in aeromedical transfers must have appropriate training including aeromedical transport medicine, safety and evacuation procedures and on board communication skills.

Aeromedical transport related considerations:

- High altitude is associated with decreased barometric pressure, partial pressure of oxygen and temperature that may lead to hypoxemia and hypothermia. Oxygen must be supplemented to maintain normal oxygen saturation and patient adequately wrapped in insulating blankets
- Decreased barometric pressure increases the volume of gas-filled cavities. Pneumothoraces must be drained and decompressive nasogastric and urinary catheters inserted
- Vibration and noise may cause nausea, pain and monitor artefacts and interfere with communication, auscultation and recognition of auditory alarms

Further reading

Fanara B, Manzon C, Barbot O, Desmettre T, Capellier G. Recommendations for the intra-hospital transport of critically ill patients. Crit Care 2010; 14:R87.

The Intensive Care Society (ICS). Guidelines for the transport of the critically ill adult, 3rd edn. London: ICS, 2011.

College of Intensive Care Medicine of Australia and New Zealand (CICM), Australian and New Zealand College of Anaesthetists, Australasian College for Emergency Medicine. Minimum standards for transport of critically ill patients. Prahran: CICM, 2010.

Related topics of interest

- Airway management in an emergency (p 21)
- Pre-hospital care (p 277)
- Respiratory support – invasive (p 306)

Trauma – primary survey

Key points

- Major trauma is the commonest cause of death under 40 years
- In-hospital resuscitation of the severely injured patient is best undertaken by a team of medical and nursing staff co-ordinated by an experienced trauma team leader
- The primary survey and resuscitation phases are undertaken simultaneously
- Unless the patient needs to go immediately to the operating room, try to obtain a CT scan within 30 min of patient arrival in the ED

Epidemiology

Major trauma kills 5400 people in England annually; it is the commonest cause of death in those under 40 years and an average of 36 life years are lost for each trauma death. Road trauma accounts for over a third of all injury-related deaths. There are two survivors with serious or permanent disability for each trauma fatality. The incidence of severe trauma, defined as an injury severity score (ISS) of $\geq$ 16, is 4 per million per week, which equates to 240 severely injured patients in the United Kingdom each week. Hypoxia and hypovolaemia are common causes of preventable trauma deaths. Severely injured patients admitted to an emergency department (ED) will require the immediate attention of the critical care team.

Pathophysiology

Several mechanisms are involved in the development of cellular injury after severe trauma. The commonest is haemorrhage, causing circulatory failure with poor tissue perfusion and generalised hypoxia (hypovolaemic shock). Myocardial trauma may cause cardiogenic shock, while spinal cord trauma may cause neurogenic shock. Severe trauma is a potent cause of the systemic inflammatory response syndrome (SIRS) and this may progress to multiple organ failure.

Physiological response to haemorrhage

Trauma compromises tissue oxygenation because haemorrhage reduces oxygen delivery, and tissue injury and inflammation increase oxygen consumption. Compensatory responses to haemorrhage are categorised into immediate, early and late. The loss of blood volume is detected by low-pressure stretch receptors in the atria and arterial baroreceptors in the aorta and carotid artery. Efferents from the vasomotor centre increase release of catecholamines, which causes arteriolar constriction, venoconstriction and tachycardia. Early compensatory mechanisms (5–60 min) include movement of fluid from the interstitium to the intravascular space and mobilisation of intracellular fluid. Long-term compensation to haemorrhage is by several mechanisms: reduced glomerular filtration rate, salt and water re-absorption (aldosterone and vasopressin), thirst and increased erythropoiesis.

Hypovolaemic shock is divided into four classes according to the percentage of the total blood volume lost, and the associated symptoms and signs (**Table 62**). A decrease in systolic pressure suggests a loss of >30% of total blood volume (approximately 1500 mL in a 70 kg adult). Pure haemorrhage without the presence of significant tissue injury may not cause this typical pattern of a stepwise increase in heart rate. Occasionally, the heart rate may remain relatively low until the onset of cardiovascular collapse.

Haemorrhagic shock causes a significant lactic acidosis: once the mitochondrial PO_2 is less than 2 mmHg, oxidative phosphorylation is inhibited and pyruvate is unable to enter the Krebs cycle. Instead, pyruvate undergoes anaerobic metabolism in the cytoplasm, a process that is relatively inefficient for adenosine triphosphate (ATP) generation. ATP depletion causes cell membrane pump failure and cell death. Resuscitation must restore oxygen delivery rapidly if irreversible haemorrhagic shock and death of the patient is to be prevented.

Table 62　A classification of haemorrhage (adapted from the Advanced Trauma Life Support manual)				
	Class 1	Class 2	Class 3	Class 4
Blood loss (% of TBV)	< 15%	15–30%	30–40%	> 40%
Blood loss/70 kg (mL)	750	750–1500	1500–2000	> 2000
Systolic BP	Normal	Normal	Reduced	Very low
Diastolic BP	Normal	Raised	Reduced	Very low
Heart rate	< 100	> 100	> 120	> 140
Respiratory rate	14–20	20–30	30–40	30–40
Urine output (mL h^{-1})	> 30	20–30	10–20	0
Mental state	Alert	Anxious or aggressive	Confused	Drowsy or unconscious

Systemic inflammatory response syndrome

Crushed and wounded tissues activate complement, which triggers a cascade of inflammatory mediators [C3a, C5a, tumour necrosis factor α (TNF-α), interleukin 1 (IL-1), IL-6 and IL-8] that results in SIRS. The metabolic response to severe trauma was thought to be biphasic with a pro-inflammatory early innate immune response lasting 3–5 days (SIRS) followed by the compensatory anti-inflammatory response syndrome resulting in suppression of adaptive immunity for perhaps 10–14 days, during which the patient is prone to infection. Following the study of leucocyte genomic expression patterns, it now seems as though there is simultaneous induction of innate and suppression of adaptive immunity genes so that inflammation and immunosuppression occur in parallel.

Pre-hospital management

In the United Kingdom (UK), the pre-hospital management of severely injured patients is performed mainly by paramedics, although doctors are increasingly involved, particularly with helicopter emergency medical services (see Pre-hospital care). Paramedics are trained to minimise on-scene time; a prolonged time to definitive care will increase mortality. Unless the patient is trapped, on-scene interventions are restricted to control of haemorrhage (direct pressure, pelvic binder), the airway and ventilation, and stabilisation of the spine. The pre-hospital presence of a doctor enables rapid sequence induction and intubation to be undertaken in patients with severe traumatic brain injury and others in whom control of the airway and ventilation is considered important before transfer to hospital. The receiving hospital is given advanced warning of the impending admission of a severely injured patient. Concise and essential information on the patient's condition and estimated time of arrival must be given. ED staff can then decide whether to alert the trauma team.

Trauma networks

Severely injured patients who are treated in specialised trauma centres have better outcomes than those treated in smaller hospitals that treat relatively few patients. Severely injured patients are transferred directly to a major trauma centre (MTC) unless they have immediately life-threatening injuries that require initial stabilisation at the nearest trauma unit (usually a district general hospital) before secondary transfer to the MTC.

The trauma team

With advance warning, medical and nursing staff can prepare a resuscitation bay in readiness for the patient's arrival.

Resuscitation is best undertaken by a team of medical and nursing staff co-ordinated by an experienced trauma team leader. The initial management of the trauma patient is consider in four phases:

- Primary survey
- Resuscitation
- Secondary survey
- Definitive care

The primary survey and resuscitation

Although the first two phases are listed consecutively, they are performed simultaneously. The aim of the primary survey is to look sequentially for immediately life-threatening injuries, using an ABCDE sequence:

1. Airway with cervical spine control.
2. Breathing.
3. Circulation and haemorrhage control.
4. Disability – a rapid assessment of neurological function.
5. Exposure – while considering the environment, and preventing hypothermia.

Life-threatening problems are treated immediately (resuscitate) before proceeding to the next step of the primary survey. In the presence of exsanguinating external haemorrhage, a CABC sequence is used – external bleeding is first controlled with external pressure or, if a limb is involved, by the application of a tourniquet.

Airway and cervical spine control

High concentration oxygen is given by facemask with a reservoir bag. The cervical spine is stabilised with manual in-line cervical stabilisation (MILS) or a rigid cervical collar with lateral blocks. Place a pulse oximeter probe on the patient's finger. If the airway is obstructed, immediate basic manoeuvres such as suction, chin lift and jaw thrust may clear it temporarily. A soft nasopharyngeal airway (size 6.0–7.0 mm) may be particularly useful in the semiconscious patient who will not tolerate an oropharyngeal airway.

Tracheal intubation will be required if the airway is at risk (comatose, haemorrhage or oedema). Unless the patient is in extremis, intubation will necessitate rapid sequence induction of anesthesia, MILS and cricoid pressure.

Breathing

Immediately life-threatening chest injuries require urgent treatment at this stage:

- **Tension pneumothorax:** Reduced chest movement, reduced breath sounds and a resonant percussion note on the affected side, along with respiratory distress, hypotension and tachycardia, indicate a tension pneumothorax. Deviation of the trachea to the opposite side is a late sign, and neck veins may not be distended in the presence of hypovolaemia. Treatment is immediate decompression with either a large cannula placed in the second intercostal space, in the mid-clavicular line on the affected side or a rapid thoracostomy (small incision into the pleural space) in the fifth intercostal space in the anterior axillary line. Once intravenous access has been obtained, insert a large chest drain (32 F) in the fifth intercostal space in the anterior axillary line, and connect to an underwater seal drain
- **Open pneumothorax:** Cover an open pneumothorax with an occlusive dressing and seal on three sides: the unsealed side should act as a flutter valve. Insert a chest drain away from the wound in the same hemithorax
- **Flail chest:** Multiple fractures in adjacent ribs will cause a segment of the chest wall to lose bony continuity with the thoracic cage. This flail segment will move paradoxically with inspiration. The immediately life-threatening problem is the underlying lung contusion, which can cause severe hypoxia. The patient must be given effective analgesia – in the cardiovascularly stable patient a thoracic epidural is ideal. Assisted ventilation, via a tracheal tube or by a non-invasive technique, is required if hypoxia persists despite supplemental oxygen

- **Massive haemothorax:** A massive haemothorax is defined as more than 1500 mL blood in a hemithorax, and it will cause reduced chest movement, a dull percussion note and hypoxaemia. Start fluid resuscitation and insert a chest drain. The patient is likely to require a thoracotomy if blood loss from the chest drain exceeds 200 mL per hour, but this decision will depend also on the patient's general physiological state
- **Cardiac tamponade:** Whilst not a disorder of breathing, it is logical to consider the possibility of cardiac tamponade while examining the chest, particularly if the patient has sustained a penetrating injury to the chest or upper abdomen. Distended neck veins in the presence of hypotension are suggestive of cardiac tamponade although, after rapid volume resuscitation, myocardial contusion will also present in this way. Ultrasound examination in the resuscitation room is the best way to make the diagnosis and focussed assessment sonogram in trauma scanning is becoming routine in most EDs. If cardiac tamponade is diagnosed and the patient is deteriorating a resuscitative thoracotomy and pericardiotomy is indicated. Needle pericardiocentesis is often unsuccessful because the pericardial blood is often clotted or re-accumulates rapidly once aspirated

Circulation

Control any major external haemorrhage with direct pressure. Severe haemorrhage from open limb injuries may be controlled with a properly applied tourniquet. Rapidly assess the patient's haemodynamic state and attach ECG leads. Until proven otherwise, assume hypotension is caused by hypovolaemia; less likely causes include blunt cardiac injury, cardiac tamponade, tension pneumothorax, neurogenic shock and sepsis. In the absence of obvious external haemorrhage, the likely sources of severe haemorrhage are the chest, abdomen including retro-peritoneum or pelvis. Explore these possibilities and treat them during the primary survey. Careful examination of the chest should exclude massive haemothorax. Obvious abdominal distension mandates a laparotomy, while an equivocal abdominal examination is an indication for computerised tomograpy (CT) or ultrasound. If significant pelvic injury is suspected, apply a pelvic binder. Springing the iliac crests to detect stability is not recommended because it aggravates bleeding. Angioembolisation and other endovascular techniques are increasingly used to stop bleeding associated with abdominal and pelvic injuries. Some major trauma centres now have specialised resuscitation with angiography, percutaneous techniques and operative repair suites that enable advanced interventional radiology techniques to be undertaken simultaneously with open surgery.

Intravenous access: Insert two short, large-bore intravenous cannulae (14 gauge or larger) into a peripheral vein. Insertion of central lines may not be easy in the hypovolaemic patient and there is a risk of creating a pneumothorax. The femoral vein provides a good route for a large-bore cannula. In the severely-injured patient, central venous access is valuable because it enables delivery of multiple drug infusions as well as central venous pressure monitoring. The intra-osseous route (usually via the proximal tibia) is useful in adults and children if intravenous access fails and modern devices enable infusion of fluids at up to 200 mL min^{-1}. Insert an arterial cannula for continuous direct blood pressure monitoring and send a sample for blood gas analysis – severely injured patients will have a marked base deficit, and its correction will help to confirm adequate resuscitation.

Fluids: Aggressive fluid resuscitation before surgical control of the bleeding is harmful: in the presence of active bleeding, increasing the blood pressure with fluid accelerates the loss of red blood cells and clotting factors. However, untreated hypovolaemic shock is associated with microvascular hypoperfusion and hypoxia, leading to multiple organ failure. The balance is between the risk of inducing organ ischaemia and the risk of accelerating haemorrhage: until haemorrhage control is achieved, the current recommendation is to give 250 mL boluses of crystalloid to maintain systolic blood pressure of 80 mmHg. Older patients and those with a significant head injury may require a higher blood pressure. In an attempt to avoid high volumes of crystalloid in hypovolaemic trauma patients, blood and blood products are given much earlier. Observational data from both military and civilian settings have documented increased survival rates associated with earlier use of platelets and FFP particularly when given with blood in ratios approximating 1:1:1. More recently, it has been suggested that a blood:FFP ratio of 2:1–1.5:1 may be optimal. Tranexamic acid (1 g over 10 min given within 3 h of injury and then an infusion of 1 g over 8 h) reduces mortality from bleeding in trauma patients. The use of recombinant factor VII may be considered if coagulopathy persists despite adequate treatment with other blood products, but the initial enthusiasm for this expensive product has waned following a randomised controlled trial that showed no mortality benefit.

Fluid warming: Warm all intravenous fluids, especially blood products. A high-capacity fluid warmer will be required to cope with the rapid infusion rates used during trauma patient resuscitation. Hypothermia (core temperature less than 35 °C) is a serious complication of severe trauma and haemorrhage and is an independent predictor of mortality.

Resuscitation end points: Simply returning the heart rate, blood pressure and urine output to normal does not represent a suitable resuscitation end point for the trauma patient. Plasma lactate and base deficit are better end points to use.

Disability

Record the size of the pupils and their reaction to light, and rapidly assess the Glasgow coma scale score (see Venous thromboembolism). If the patient requires urgent induction of anaesthesia and intubation, a rapid neurological assessment should be performed first.

Exposure/environment

If the patient's clothes have not been removed, undress them completely and apply a forced-air warming blanket to keep the patient warm.

Tubes

Insert a urinary catheter – urine output is an excellent indicator of the adequacy of resuscitation. Before inserting the catheter, check for indications of a ruptured urethra such as scrotal haematoma, blood at the meatus or a high prostate. If any of these signs are present, ask a urologist to assess the patient – the specialist may make one attempt to gently insert a urethral catheter before using the supra-pubic route. Insert a gastric tube to drain the stomach contents and reduce the risk of aspiration. If there is any suspicion of a basal skull fracture, use of the orogastric route will eliminate the possibility of passing a nasogastric tube through a basal skull fracture and into the brain.

Radiology

Advances in the image quality and speed of CT, combined with increasing recognition of the limitations of plain radiographs, has led to a much greater reliance on whole body CT as the primary radiological investigation in severely injured patients. Today's standard is to obtain a CT scan within 30 min of patient arrival in the ED. Chest and pelvic X-rays are considered if the patient is going directly to the operating room or they are haemodynamically very unstable (e.g. systolic blood pressure < 90 mmHg or heart rate > 120 min⁻¹ despite 2 units of Group O negative blood). Any X-rays must be taken without interrupting the resuscitation process – this is achievable if members of the trauma team are wearing lead protection. In the severely injured patient, plain X-rays of the cervical spine have been replaced by helical CT scanning.

Further reading

Gentile LF, Cuenca AG, Efron PA, et al. Persistent inflammation and immunosuppression: a common syndrome and new horizon for surgical intensive care. J Trauma Acute Care Surg 2012; 72:1491–1501.

Gruen RL, Brohi K, Schreiber M, et al. Haemorrhage control in severely injured patients. Lancet 2012; 380:1099–1108.

Harris T, Rhys Thomas GO, Brohi K. Early fluid resuscitation in severe trauma. Br Med J 2012; 345:e5752.

Harris T, Davenport R, Hurst T, Jones J. Improving outcome in severe trauma: trauma systems and initial management – intubation, ventilation and resuscitation. Postgrad Med J 2012; 88:588–594.

Findlay G, Martin IC, Carter S, et al. Trauma: who cares? A report of the National Confidential enquiry into patients' outcome and death 2007.

Rossaint R, Bouillon B, Cerny V, et al. Management of bleeding following major trauma: an updated European guideline. Crit Care 2010; 4:R52.

Tobin JM, Varon AJ. Review article: update in trauma anesthesiology: perioperative resuscitation management. Anesth Analg 2012; 115:1326–1333.

American College of Surgeons Committee on Trauma. Advanced Trauma Life Support for Doctors. Student Course Manual, 9th edn. Chicago: American College of Surgeons, 2012.

Related topics of interest

Trauma – secondary survey

Key points

- A detailed head-to-toe survey is not undertaken until resuscitation is well under way and the patient's vital signs are stable
- There are six potentially life-threatening injuries (two contusions and four ruptures) that can be identified during the secondary survey
- The patient with chest trauma requires appropriate fluid resuscitation, but avoid fluid overload which will worsen lung contusion

Objectives of the secondary survey

A detailed head-to-toe survey is not undertaken until resuscitation is well under way and the patient's vital signs are stable. Re-evaluate the patient continually, so that ongoing bleeding is detected early. Patients with exsanguinating haemorrhage may need a laparotomy as part of the resuscitation phase. They should be transferred directly to the operating room (within 30 min of emergency department arrival); the secondary survey is postponed until the completion of life-saving surgery. The objectives of the secondary survey are: to examine the patient from head-to-toe and front-to-back; to take a complete medical history; to gather all clinical, laboratory and radiological information; and to devise a management plan.

Head

Inspect and feel the scalp for lacerations, haematomas or depressed fractures. Look for evidence of a basal skull fracture:
- Panda (raccoon) eyes
- Battle's sign (bruising over the mastoid process)
- Subhyaloid haemorrhage
- Scleral haemorrhage without a posterior margin

- Haemotympanum
- CSF rhinorrhoea and otorrhoea

Primary brain injury (concussion, contusion and laceration) occurs at the moment of impact; secondary brain injury is compounded by hypoxia, hypercarbia and hypotension. The conscious level is assessed using the Glasgow Coma Scale (GCS); the pupillary response and the presence of any lateralising signs are recorded. A GCS score of less than 9 is generally cited as the primary indication for intubating the head-injured but in practice virtually all patients with a moderate head injury are normally intubated and ventilated to enable a CT scan to be undertaken.

Face and neck

Palpate the face and look for steps around the orbital margins and along the zygoma. Check for mobile segments in the mid-face or mandible. While an assistant maintains the head and neck in neutral alignment, inspect the neck for swelling or lacerations. Carefully palpate the cervical spinous processes for tenderness or deformities. In the patient who is awake, alert, sober, neurologically normal and without distracting injuries, the cervical spine may be cleared if there is no pain at rest and, subsequently, on flexion and extension. All other patients who have head injuries or multi-system trauma will require a CT scan of their cervical spine (occiput to T1). Most of these patients will have also have scans of their chest, abdomen and pelvis, which will include the entire spine. Obtunded patients will have their spines cleared (and spinal immobilisation removed) using the CT images alone; however, if a reliable clinical examination is considered possible within 24 h, some clinicians will continue spinal immobilisation until this examination is completed (there is a very small possibility of clinically significant ligamentous injury that is not detected by CT scan).

Thorax

There are six potentially life-threatening injuries (two contusions and four 'ruptures') that can be identified by careful examination of the chest during the secondary survey:

- Pulmonary contusion
- Cardiac contusion/blunt cardiac injury
- Aortic rupture (blunt aortic injury)
- Ruptured diaphragm
- Oesophageal rupture
- Rupture of the tracheobronchial tree

Pulmonary contusion

Inspect the chest for signs of major deceleration, such as seat belt bruising. Even in the absence of rib fractures, pulmonary contusion is the commonest potentially lethal chest injury. Young adults and children have compliant ribs and considerable energy can be transmitted to the lungs in the absence of rib fractures. The earliest indication of pulmonary contusion is hypoxaemia (reduced Pao_2/Fio_2 ratio). The chest radiograph will show patchy infiltrates over the affected area but it may be normal initially. Increasing the Fio_2 alone may provide sufficient oxygenation but, failing that, the patient may require continuous positive airway pressure by facemask, or tracheal intubation and positive pressure ventilation. Check the ventilator settings continually. Use a small tidal volume (5–7 mL kg^{-1}) and keep the peak inspiratory pressure below 35 cmH$_2$O to minimise volutrauma and barotrauma. The patient with chest trauma requires appropriate fluid resuscitation, but fluid overload will worsen lung contusion.

Cardiac contusion

Consider cardiac contusion/blunt cardiac injury in any patient with severe blunt chest trauma, particularly those with sternal fractures. A normal ECG on admission virtually eliminates the possibility of significant cardiac injury. Cardiac arrhythmias and ST changes on the ECG may indicate myocardial contusion, coronary artery injury or septal or valve injury. Echocardiography is the investigation of choice if there is suspicion of a cardiac injury and haemodynamic instability. Some patients will require coronary angiography to assess and treat coincident or trauma related coronary occlusion. Cardiac enzyme values will not determine clinical significance. The right ventricle is most frequently injured because it is predominantly an anterior structure. The severely contused myocardium is likely to require inotropic and/or mechanical support.

Blunt aortic injury

The thoracic aorta is at risk in any patient subjected to a significant decelerating force, e.g. a fall from a height or a high-speed road traffic crash. Only 10–15% of these patients will reach hospital alive. The commonest site for aortic injury is at the aortic isthmus, just distal to the origin of the left sub-clavian artery at the level of the ligamentum arteriosum. Deceleration produces huge shear forces at this site because the relatively mobile aortic arch travels forward relative to the fixed descending aorta. The tear in the intima and media may involve part of, or the entire, circumference of the aorta, and in survivors the haematoma is contained by an intact aortic adventitia and mediastinal pleura. Patients sustaining traumatic aortic rupture usually have multiple injuries and may be hypotensive at presentation. However, upper extremity hypertension is present in 40% of cases as the haematoma compresses the true lumen, causing a pseudo-coarctation. The supine chest radiograph will show a widened mediastinum in the vast majority of cases but the diagnosis is usually achieved with urgent CT angiography. If a rupture of the thoracic aorta is suspected, maintain the blood pressure at 80–100 mmHg systolic (using a beta-blocker such as esmolol) to reduce the risk of further dissection or rupture. Pure vasodilators, such as sodium nitroprusside, increase the pulse pressure and will not reduce the shear forces on the aortic wall. The majority of these blunt aortic injuries are now treated with endovascular stents.

Rupture of the diaphragm

Rupture of the diaphragm occurs in about 5% of patients sustaining severe blunt trauma to the trunk. It can be difficult to diagnose initially, particularly when other severe injuries dominate the patient's management, and consequently the diagnosis may be made late. Early detection has been improved by the routine use of high quality CT in all severely injured patients. Approximately 75% of ruptures occur on the left side. The stomach or colon commonly herniates into the chest, and strangulation of these organs is a significant complication. Signs and symptoms detected during the secondary survey may include diminished breath sounds on the ipsilateral side, pain in the chest and abdomen, and respiratory distress. Diagnosis can be made on a plain radiograph (elevated hemi-diaphragm, gas bubbles above the diaphragm, shift of the mediastinum to the opposite side, nasogastric tube in the chest) but is more usually made with CT. Once the patient has been stabilised, the diaphragm will require surgical repair.

Oesophageal rupture

A severe blow to the upper abdomen may result in a torn lower oesophagus, as gastric contents are forcefully ejected. The conscious patient will complain of severe chest and abdominal pain, and mediastinal air may be visible on the chest X-ray. Gastric contents may appear in the chest drain. The diagnosis is confirmed by contrast study of the oesophagus, CT and endoscopy. Urgent surgery is essential, since accompanying mediastinitis carries a high mortality.

Tracheobronchial injury

Laryngeal fractures are rare. Signs of laryngeal injury include hoarseness, subcutaneous emphysema, haemoptysis and palpable fracture crepitus. Total airway obstruction or severe respiratory distress will have been managed by intubation or surgical airway during the primary survey and resuscitation phases. This is the one situation where tracheostomy, rather than cricothyroidotomy, is indicated. Less severe laryngeal injuries are assessed by CT before any appropriate surgery. Transections of the trachea or bronchi proximal to the pleural reflection cause massive mediastinal and cervical emphysema. Injuries distal to the pleural sheath lead to pneumothoraces. Typically, these will not resolve after chest drainage because the bronchopleural fistula causes a large air leak. Most bronchial injuries occur within 2.5 cm of the carina and the diagnosis is confirmed by bronchoscopy. Tracheobronchial injuries require urgent repair through a thoracotomy.

Abdomen

The priority is to determine quickly the need for laparotomy and not to spend considerable time trying to define precisely what is injured. Inspect the abdomen for bruising, lacerations and distension. Careful palpation may reveal tenderness. Focused assessment sonogram in trauma scanning will detect significant free fluid in the regions defined by the four Ps: pericardial, perihepatic, perisplenic and pelvic. While ultrasound is good for detecting blood, CT will provide information on specific organ injury; however, CT may miss some gastrointestinal, diaphragmatic and pancreatic injuries. In patients with multiple injuries 'damage control' surgery is often undertaken. This emphasises rapid but definitive haemostasis, closure of all hollow-viscus injuries or performing only essential bowel resections, and delaying the reconstruction until after the patient has been stabilised and their physiology have been corrected. Major pelvic trauma resulting in exsanguinating haemorrhage is managed during the resuscitative phase.

Extremities

Inspect all limbs for bruising, wounds and deformities, and examine for vascular and neurological defects. Correct any neurovascular impairment by realignment of any deformity and splintage of the limb.

Spinal column

A detailed neurological examination at this stage should detect any motor or sensory deficits. The patient will need to be log rolled to enable a thorough inspection and palpation of the whole length of the spine. A safe log roll requires a total of five people: three to control and turn the patient's body, one to maintain the cervical spine in neutral alignment with the rest of the body, and one to examine the spine. The person controlling the cervical spine commands the team. Re-construction in the coronal and sagittal planes of the images obtained from the CT scan of the chest, abdomen and pelvis will provide scanograms, which enable clearance of the thoracolumbar spine.

Burns

The management of burns is discussed in the Burns section.

Medical history

Obtain a medical history from the patient, relatives and/or the ambulance crew. A useful mnemonic is:

A   Allergies
M   Medications
P   Past medical history
L   Last meal
E   Event leading to the injury and the environment

It is possible that a patient's pre-existing medical problem contributed to or precipitated an accident, e.g. myocardial infarction while driving a car. The paramedics will be able to give in valuable information about the mechanism of injury. The speed of a road traffic crash and the direction of impact will dictate the likely injury patterns.

Analgesia
Systemic analgesia

Give effective analgesia as soon as practically possible. If the patient needs surgery imminently, then immediate induction of general anaesthesia is a logical and very effective solution to the patient's pain. If not, titrate intravenous opioid (e.g. fentanyl or morphine) to the desired affect. Head-injured patients will require adequate pain relief for any other injuries. Careful titration of intravenous morphine or fentanyl will provide effective pain relief without serious respiratory depression. Non-steroidal anti-inflammatory drugs (NSAIDs) provide moderate analgesia but are relatively contraindicated in patients with hypovolaemia; these patients depend on renal prostaglandins to maintain renal blood flow. In normovolaemic trauma patients, use of regular paracetamol and NSAIDs reduce the need for opioids.

Local and regional analgesia

Local anaesthetic blocks are ideal in the acute trauma patient. Unfortunately, there are relatively few blocks that are both simple and effective. A femoral nerve block provides useful analgesia for a fracture of the femoral shaft. Regional analgesia has a useful role in some acute trauma patients. Exclude hypovolaemia and coagulopathy before attempting epidural analgesia in the acute trauma patient. In patients with multiple rib fractures, including flail segments, a thoracic epidural will provide excellent analgesia. This will help the patient to tolerate physiotherapy and to maintain adequate ventilation.

Further reading

Como JJ, Diaz JJ, Dunham CM, et al. Practice management guidelines for identification of cervical spine injuries following trauma: update from the Eastern Association for the Surgery of Trauma Practice Management Guidelines Committee. J Trauma 2009; 67:651–659.

Plumb JOM, Morris CG. Clinical review: Spinal imaging for the obtunded blunt trauma patient: update from 2004. Intensive Care Med 2012; 38:752–771.

Zeally IA, Chakraverty S. The role of interventional radiology in trauma. Br Med J 2010; 340:c497.

Propper BW, Clouse WD. Thoracic aortic endografting for trauma. Arch Surg 2010; 145:1006–1011.

Simon B, Ebert J, Bokhari F, et al. Management of pulmonary contusion and flail chest: an Eastern Association for the Surgery of Trauma practice management guideline. J Trauma Acute Care Surg 2012; 73:S351–361.

Related topics of interest

Trauma – anaesthesia and critical care

Key points

- The technique of choice for emergency intubation of a patient with a potential cervical spine injury is rapid sequence induction (RSI), direct laryngoscopy and oral intubation with manual in-line stabilisation of the cervical spine
- There is no ideal induction drug and individual practice is determined by operator experience; however, ketamine is becoming more popular for induction of anaesthesia in the shocked trauma patient
- Intra-operatively, the combination of hypothermia, acidosis, tissue injury, and massive transfusion can cause profound coagulopathy

In-hospital airway management for the trauma patient

Depending on use of pre-hospital intubation, approximately 10–25% of major trauma patients will require intubation in the emergency department. Altered mental state, hypoventilation/hypoxaemia, combativeness and preoperative pain management are among the most common indications.

The technique of choice for emergency intubation of a patient with a potential cervical spine injury is direct laryngoscopy and oral intubation with manual in-line stabilisation (MILS) of the cervical spine, following a period of pre-oxygenation, intravenous induction of anaesthesia, paralysis with suxamethonium and application of cricoid pressure. Successful intubation must be confirmed with waveform end-tidal carbon dioxide ($ETCO_2$) as well as clinical examination. Severely injured patients requiring intubation fall generally into one of three groups:

(a) Stable and adequately resuscitated. These patients should receive a standard or slightly reduced dose of induction drug.

(b) Unstable or inadequately resuscitated but require immediate intubation. These patients should receive a reduced, titrated dose of induction drug.

(c) In extremis – severely obtunded and hypotensive. Induction drugs would be inappropriate, but muscle relaxants may be used to facilitate intubation. Give anaesthetic and analgesic drugs as soon as adequate cerebral perfusion is achieved.

Cervical spine protection

MILS reduces neck movement during intubation, axial traction must be avoided. An assistant kneels at the head of the patient and to one side to leave room for the intubator. The assistant holds the patient's head firmly down on the trolley by grasping the mastoid processes. The tape or straps, lateral blocks and front of the collar are removed. The front of a single-piece collar can be folded under the patient's shoulder, leaving the posterior portion of the collar in situ behind the head. Do not attempt laryngoscopy and intubation with the anterior collar in place – it will make it very difficult to get an adequate view of the larynx.

The evidence base for MILS is extremely limited with data originating from studies on uninjured volunteers, cadaveric models and small and uncontrolled case series. Appreciation of the potential detrimental effect of MILS has been emerging gradually, e.g. significant worsening of laryngoscopic view, increased time to intubation and increased likelihood of failed intubation. As only 4% of trauma patients have cervical spine injuries, and unstable injuries with recoverable cord function occur in only a minority of these, neurological deterioration during airway manipulation is likely to be extremely rare. Animal data indicate that compression in excess of 50% of the cord diameter for greater than one hour is required for permanent injury to occur. There have been few, if any, reliable reports of intubation causing a secondary spinal cord injury. Maintenance of spinal cord perfusion pressure and tissue oxygenation is more important factors in preventing secondary injury than minor cervical spine movement.

Placing the patient's head and neck in neutral alignment will make the view at laryngoscopy worse – Grade 3 (epiglottis only) or worse in approximately 20% of patients. Intubation is aided greatly by the use of a gum-elastic bougie – it enables less force to be applied to the laryngoscope because intubation can be achieved despite a relatively poor view. The McCoy levering laryngoscope may also be useful: it reduces the incidence of Grade 3 or worse views to 5%. A variety of videolaryngoscopes are now available and use of these devices in the trauma setting is likely to become the standard of care.

Failed intubation

If intubation of the patient proves impossible the airway should be secured by surgical cricothyroidotomy. A supraglottic airway device (SAD) may provide a temporary airway, but does not guarantee protection against aspiration. A second generation SAD, such as the ProSeal LMA, is better than a classic LMA under these circumstances. The laryngeal tube and i-gel are reasonable alternatives. Needle cricothyroidotomy and jet insufflation of oxygen from a high-pressure source (400 kPa) is an alternative method of providing temporary oxygenation but seemed less successful than surgical cricothyroidotomy in the National Audit Project 4 study. Standard cannulae may kink and become obstructed so use a device manufactured specifically for needle cricothyroidotomy.

Induction drugs in the haemodynamically compromised trauma patient

The ideal induction drug does not exist and individual practice is determined often by operator experience. Etomidate has long been considered safe and reliable for emergency intubation and has become one of the most widely used drugs for RSI in trauma patients worldwide. However, the adrenocortical suppression produced by etomidate and its association with increased mortality in septic patients has brought its use in trauma patients into question. Even when injected as a single bolus dose, etomidate causes adrenal suppression in the critically ill for at least 24 h, and possibly up to 72 h. There is an association between use of etomidate and pneumonia in trauma patients. Ketamine is the most favourable alternative to etomidate in the treatment of the haemodynamically compromised patient because its sympathomimetic action maintains cardiovascular stability. Initial concerns about the use of ketamine in traumatic brain injury have been re-evaluated – when given as part of a well conducted RSI, it does not cause a significant increase in intracranial pressure.

Neuromuscular blocking drugs

Suxamethonium remains the neuromuscular blocker with the fastest onset of action and remains popular to assist intubation of the acute trauma patient. In the presence of adequate anaesthesia, suxamethonium does not increase intracranial pressure in severe head-injured patients. Rocuronium is almost as fast in onset (1 mg kg^{-1}) and is favoured by some trauma anaesthetists, particularly as it can be reversed rapidly with sugammadex. In practice, if airway management is difficult, waking the patient is up is often not feasible because these patients need urgent resuscitation, assessment and definitive surgery.

Cricoid pressure

The precise role of cricoid pressure during airway management of the trauma patients is controversial. The optimal method, timing and force applied remain unclear; the only consistent data relating to cricoid pressure indicate that the majority of personnel apply it incorrectly and this can result in either incomplete occlusion or airway compression and limited laryngeal visualisation. Magnetic resonance imaging (MRI) imaging indicates that cricoid pressure occludes the hypopharynx, which makes the position of the oesophagus irrelevant for the success of cricoid pressure in preventing regurgitation. Higher rates of aspiration are associated with repetitive attempts at laryngoscopy and poor application of cricoid pressure will make multiple attempts more likely. The risk of aspiration versus the risk of hypoxaemia should be considered case-by-case and if there is difficulty with intubation or ventilation, remove the cricoid pressure.

Bag-mask ventilation during rapid sequence induction and intubation

The traditional teaching is that mask ventilation is avoided during RSI and intubation but in the United States it is common practice to ventilate the lungs during RSI. In the patient with a significant chest injury, hypoxaemia will ensue rapidly after inducing anaesthesia and gentle mask ventilation before onset of neuromuscular blockade will prolong the time to de-saturation without increasing the risk of aspiration.

Intra-operative management

Considerations of relevance to the anaesthetist during surgery for the severely injured patient include:

- Prolonged surgery – the patient will be at risk from heat loss and the development of pressure sores. Anaesthetists (and surgeons) should rotate to avoid exhaustion
- Fluid loss – be prepared for heavy blood loss. The combination of hypothermia, acidosis, tissue injury and massive transfusion will result in profound coagulopathy. Expect to see a significant metabolic acidosis in patients with major injuries. This needs frequent monitoring (arterial blood gases) and correction with fluids, blood and inotropes, as appropriate. Massive haemorrhage is initially treated with empiric transfusion of blood, fresh frozen plasma, platelets and cryoprecipitate, and later guided by coagulation tests and clinical evidence of coagulopathy. Give cryoprecipitate if the fibrinogen concentration is < 1.5 g L^{-1}. Give tranexamic acid as early as possible and certainly within 3 h of injury. Consider the use of recombinant factor VIIa if

coagulopathy persists despite adequate treatment with other blood products

- Multiple surgical teams – it is more efficient if surgical teams from different specialties are able to work simultaneously. However, this may severely restrict the amount of space available to the anaesthetist
- Acute lung injury – trauma patients are at significant risk of hypoxia caused by acute lung injury. This may be secondary to direct pulmonary contusion or due to fat embolism from orthopaedic injuries. Advanced ventilatory modes may be required to maintain appropriate oxygenation. The ability to provide positive end-expiratory pressure is essential

Management of the trauma patient on the critical care unit

The initial management of the trauma patient on the critical care unit includes continuation of resuscitation and correction of metabolic acidosis. Once haemodynamic stability has been achieved the focus shifts to the prevention of complications and exclusion of injuries missed in the emergency department (tertiary survey).

Major trauma patients will develop the systemic inflammatory response syndrome. Secondary infection will compound the risk of developing multiple organ failure. Careful application of the ventilator bundle will reduce the risk of ventilator-associated pneumonia. Ventilation is undertaken using lung-protective strategies to minimise barotrauma and volutrauma.

Early long bone fracture fixation enables the patient to be mobilised and reduces respiratory complications. It may reduce the risk of developing fat embolism syndrome, although this has not been proven. The counter argument is that early fixation may exacerbate secondary brain injury and increase pulmonary complications after thoracic trauma. Timing should be individualised to each patient with the treatment and stabilisation of life-threatening injuries taking priority over limb-threatening injuries.

Enteral feeding reduces the incidence of septic complications.

Venous thromboembolism

Pulmonary embolism is a common late cause of death in trauma patients. Patients with lower limb fractures and/or spinal injuries are at high risk. Preventative measures include early mobilisation (if feasible), mechanical prophylaxis (external compression devices), pharmacological prophylaxis, insertion of an inferior vena cava (IVC) filter and avoidance of dehydration. Pharmacological venous thromboembolism (VTE) prophylaxis is used in the polytrauma patient unless there are clear contraindications; these include – intraocular haemorrhage, intracranial bleeding, incomplete spinal cord injury associated with paraspinal haematoma, ongoing uncontrolled bleeding and uncorrected coagulopathy. Following traumatic brain injury, pharmacological VTE prophylaxis can be considered after 24 h if a repeat CT confirms no ongoing intracranial bleeding.

Fat embolism syndrome

Fat embolism syndrome is associated typically with a fracture of a long bone or the pelvis. The pathogenesis of fat embolism syndrome is not absolutely certain but the most likely mechanism is that intra-medullary fat and other particulate matter (microemboli) enters the circulation through venous sinusoids that have been disrupted by the fracture. This material lodges in the small blood vessels in the lung. This phenomenon is extremely common after long bone fractures and occurs routinely during the course of hip-replacement surgery. In the majority of cases it produces no clinically significant effect. However, in some cases, the fat provokes a significant inflammatory response causing lung injury and hypoxia. This process takes several hours to develop and probably accounts for the typical delay of at least 6–12 h after injury before the onset of fat embolism syndrome.

The cerebral manifestations of fat embolism syndrome may be secondary to hypoxia or to the effects of fat emboli in the cerebral circulation or, more likely, a combination of both. Fat emboli access the cerebral circulation by passing through the pulmonary capillaries, or through shunts in the lungs, or through a potentially patent foramen ovale (present in 20% of the population). Cerebral fat emboli cause perivascular oedema or may provoke local platelet aggregation, which then produces microvascular thrombosis. This, along with any accompanying hypoxia is responsible for the reduction in conscious level. Cerebral fat embolism can be identified by MRI.

A petechial rash on the anterior part of the thorax and neck, mucous membranes and conjunctiva is seen in about 50% of patients with fat embolism syndrome. The diagnosis of fat embolism depends on the presence of at least two of the three main signs of hypoxia, reduced conscious level and petechial rash. In addition, fever is often present. A chest X-ray will usually show infiltrates consistent with acute respiratory distress syndrome, but it may be normal initially. Treatment of fat embolism syndrome is supportive. Some patients can be managed with high flow oxygen or CPAP, but more severe cases will require tracheal intubation and positive pressure ventilation using a protective strategy.

Further reading

Jansen JO, Thomas R, Loudon MA, Brooks A. Damage control resuscitation for patients with major trauma. Br Med J 2009; 338:b1778.

Kidane B, Madini AM, Vogt K, et al. The use of prophylactic inferior vena cava filters in trauma patients: a systematic review. Injury 2012; 43:542–547.

Habashi NM, Andrews PL, Scalea TM. Therapeutic aspects of the fat embolism syndrome. Injury 2006; 37:S68–73.

Husebye EE, Lyberg T, Røise O. Bone marrow fat in the circulation: clinical entities and pathophysiological mechanisms. Injury 2006; 37:S8–18.

Mayglothling J, Duane TM, Gibbs M, et al. Emergency tracheal inubation following traumatic injury: an Eastern Association for the Surgery of Trauma practice management guideline. J Trauma Acute Care Surg 2012; 73:S333–340.

Morris C1, Perris A, Klein J, Mahoney P. Anaesthesia in haemodynamically compromised emergency patients: does ketamine represent the best choice of induction agent? Anaesthesia 2009; 64:532–539.

Sise MJ, Shackford SR, Sise CB, et al. Early intubation in the management of trauma patients: indications and outcomes in 1,000 consecutive patients. J Trauma 2009; 66:32–39.

Weingart SD, Levitan RM. Preoxygenation and prevention of desaturation during emergency airway management. Ann Emerg Med 2012; 59:165–175.

Related topics of interest

Traumatic brain injury

Key points

- Rapid assessment and resuscitation aim to identify and manage secondary brain injury
- Hypoxaemia and hypotension must be avoided as they markedly increase mortality
- Urgent CT scanning identifies patients that require neurosurgery

Epidemiology

Head injury accounts for approximately a third of all trauma deaths and is the leading cause of death and disability in young adults; however, severe head injury may still be compatible with a good outcome. Only preventative measures will help to address the primary brain injury. The role of critical care is to assess and resuscitate, identify intra-cranial pathology that can be improved by surgery, prevent secondary brain injury through monitoring and intervention (**Table 63**), and prevent other complications that will reduce the chances of the best possible recovery.

Table 63 Causes of secondary brain injury and therapeutic aims	
Cause	Aim
Hypotension	Avoid hypotension: SBP <90 mmHg doubles mortality; maintain cerebral perfusion pressure > 50–70 mmHg
Hypoxia	Spo_2 > 95%
Hypo/hypercapnia	Low normocarbia ($Paco_2$ 4.5 kPa, 35 mmHg)
Raised intra-cranial pressure (ICP)	Treat to maintain ICP < 20 mmHg
Seizures	Treat convulsions with lorazepam and phenytoin
Hyperthermia	Core temperature 35–37 °C (avoid hyperthermia)
Hyperglycaemia	Normoglycaemia: Blood sugar 4–10 mmol lL^{-1}

Pathophysiology of secondary brain injury

Immediate assessment and resuscitation

Initial resuscitation of patients with severe head injury follows the ABCDE format. Hypoxaemia (Spo_2 < 90%) and hypotension (SBP < 90 mmHg) independently increase mortality after severe head injury and are treated aggressively. A rapid neurological assessment, including response to commands and any focal signs, is made before giving any sedative/paralysing drugs.

Management of intubation

Patients with head injuries should be sedated, paralysed, intubated and ventilated if there is airway compromise, ventilatory failure, a Glasgow Coma Score (GCS) ≤8 or if warranted because of another injury. The airway is also secured if there is any doubt that there may be airway compromise, or agitation requiring sedation for a computed tomography (CT) scan. It is appropriate to sedate and intubate patients with GCS scores >8 to ensure optimal conditions for CT scanning and prevention of secondary brain injury. Do not sedate a head-injured adult or child for a CT scan without control of the airway, even if this is to be reversed immediately afterwards.

Assume an unstable cervical spine injury until it is excluded. Oral tracheal intubation follows a rapid sequence induction of anaesthesia and neuromuscular blockade with in-line stabilisation of the cervical spine and cricoid pressure. Avoid hypotension during induction of anaesthesia – all intravenous anaesthetics are cardiovascular depressants (ensure a vasopressor, e.g. metaraminol is ready for immediate injection). Once intubated, maintain sedation (+/– paralysis) and insert a gastric tube. The oral route is initially preferred because of the risk of intra-cranial passage of a nasogastric tube in the presence of a base of skull fracture.

Breathing

All head-injured patients requiring intubation will need ventilatory support. Monitor ventilation by arterial blood gas analysis and capnography. In most cases, the patient should be ventilated to normocapnia. In the early stages after head injury, the patient should not be hyperventilated excessively because it induces vasoconstriction, which reduces cerebral blood flow (CBF). Long-term outcome is worse following prolonged hyperventilation ($Pa_{CO_2} < 3.4$ kPa). If used, hyperventilation is titrated against the ICP and jugular bulb oxygen saturation (Sj_{O_2}).

Circulation

Control haemorrhage by whatever means is required. Blood pressure is maintained with intravenous fluids, blood products and vasopressors if required. Avoid hypotonic solutions. In the adult, avoid hypotension (SBP <90 mmHg) aiming for a SBP >120 mmHg systolic is reasonable (children >90 mmHg systolic). Once hypovolaemia has been excluded, a vasopressor may be needed to counteract the vasodilatory effects of anaesthetic drugs. In the multi-trauma patient, persistent hypotension and tachycardia implies blood loss from extra-cranial injuries. Keep the haemoglobin concentration >100 g L^{-1} to ensure adequate cerebral oxygen delivery. Circulatory monitoring includes ECG, pulse oximetry, invasive blood pressure measurement and urinary output. Do not move or transfer severely head-injured patients until life-threatening injuries are stable and an adequate blood pressure has been achieved.

Disability

Undertake a rapid assessment of the GCS before anaesthesia is induced. An accurate assessment of the GCS and pupil abnormalities takes a few seconds and has therapeutic and prognostic implications [see Scoring systems (p. 316)].

Exposure

Fully examine all patients. Head injuries are often associated with other injuries. This exposure includes a log-roll. Assess and treat fully any life-threatening extra-cranial injuries simultaneously while prioritizing head and cervical spine CT. Whole body CT is increasingly seen as a reasonable approach to the initial assessment of the multi-trauma patient. If whole body CT is not done, obtain X-rays of spine, chest and pelvis in multitrauma patients and also insert a urinary catheter.

Management of critically raised intra-cranial pressure

Critically high ICP secondary to a CT-proven or clinically suspected intra-cranial haematoma is treated with sedation +/- neuromuscular blockade and a mannitol bolus (0.25–0.5 g kg^{-1}). Mannitol is effective in lowering an acute rise in ICP, but the hyper-osmolality and dehydration may cause hypotension. Give mannitol as a bolus and not as an infusion. The use of mannitol before ICP monitoring or CT scanning is based on evidence of intracranial hypertension (pupil dilation, motor posturing or progressive neurological deficit). Adequate sedation is essential. Serum osmolality may be used as a guide for further mannitol therapy. Ensure that the osmolality does not exceed 310 mosmol kg^{-1}. Furosemide (frusemide) or hypertonic saline may be given instead of, or in conjunction with, mannitol.

Patients with severe head injury are nursed approximately 30° head-up. This enables adequate venous drainage and also reduces the risk of nosocomial pneumonia. Cervical collars impede venous return and increase ICP so use alternate immobilization techniques.

Emergency craniectomy and evacuation of haematoma with insertion of an external ventricular drain to enable CSF drainage are the most appropriate surgical procedures in this setting. Decompressive craniectomy was not found to improve outcome in a randomized controlled clinical trial (the Decompressive Craniectomy in Diffuse Traumatic Brain Injury trial).

Steroids

The CRASH study demonstrated that steroids do not have a role in patients with traumatic brain injury because they increase mortality.

Management of seizures

Treat seizures aggressively because they increase the cerebral metabolic rate and may increase ICP. Recheck the ABC sequence and then give a bolus of lorazepam, thiopental or propofol. This is usually followed by a loading dose of phenytoin ($15-18$ mg kg^{-1}).

Identifying head-injured patients who require immediate life-saving neurosurgery

Patients who have an expanding intracranial haematoma and a critically rising ICP, as shown by a deteriorating level of consciousness and/or progressive focal signs, require immediate neurosurgery. If it is necessary to transfer the patient to another centre for neurosurgery, do not delay the transfer for a CT scan if it can be performed more rapidly at the neurosurgical centre. Surgery may also be required for hydrocephalus and elevation of a depressed skull fracture.

Reducing cerebral metabolic requirements

If conventional therapy fails to control ICP adequately, an infusion of thiopental or propofol will reduce cerebral oxygen requirement (CMRO$_2$). Thiopental is given by infusion while monitoring the EEG to produce burst suppression. Increased temperature increases metabolic requirements and cerebral blood flow. Therapeutic hypothermia to temperatures of around 33 °C has been used but studies suggest no significant differences in neurological outcomes between those treated with 48 h of therapeutic moderate hypothermia and those kept at normal temperature. Rapid rewarming of patients with head injuries is probably harmful and hyperthermia must be avoided. Temperatures of less than 34 °C can be associated with coagulopathy and may have a negative effect on outcome, particularly in those patients with multi-trauma.

Investigations

- Blood glucose, urea, creatinine, electrolytes and osmolality
- Full blood count and coagulation screen
- Blood alcohol level
- Arterial blood gases

Computed tomography

CT scanning is needed to exclude lesions that require surgical intervention; the scans obtained have therapeutic and prognostic significance. With modern multislice helical CT scanners the opportunity should also be used to scan the cervical spine and any other areas that warrant assessment (pan scanning: head neck thorax, abdomen and pelvis with spine reconstructions may be appropriate for major trauma victims and if obtained with minimal delay may negate the need for any other X-rays). Adequate access to the patient, monitoring and sedation must be ensured during CT scanning.

Monitoring

1. **ICP monitoring** is undertaken in all patients with severe head injury who are being managed actively. The gold standard remains a surgically placed intraventricular catheter, which also enables the removal of CSF to reduce ICP. Prolonged periods with ICP > 25 mmHg are associated with a poor outcome. Monitoring ICP enables cerebral perfusion pressure (CPP) to be measured (CPP = MAP − ICP). A CPP <50–70 mmHg is associated with a poor outcome. Therefore, CPP is maintained at >50–70 mmHg and this often necessitates a vasopressor such as noradrenaline.

2. **Sjo$_2$:** Jugular bulb saturation is measured by a retrograde fibreoptic catheter placed in the internal jugular vein at the level of the C$_1$ vertebral body. Sjo$_2$ measurements

enable assessment of global cerebral ischaemia or hyperaemia. Monitoring enables targeted hyperventilation, CPP management and osmotherapy. Saturations <50% is a threshold for intervention.

3. **Transcranial Doppler:** This technique enables assessment of CBF velocity. A pulsatility index (systolic velocity-diastolic velocity/mean velocity) can be derived, which, with Sjo_2 (normal range 50–75%) can be used to define the optimum CPP.

4. **Intra-parenchymal cerebral monitors.** Microdialysis techniques and improved catheter technology enable multiple intra-cerebral measurements, including Pao_2, pH and lactate. The precise role of these monitors remains to be defined but brain tissue oxygen tension (<15 mmHg) may be a threshold for intervention.

5. **Evoked potentials and the electroencephalogram (EEG):** In selected patients, these are used to assess activity and gauge the level of sedation in thiopental coma. Regular assessment of GCS is mandatory. Deterioration in the GCS and/or the onset of lateralising signs necessitates urgent investigation.

Adjunctive therapy

- Carefully adjust fluid balance; avoid large osmolar shifts, hyponatraemia and fluid overload
- Electrolyte disturbances are common in severe head injury patients and are caused by inappropriate fluid therapy, the stress response, osmotic and loop diuretics and diabetes insipidus
- Physiotherapy is important in preventing chest infection and limb contractures but adequate sedation is required to prevent increases in ICP
- Prophylactic antibiotics are required only for invasive procedures
- Prophylactic anti-convulsants are often commenced in severe head injury; however, there is little evidence that anticonvulsant therapy has an impact on the development of late seizures. The relationship of early seizures to outcome is unclear
- Early enteral nutrition reduces the incidence of gastric erosions and nosocomial chest infection and reduces the negative nitrogen balance that accompanies severe head injury
- Start DVT prophylaxis early. Compression stockings and calf compression devices may be used shortly after admission. Heparin therapy is often delayed for 24–48 h because of the presence of intra-cerebral blood and the risk of further bleeding

Outcome

Outcome is determined largely by the initial mechanism of injury. The post-injury GCS provides a prognostic guide. Roughly a third of patients who survive a head-injury with an initial GCS of less than 9 never regain independent activity. The remaining survivors can be expected to be independent or requiring some assistance.

Further reading

Brain Trauma Foundation (BTF). http://www.braintrauma.org/.

European Brain Injury Consortium. http://www.ebic.nl/.

Roberts I, Yates D, Sandercock P, et al. Effect of intravenous corticosteroids on death within 14 days in 10,008 adults with clinically significant head injury (MRC CRASH trial): randomised placebo-controlled trial. Lancet 2004; 364:1321–1328.

Cooper JD, Rosenfeld JV, Murray L, et al. Decompressive Craniectomy in Diffuse Traumatic Brain Injury. N Engl J Med 2011; 364:1493–15021.

Related topics of interest

Upper gastrointestinal bleeding

Key points

- Upper gastrointestinal bleeding occurs from the oesophagus, stomach, duodenum, liver or pancreas and is multi-factorial in origin
- Timely endoscopy is the mainstay of both diagnosis and treatment
- When endoscopy fails, radiological or surgical intervention may be required

Epidemiology

The incidence of acute upper gastrointestinal (UGI) haemorrhage is approximately 100/100,000 adults per year in the United Kingdom. Incidence rises with age and is more common in men. Mortality is higher in those with significant co-morbidities and in patients who have an UGI bleed as an in-patient rather than an emergency admission.

Pathophysiology

UGI haemorrhage is defined as any bleeding that occurs proximal to the ligament of Treitz (duodenojejunal flexure), i.e. the oesophagus, stomach or duodenum. It may also occur from the liver or pancreas causing haemobilia (bleeding into the biliary tract). Bleeding may be caused by inflammation of the gastrointestinal tract (oesophagitis, gastritis and duodenitis), overt peptic ulceration, oesophageal or gastric varices, oesophageal trauma (Mallory–Weiss tear or iatrogenic), or malignancy.

Inflammation and ulceration occurs when there is an imbalance of gastric protective factors and gastric acid. This is precipitated by direct trauma (endoscopy/NG tubes), drugs, alcohol or critical illness. Causative drugs include aspirin, NSAIDs, bisphosphonates, anticoagulants and steroids. Critical illness is thought to cause inflammation and ulceration through tissue hypoperfusion rather than as a result of acid production which is often normal or even reduced. The bacterium *Helicobacter pylori* (*H. pylori*) is the commonest cause of ulceration.

Clinical features

The patient may present with obvious or concealed bleeding and may be clinically stable or compromised cardiovascularly.

Haematemesis is vomiting of frank blood, and usually indicates active bleeding. Altered blood from recent bleeding is seen as coffee-ground vomiting. Melaena is black tarry stools and is most often associated with upper GI haemorrhage, but may be seen in slow colonic bleeds. Fresh bleeding per rectum (haematochezia) may be seen in profuse upper GI haemorrhage, but usually indicates lower GI bleeding.

When the bleeding is concealed and the patient is stable, anaemia may be the only clinical feature. Major bleeding may present with hypovolaemic shock and organ failure. If conscious level is impaired, there is a high risk of aspiration.

Investigations

Endoscopy is the mainstay of investigation, diagnosis and treatment for UGI bleeding. Current NICE guidelines recommend endoscopy immediately after initial resuscitation for all patients with haemodynamic compromise. Endoscope stable patients within 24 h.

Blood tests are used to monitor the haemoglobin, platelet and clotting function, and to help evaluate the underlying liver function. An elevated urea may suggest a concealed upper intestinal haemorrhage.

Ultrasound is the best method to evaluate cirrhosis and liver injury, but computed tomography (CT) is used with suspected peptic ulcer perforation or neoplasm, provided the patient is physiologically stable. CT angiography is invaluable when the precise bleeding point is more difficult to locate.

Diagnosis

Diagnosis is made through a combination of history and endoscopic findings. Further information may be obtained by performing biopsies. Risk stratify the patient using the Blatchford Score and/or Rockall score (based on age, co-morbidity, presence of shock, underlying pathology and stigmata of recent haemorrhage on endoscopy).

Treatment

Major haemorrhage necessitates an ABC approach to resuscitation with attention to replacing lost circulating volume and coagulation factors through wide bore IV cannulae. Stop and, where possible, reverse antiplatelet drugs and anticoagulants. Undertake endoscopy as soon as possible, both for diagnosis and treatment.

Endoscopic treatment options include injection of adrenaline or thermal coagulation (ulcers and inflammation), sclerotherapy or banding (varices) and clipping (bleeding vessels). Hepatic or pancreatic bleeding is generally treated with radiological embolisation. Where endoscopic measures fail, interventional radiology with embolisation of the culprit vessels or surgical intervention is required. Bleeding varices may require a Minnesota tube. Once the variceal patient is stabilised, consider referral for a TIPSS (Transjugular Intrahepatic PortoSystemic Shunt) procedure.

Prevention of UGI bleeding in critically ill patients centres on early enteral feeding, and prophylaxis with proton pump inhibitors (PPIs) or H_2-receptor antagonists in high-risk patients or in those for whom enteral feeding is not possible. High-risk patients include those patients mechanically ventilated for more than 48 h, those with a coagulopathy and patients with a past history of ulcer disease.

In patients with non-variceal haemorrhage, start PPIs after endoscopy, aiming to maintain gastric pH above 6 to stabilise the clot and prevent re-bleeding. Infuse a PPI for 72 h if there is major bleeding. Where *H. pylori* is strongly suspected or proven, start eradication treatment.

Drugs used to treat variceal haemorrhage include terlipressin, a synthetic analogue of vasopressin, which reduces the hepatic venous pressure gradient, variceal pressure and azygous blood flow. Use of terlipressin reduces mortality and improves haemostasis at endoscopy. Propranolol is used for long-term prevention of bleeding but is not used acutely. Concurrent infection (most commonly Gram-negative bacteria) occurs in up to 66% of cirrhotic patients with GI bleeding; therefore, give broad spectrum antibiotics.

Complications

Complications from haemorrhage include anaemia, coagulopathy, cardiovascular compromise and haemodynamic shock which can lead to multi-organ failure. Ulceration can lead to perforation and peritonitis.

Risk factors associated with a poor outcome following an upper GI bleed include increasing age, significant co-morbidities, liver disease, initial presentation with hypovolaemic shock, haematemesis or haematochezia, continued bleeding or re-bleeding after treatment.

Further reading

Rockall TA1, Logan RF, Devlin HB, Northfield TC. Incidence of and mortality from acute upper gastrointestinal haemorrhage in the United Kingdom. Steering Committee and members of the National Audit of Acute Upper Gastrointestinal Haemorrhage. Br Med J 1995; 311:222–226.

Hearnshaw SA, Logan RF, Lowe D, et al. Acute Upper Gastrointestinal Bleeding in the UK: patient characteristics, diagnoses and outcomes in the 2007 UK Audit. Gut 2011; 60:1327–1335.

National Institute for Health and Clinical Excellence (NICE). Acute upper gastrointestinal bleeding, Quality Standard 38. London: NICE, 2013.

Barkun AN, Bardou M, Kuipers EJ, et al. International Consensus Recommendations on the Management of Patients with Upper Nonvariceal Upper Gastrointestinal Bleeding. Ann Intern Med 2010; 152:101–113.

Related topics of interest

- Blood transfusion and complications (p 58)
- Liver failure – chronic (p 209)
- Stress ulceration prophylaxis (p 353)

Vasculitides

Key points

- Vasculitides are uncommon and often undiagnosed
- Delayed treatment can lead to multi-organ dysfunction with high mortality
- Consider systemic vasculitis in unexplained respiratory or renal failure or multi-organ dysfunction with unusual features

Epidemiology

Systemic vasculitides are rare, with an annual incidence of 20–100 cases per million and prevalence of 150–450 per million. The commonest systemic vasculitides leading to intensive care unit (ICU) admission are polyarteritis nodosa (PAN), prevalence 30 cases per million; granulomatosis with polyangiitis (GPA; previously known as Wegener's granulomatosis), prevalence 23 cases per million; microscopic polyangiitis (MPA), prevalence 25 cases per million and eosinophilic granulomatosis with polyangiitis (EGPA; previously known as Churg–Strauss syndrome), prevalence 10 cases per million. Systemic vasculitides can be classified according to aetiology and size of vessel affected (see **Table 64**).

Table 64 The classification of systemic vasculitides according to aetiology and size of vessel affected		
Primary idiopathic	Large vessel	PMR
		GCA
		Takayasu's arteritis
	Medium vessel	PAN
		Kawasaki disease
	Small vessel	GPA
		EGPA
		MPA
		Pauci-immune glomerulonephritis
Primary immune-complex mediated		Goodpasture syndrome
		HSP
		IgA nephropathy
Secondary	Inflammatory	SLE
		Rheumatoid arthritis
		Scleroderma
		Polymyositis/dermatomyositis
		Inflammatory bowel disease
	Infective	Bacterial endocarditis
	Malignant	Leukaemia/lymphoma
		Paraneoplastic
PMR = polymyalgia rheumatica, GCA= giant cell arteritis, HSP = Henoch-Schönlein purpura, SLE = systemic lupus erythematosus.		

Pathophysiology

The core pathological feature of vasculitis is inflammation within or through blood vessel walls with either fibrinoid necrosis or granuloma formation. The clinical manifestations are due to ischaemia or necrosis of tissues and organs, with the pattern of disease depending on the type, size and location of vessels affected.

Clinical features

At presentation, vasculitides exhibit systemic and organ-specific features, some of which are more likely to be found in some conditions, although there are few pathognomonic features. **Table 65** summarises the symptoms and signs associated with the different vasculitides.

Polyarteritis nodosa

A systemic necrotising vasculitis involving medium-sized vessels, often at branches or bifurcations. Unknown pathogenesis but may be associated with hepatitis B. Affects any organ, mainly skin, peripheral nerves, kidneys, GI tract and joints. Cardiac disease (pericarditis, heart failure and myocardial infarction) affects up to 60%, which may be silent.

Granulomatosis with polyangiitis: previously known as Wegener's granulomatosis

Disease of small vessels with vasculitic granulomata of the respiratory tract but particularly ears, nose and sinuses, with necrotising glomerulonephritis, leading to pneumonitis and/or renal failure. Aetiology is unknown but up to 90% are c-anti-neutrophil cytoplasmic antibody (cANCA) positive (usually PR3), the rest being pANCA (MPO) positive.

Microscopic polyangiitis

Necrotising vasculitis of small vessels, primarily causing glomerulonephritis with

Table 65 Symptoms and signs associated with the different vasculitides		
System	**Symptom/sign**	**Associated diseases**
Systemic	Malaise	All
	Weight loss	All
	Fever	All
Renal	Proteinuria/haematuria	GPA, MPA
Respiratory	Sinusitis/epistaxis	GPA, MPA, EGPA
	SOB/cough	GPA, MPA, EGPA
	Haemoptysis/haemorrhage	GPA, MPA, rarely EGPA, BS
	Asthma	EGPA
Neurological	Mononeuritis multiplex	GPA, PAN, MPA
Cardiovascular	Hypertension	PAN, TA
	Pericarditis	EGPA, PAN, GPA, TA
	Cardiac failure	EGPA, PAN, GPA, TA
	Bruits/absent pulses	PAN, TA
Gastrointestinal	Abdominal pain/GI bleeding	PAN, EGPA, BS, MPA
Others	Rash (purpuric/maculopapular)	GPA, PAN, MPA, EGPA, BS
	Arthritis/arthralgia	GPA, EGPA, MPA, PAN
	Scleritis/episcleritis	GPA, BS, GCA, TA

pulmonary involvement in around 30% of cases. Cutaneous and neuronal involvement in 50% of cases. Pathological findings are similar to granulomatosis with polyangiitis (GPA), although microscopic polyangiitis (MPA) is usually pANCA (MPO) positive (75% of cases).

Eosinophilic granulomatosis with polyangiitis: previously known as Churg-Strauss syndrome

Eosinophilic systemic small vessel vasculitis, characterised by asthma and rhinitis followed (sometimes years later) by granulomatous vasculitis of lungs, peripheral nerves and skin. Cardiac and gastrointestinal systems can be affected (50% of eosinophilic granulomatosis with polyangiitis (EGPA) deaths are due to cardiac disease), but renal involvement is rare. Eosinophil count is usually high and pANCA is positive in 50% of cases.

Behçet's syndrome

Systemic vasculitis of unknown cause, particularly affecting people from Turkey, Iran and Japan. It is characterised by oral ulceration with uveitis, arthritis, and gastrointestinal, pulmonary and renal involvement.

Giant cell arteritis

Inflammation of large arteries often associated with PMR. Headaches, jaw claudication and tender arteries associated with general malaise. Can cause unilateral painless blindness or stroke.

Takayasu's arteritis

Rare outside Japan, Takayasu's arteritis (TA) causes vasculitis of the aortic arch and its branches leading to hypertension, heart failure and stroke. Characterised by absent pulses and tenderness over arteries.

Other autoimmune disorders associated with vasculitis

Rheumatoid arthritis: Rheumatoid arthritis (RA) is associated with a number of extra-articular complications including pericarditis, pleural effusion, anaemia, lymphadenopathy, carpal tunnel syndrome, atlantoaxial subluxation, Sjögren's syndrome, fatigue, ischaemic heart disease, skin nodules and ulcers, lung fibrosis and lung nodules. Rheumatoid vasculitis is rare and affects approximately 1% of those with the disease. It affects medium and small sized arteries. Rheumatoid factor levels are usually extremely high, anti-nuclear antibody (ANA) and ANCA are often positive, complement levels are low. A tissue biopsy can confirm the diagnosis.

Scleroderma: A disorder associated with overproduction of collagen. It can cause localised disease (morphoea) affecting the skin and underlying tissues only, or can be systemic (systemic sclerosis) affecting the skin, gastrointestinal tract, lungs, heart, kidneys, blood vessels, muscles and joints. Raynaud's phenomenon is commonly associated.

It affects females four times more than men. The presence of ANA, extractable nuclear antigens (ENA), anti-topoisomerase-1 (Scl70) antibody, anti-centromere antibody (ACA), anti-RNA polymerase I and III antibody, anti-fibrillarin (U3RNP) antibody, anti-PM-Scl antibody and anti-U1RNP (nRNP) antibody support the diagnosis of the various forms of scleroderma. Nail fold capillaroscopy can identify patients at risk of scleroderma in its early stages.

Systemic lupus erythematosus (SLE): A disorder that causes inflammation of the skin, joints, heart and kidneys with a variable and multi-system presentation. Symptoms include a photosensitive rash, Raynaud's phenomenon, flitting pains in the small joints of the hands and feet, anaemia, arterial and venous clots usually associated with anti-phospholipid syndrome, seizures and other neurological symptoms, pericarditis, pleurisy and glomerulonephritis. It is a disease of young women, usually presenting before the age of 50 and affecting women nine times more often than men. Complement levels are low. ANA, anti-double stranded DNA (anti-dsDNA) antibody, anti-Ro antibody and anti-phospholipid antibody tests may be positive.

Sjögren's syndrome: A disorder that affects the glands that produce saliva, tears and other bodily fluids. It is classically associated with dry mouth and eyes. It can be a primary disorder or associated with other autoimmune disorders including rheumatoid arthritis, scleroderma and SLE. It mainly affects women between the ages of 40–60 years. Tests include tear and saliva production tests. Anti-Ro and Anti-La antibodies are found in the majority of primary Sjögren's.

Goodpasture's syndrome: A pulmonary-renal disease with glomerulonephritis and pulmonary haemorrhage can be rapidly progressive and fatal. Diagnosis is made with anti-glomerular basement membrane antibodies (anti-GBM antibody). A renal biopsy may be required.

Polymyositis: A disorder involving inflammation of muscles. It usually involves the large muscles of the shoulders, hips and thighs. Symptoms are of weakness and pain but can also include malaise, night sweats, weight loss, arthritis, Raynaud's phenomenon and dysphagia. Creatine phosphokinase values are increased. ANA, ENA and anti-Jo-1 antibodies can support the diagnosis. A muscle biopsy may be required. With dermatomyositis, there is an associated rash to the face, neck and hands.

Henoch–Schönlein purpura (HSP): The most common vasculitis in children. Usually occurs after an upper respiratory tract infection can affect adults but is usually a more severe disease if so. Classically associated with a purpuric rash, it can also cause arthritis, renal involvement and abdominal pain. A biopsy reveals IgA infiltration and deposition in blood vessel walls.

Investigations

There are few diagnostic tests for specific vasculitides, but non-specific findings often suggest vasculitis and exclusion of other diagnoses is usually sufficient to commence appropriate treatment. Biopsies of affected organs should be performed, but if impractical, biopsies of skin lesions, kidney or lung may yield meaningful histological specimens.

Urinalysis
- Blood and protein – glomerulonephritis
- Microscopy – casts

Blood tests
- Raised urea and creatinine
- Raised CRP/ESR
- FBC – Normocytic anaemia
     Eosinophilia
- Antibody screen

Imaging
- CXR – Nodules, infiltrates or haemorrhage
- HRCT - Pulmonary vessel changes
- Angiography – Aneurysms, constrictions and occlusions

Histology
- Skin lesion – leucocytoclastic vasculitis
- Renal – Pauci-immune segmental GN
- Necrotic inflammation of medium-sized arteries
- Nasopharyngeal granulomata
- Lung granulomata

Diagnosis

Identification of a particular vasculitis is usually less important than the exclusion of alternative diagnoses and recognition of a primary vasculitic process. The principle differential diagnoses are infection, collagen vascular disease, malignancy and immune-mediated disease. **Table 66** summarises the different investigations required to diagnose the different vasculitides.

Treatment

The commonest autoimmune disorders to be admitted to ICU are SLE, rheumatoid arthritis and systemic vasculitis. The commonest reasons for patients with autoimmune disorders to be admitted to ICU are for infection; associated respiratory complications including pneumonia, alveolar haemorrhage and interstitial lung disease; as well as exacerbation of the underlying disease. Some patients will be admitted for reasons unassociated to their vasculitis and

Table 66　Investigations required to diagnose the different vasculitides		
Pathology	**Disease**	**Tests**
Primary idiopathic vasculitis	GPA, MPA, EGPA, PAN, etc.	Histology, ANCA
Immune-complex mediated	Goodpasture's, HSP, IgA nephropathy	Complement levels (low), renal biopsy
Infection	Systemic sepsis (e.g. meningococcus)	Repeated cultures
	Bacteria (Endocarditis, Legionella, Leptospirosis, Lyme disease)	Repeated cultures Immunological tests (e.g. antigens; PCR) Imaging
	Mycobacteria (TB, MAI)	Repeated cultures Immunological tests (e.g. antigens; PCR) Imaging
	Viruses (Hepatitis B and C, HIV)	Repeated cultures Immunological tests (e.g. antigens; PCR) Imaging
Malignancy	Haematological (lymphoma, leukaemia)	Blood film, bone marrow
	Paraneoplastic	Imaging (e.g. CT)
Collagen vascular disease	RA, SLE, scleroderma, anti-phospholipid syndrome, inflammatory bowel disease	Autoantibody assays, imaging, biopsies
Drug-induced vasculitis	Propylthiouracil, hydralazine, allopurinol, D-penicillamine, phenytoin, methotrexate	
Other	Sarcoidosis	
	Cholesterol emboli	

autoimmune disorder but an understanding of their disease and the management required is vital to ensure a holistic approach to their care.

Patients admitted to ICU with vasculitis usually require multiorgan support, particularly of respiratory and renal systems. Disease-specific problems include subglottic stenosis (GPA), pulmonary haemorrhage (GPA, EGPA), hypertension (PAN) and gastrointestinal haemorrhage or perforation.

Immunosuppressive therapy is the mainstay of treatment of vasculitis. While corticosteroids alone may be sufficient for initial treatment of mild disease, patients admitted to ICU with vasculitic disease will usually require the addition of other immunosuppressive treatment including methylprednisolone and cyclophosphamide. Other options include plasma exchange, intravenous immunoglobulins or specific antibodies to TNF or lymphocytes, although little evidence exists to support their use.

Complications

Prognosis has improved markedly in recent times, and 5-year survival for primary vasculitides is around 70–80%. However, fulminant vasculitis requiring ICU admission has a much lower survival rate of 20–50%.

There are complications associated with treatment, such as opportunistic infections and sequelae of long-term steroid use (osteoporosis, GI ulceration, diabetes, hypertension and Cushing's syndrome).

Further reading

Irwin RS, Rippe JM. Intensive Care Medicine, 6th edn. Philadelphia: Lippincott, Williams & Wilkins, 2008: 2276–2285.

Semple S, Keogh J, Forni L, Venn R. Clinical review: Vasculitis on the intensive care unit – part 1: diagnosis. Crit Care 2005; 9:92–97.

Semple S, Keogh J, Forni L, Venn R. Clinical review: Vasculitis on the intensive care unit – part 2: treatment and prognosis. Crit Care 2005; 9:193–197.

Frankel SK, Schwarz MI. The pulmonary vasculitides. Am J Respir Crit Care Med 2012; 186:216–224.

Wilfong EM, Seo P. Vasculitis in the intensive care unit. Best Pract Res Clin Rheumatol 2013; 27:95–106.

Quintero OL, Rojas-Villarraga A, Mantilla RD, Anaya JM. Autoimmune diseases in the intensive care unit – An update. Autoimmun Rev 2013; 12:380–395.

Related topics of interest

- Acute respiratory distress syndrome (ARDS) – diagnosis (p 8)
- Renal – acute kidney injury (p 298)
- Sepsis and SIRS (p 336)

Venous thromboembolism

Key points

- Venous thromboembolism is an important patient safety issue in modern hospitals
- PEs and DVTs in the critical care patient often present with non-classical symptoms
- There is a paucity of evidence about the effectiveness of thromboprophylaxis in the critical care population

Epidemiology

- The estimated incidence of Deep Vein Thrombosis (DVT) is between 9% and 40% during the course of an ICU stay, depending on the screening tool and diagnostic criteria used
- There is a 40–50% risk of pulmonary embolism (PE) from proximal thrombi in the thigh
- Untreated PE have a 25% mortality
- One to five percent of DVTs may progress to fatal PE

Pathophysiology

Clinically significant PEs come from the deep veins, commonly the femoral or iliac veins. An untreated calf vein DVT may extend into the popliteal and femoral veins, causing proximal DVT (20–30%) and PE. This is unlikely to occur when asymptomatic popliteal clot is discovered in patients who are progressively ambulatory after surgery.

Clinical features

Trials have shown that history and physical examination (including Well's criteria) are not useful diagnostic tools in the critical care population. As a result of recumbence, they do not develop unilateral symptoms, nor are they able to express symptoms unless they have the ability to communicate.

- Symptoms may present as difficulty weaning from mechanical ventilation, sudden episodes of hypotension, tachycardia or hypoxia
- Even a small PE can have severe or fatal consequences among patients with impaired cardiopulmonary reserve
- Venous thromboembolism (VTE) increases the length of stay on ICU and the duration of ventilation, but has no clear influence on mortality

Risk factors

- Virchow's triad:
  Venous stasis
  Activation of the coagulation cascade
  Vascular damage
- The most common risk factors are previous VTE, prolonged immobilization, underlying malignancy, recent surgery, pregnancy, obesity, smoking, varicose veins and acquired thrombophilic conditions
- VTE risk increases in the critical care patient because of their acute illness (e.g. trauma or sepsis) and the increased need for mechanical ventilation, sedation, paralysis, vasopressors and an increased exposure to surgical procedures and central venous catheters

Diagnosis

Presentation depends upon the size, location, number of thrombi and the patient's underlying cardiorespiratory reserve.

- Less than 20% patients present with chest pain, dyspnoea and haemoptysis
- Ninety-seven percent of patients with PE have one of the following: pleuritic chest pain, dyspnoea or tachypnoea
- In mechanically ventilated patients, a fall in end tidal CO_2 might be useful in raising clinical suspicion of PE, whereas a decrease in the difference between $PaCO_2$ and $ETCO_2$ probably indicates effective thrombolysis

Clinical examination is often not reliable in the diagnosis of DVT, especially in the critical care population.

Investigations

See **Table 67**.

Prophylactic measures

- The risk of a patient having a DVT is far higher than that of catastrophic bleeding from use of thromboprophylaxis
- Because of the balance between risk and benefit, pharmacological thromboprophylaxis prescriptions are reviewed daily
- It should only be omitted in patients with active major bleeding or those at high risk of serious re-bleeding, e.g. very recent intracerebral haemorrhage
- When pharmacological thromboprophylaxis is contraindicated, mechanical prophylaxis should be used

Physical

- Adequate hydration, early mobilisation, frequent repositioning of immobile patient
- Graduated elastic compression stockings
  - Reduces venous stasis in the leg
  - Caution with critical limb ischaemia, limb factures, severe neuropathy and cellulitis
- Intermittent pneumatic compression
  - Sequential compression of calves enhances blood flow in the deep veins and reduces plasminogen activator inhibitor
- Regional anaesthesia
  - Data suggest that it reduces the risk of perioperative VTE

Although utilised, all these measures have little evidence in the critical care population.

Pharmacological

- Unfractionated heparin (UFH)
  - Reduces risk with no increased risk of major haemorrhage

Table 67 Investigations for suspected VTE	
Investigation	**Findings**
Chest X-ray	Usually normal but can show cardiomegaly, pleural effusion, Westermark sign (dilatation of pulmonary artery proximal to the emboli with sharp cut-off), pulmonary infiltrates (can be wedge shaped), elevated hemidiaphragm and atelectasis.
ECG	Tachycardia and non-specific ST changes. More specific signs are that of right ventricular strain – P pulmonale, S1Q3T3, right bundle branch block or right axis deviation
Echocardiogram	Sign of acute pulmonary artery hypertension – right heart dilated, tricuspid regurgitation, pulmonary artery dilatation, loss of respiratory variation in vena cava diameter and inter-ventricular septum bulge into left ventricle. Acute right ventricular dilatation with hypokinesis sparing the apex is a characteristic finding.
D-dimer	If normal, VTE ruled out, but if positive a CT angiogram/venogram (CTA/V) of the femoral and popliteal veins is recommended. Importantly, D-dimer is likely to be positive in ITU patients for a variety of different reasons.
CT Angiogram/venogram (CT A/V)	All risk groups → specificity 95%, sensitivity 90%. However, 18% false negative result in high probability patients
Ultrasound	A leg ultrasound scan may be used in combination with a negative CT A/V to enhance negative predictive power.
Ventilation/perfusion (V/Q) scan	Normal scan rules out PE, but high probability V/Q scan rules in PE in most cases. Largely superseded by high resolution CT scans in ITU.
DSA	Digital subtraction angiogram (DSA) is the gold standard in the evaluation of PE

Platelet count should be monitored due to risk of heparin-induced thrombocytopenia (HITS)

- Low molecular weight heparin (LMWH)
  - Shown to be as effective as low dose UFH but has a reduced frequency dose, it is given subcutaneously and it does not require regular monitoring
  - Lower incidence of HITS

Alternative products to UFH or LMWH have not undergone rigorous testing in the critical care population but are used under certain circumstances:

- Direct thrombin inhibitors (DTI)
  - Different types include hirudin and its derivatives (Bivalent DTI) and Argatroban (Univalent DTI)
  - Currently choice agents in HITS; more effective than LMWH in VTE prophylaxis with no alteration in risk of bleeding
- Oral anticoagulants
  - Warfarin most commonly used, but it is inappropriate for the critical care population
- Specific factor Xa inhibitor – fondaparinux
  - Synthetic heparin pentasaccharide, which inhibits factor Xa via antithrombin III without inhibiting thrombin
  - However, it may not be suitable for ICU because it has a long half life, no antidote and is dependent on renal function for clearance

Insertion of IVC filter

- Lack of trial data supporting its use as a primary prevention

Treatment

Anticoagulation

- Full anticoagulation doses of UFH or LMWH can be used
- If the patient is at high risk of bleeding, it may be preferable to use a heparin

infusion that can be stopped and reversed as necessary

IVC filter – indications for its use include:

- Patients with a PE or an acute proximal DVT who cannot receive anticoagulation, e.g. awaiting surgery, recent haemorrhagic stroke
- Patients who experience recurrent PE or proximal DVTs despite full anticoagulation

Thrombolytic

- This should be considered in a haemodynamically unstable patient with a PE (systolic BP <90 mmHg or a pressure drop of >=40 mmHg for more than 15 min not caused by other factors). Thrombolysis should be considered case by case but given if the benefit of thrombolysis outweighs the risk of bleeding
- Cather directed thrombolysis should be considered in patients with an iliofemoral DVT whose symptoms occurred in the last 14 days, who have a good functional status, are expected to survive > 1 year and have a low risk of bleeding. These patients may come to the HDU for post-intervention care

Embolectomy

- Tends to be reserved for patients who are shocked despite resuscitative measures or thrombolysis
- Mortality remains high despite procedure

Contraindications to pharmacological measures

- Platelets $<50 \times 10^9$ L^{-1}
- INR> 1.5
- Active bleeding
- Underlying coagulopathy, e.g. DIC
- Recent lumbar puncture/spinal/epidural
- New ischaemic or haemorrhagic cerebrovascular event

Further reading

The Intensive Care Society (ICS). Venous Thromboprophylaxis in Critical Care Standards and Guidelines. London: ICS, 2008.

Cook D, Meade M, Guyatt G, et al. Dalteparin versus unfractionated heparin in critically ill patients. N Engl J Med 2011; 364:1305–1314.

National Institute for Health and Care Excellence (NICE). Venous thromboembolic diseases: the management of venous thromboembolic diseases and the role of thrombophilia testing, Clinical Guidance 144. London: NICE, 2012.

Related topics of interest

Weaning from ventilation

Key points

- Prolonged ventilation is associated with increased mortality, ventilator associated pneumonia and lung injury
- Protocolised weaning and ventilator care bundles reduce duration of ventilation
- Extubation to noninvasive ventilation may be a suitable weaning strategy especially for patient with chronic obstructive pulmonary disease (COPD)

Epidemiology

Weaning from ventilation accounts for up to 50% of all ventilator days. While most patients (> 70%) requiring mechanical ventilation can be rapidly weaned to successful extubation on the first attempt, 15% are difficult to wean and require up to 7 days from their first spontaneous breathing trial (SBT), and 15% require prolonged weaning of greater than 7 days.

How to wean

1. Assess readiness to wean using the following criteria:
   - The causes of acute respiratory failure have resolved or are resolving
   - Pao_2/Fio_2 >200, pH >7.25, PEEP < 10 cmH_2O
   - The patient is haemodynamically stable and co-operative
   - Patient capable of reliable ventilatory effort
2. Evaluate while support is reduced either gradually or abruptly. Success is likely if:
   - Respiratory rate < 35 min^{-1}
   - Tidal volume > 5 $mL\,kg^{-1}$
   - Rapid shallow breathing index (RSBI): frequency/Vt:- < 65 likely to be successful, 65–105 may be successful, > 105 likely to fail
   - Airway occlusion pressure at 0.1 s ($P_{0.1}$) > 5 cmH_2O is sustainable

- Product of RSBI and $P_{0.1}$ < 450
- Maximal inspiratory pressure (PImax) < 20 cmH_2O
3. Consensus expert opinion is that daily SBTs are preferred to slow reductions in ventilatory support for most patients. Multiple daily SBTs are reasonable provided there is no clinical evidence of respiratory muscle fatigue. A spontaneous T piece trial (30 min duration) is a rapid way to assess potential to wean. CPAP of 5 cmH_2O is useful to reduce small airway closure during trials and the patient should remain stable, although some increase in $Paco_2$ is acceptable.
4. Failure of repeated SBTs should prompt consideration of:
   - whether there is a benefit to daily SBT trials for that patient (if ventilator muscles are allowed to fatigue they may require >24 h to recover)
   - identifying other reversible causes (e.g. a missed phrenic nerve injury)
   - introduction of a weaning protocol (e.g. gradually increasing duration of spontaneous breathing trials for short periods progressing to long periods)
   - a more gradual reduction of pressure support (which avoids fatigue and lessens anxiety)

Mode of ventilation support for patient who fail initial weaning

Randomised controlled trials have addressed whether synchronised intermittent mandatory ventilation (SIMV), intermittent T piece trials or assisted spontaneous breathing (ASB) (pressure support) are superior for weaning. The studies were performed on subgroups of patients who satisfied readiness criteria but failed to tolerate an initial 2 h SBT and resulted in conflicting results as to whether T-piece trials or ASB are better. The studies confirmed the unsuitability of SIMV as a weaning mode.

ASB (pressure support) at a fixed set pressure compensates poorly for the variable inspiratory flow rates seen in spontaneous breathing. Also the tolerance of a T piece trial (even if the patient fulfils weaning criteria) can be compromised by the extra work imposed by breathing unassisted through a tracheal tube. Both of these issues can be successfully mitigated by adding automatic tube compensation (ATC), which improves the predictive value of the f/Vt in a spontaneous breathing trial.

Proportional assist ventilation (PAV) and neurally adjusted ventilator assist (NAVA) improve patient/ventilator synchrony, sleep, and are better tolerated than pressure support ventilation. They both integrate the physiological concept of respiratory variability (i.e. noisy ventilation). They may each have a role in the difficult to wean patient.

Randomised controlled trials have assessed the value of extubating patients having difficulty weaning onto non-invasive ventilation (NIV). In this setting, NIV has been associated with reduced duration of mechanical ventilation, reduced duration of intensive care, reduced ventilator associated pneumonia and 60-day mortality. Patients with acute-on-COPD are particularly suitable.

Weaning protocols

Nurse-led protocols to assess criteria to wean and initiate weaning are now well proven to reduce duration of time on a ventilator. The daily sedation reduction or stoppage to assess appropriateness to wean is an important component of ventilator care bundles.

Cardiac failure

An impaired heart is susceptible to the transition from positive pressure ventilation to spontaneous (negative pressure) breathing. Patients that fail SBTs often fail to increase cardiac output sufficiently to perfuse respiratory muscles and have reduced gut blood flow. Echocardiography can be invaluable to target appropriate medical therapy, e.g. angiotensin converting enzyme (ACE) inhibitors, selective beta-blockers and diuretics. A positive fluid balance independently correlates with weaning failure.

Muscle wasting

Diaphragmatic weakness rather than fatigue is a significant reason for failure to wean. Within 48 h of controlled ventilation, diaphragm and inter-costal muscles exhibit a reduction in cross-sectional area of fast and slow muscle fibres. High PEEP and prolonged use of neuromuscular blockade can exacerbate this. Complete rest of respiratory muscles is disadvantageous. The optimum weaning strategies may be repeated episodes of spontaneous breathing, gradually increasing their duration based on physiological criteria, interspersed with adequate pressure supported breaths to reduce muscle wasting.

Tracheostomy

Tracheostomy is often performed on patients who require prolonged ventilatory weaning. Tracheostomy facilitates reduced sedation, reduces dead space and work of breathing, and improves secretion removal. The optimal timing for tracheostomy is unclear but in the face of a high likelihood of prolonged ventilation most clinicians will do an early tracheostomy. Some long-term ventilator care units are available for patients with continued ventilator dependence – 50% of such patients will eventually be weaned from the ventilator.

Further reading

MacIntyre NR, Cook DJ, Ely EW Jr, et al. Evidence-based guidelines for weaning and discontinuing ventilatory support: a collective task force facilitated by the American College of Chest Physicians; the American Association for Respiratory Care; and the American College of Critical Care Medicine. Chest 2001; 120:S375–395.

McConville JF, Kress JP. Weaning Patients from the Ventilator. N Engl J Med 2012; 367:2233–2239.

Blackwood B, Alderdice F, Burns K, et al. Use of weaning protocols for reducing duration of mechanical ventilation in critically ill adult patients: Cochrane systematic review and meta-analysis Br Med J 2011; 342:c7237.

Related topics of interest

- Respiratory support – invasive (p 306)
- Respiratory support – non-invasive techniques (p 311)
- Tracheostomy (p 368)

Index

Note: Page numbers in **bold** or *italic* refer to tables or figures, respectively.